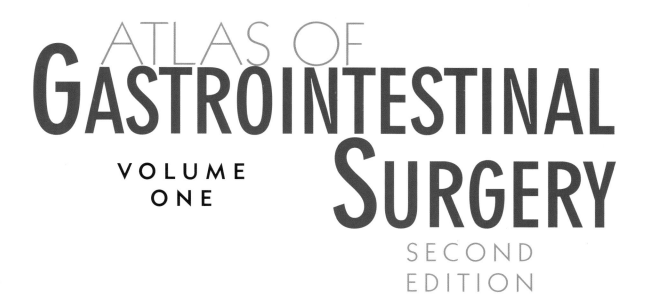

ATLAS OF GASTROINTESTINAL SURGERY

VOLUME ONE

SECOND EDITION

JOHN L. CAMERON, MD, FACS
The Alfred Blalock
Distinguished Service Professor
The Department of Surgery
The Johns Hopkins Medical Institutions
Baltimore, Maryland

CORINNE SANDONE, MA, CMI
Medical Illustrator
Associate Professor
Department of Art as Applied to Medicine
The Johns Hopkins University School of Medicine
Baltimore, Maryland

2007
PEOPLE'S MEDICAL PUBLISHING HOUSE—USA
Shelton, Connecticut

People's Medical Publishing House—USA
2 Enterprise Drive, Suite 509
Shelton, CT 06484
Tel: 203-402-0646
Fax: 203-402-0854
E-mail: info@pmph-usa.com

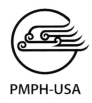

PMPH-USA

14 15 16 17 / LEGO / 9 7 8 3 2

ISBN-13 978-1-55009-270-7
ISBN-10 1-55009-270-7
eISBN   978-1-60795-056-1

Printed in Italy by Legatoria Editoriale Giovanni Olivotto.
Editor: Linda Mehta; Page Designer: Norman Reid

Library of Congress Cataloging-in-Publication Data
Cameron, John L., author.
   Atlas of gastrointestinal surgery / John L. Cameron, MD, FACS, the Alfred Blalock, Distinguished Service Professor, the Department of Surgery, the Johns Hopkins Medical Institutions, Baltimore, Maryland, Corinne Sandone, MA, CMI, Medical Illustrator, Assistant Professor, Department of Art as Applied to Medicine, Johns Hopkins University School of Medicine, Baltimore, Maryland. -- Second edition.
      pages cm
Description based on: v. 2, published in 2013.
Includes index.
ISBN-13: 978-1-60795-027-1 (v. 2 : alk. paper)
ISBN-10: 1-60795-027a-8 (v. 2 : alk. paper)
ISBN-13: 978-1-60795-235-0 (v. 2 : ebook) 1. Digestive organs--Surgery--Atlases. I. Sandone, Corinne. II. Title.
RD540.C225 2013   617.4'3--dc23   2013047568

Sales and Distribution

Canada
Login Canada
300 Saulteaux Cr., Winnipeg, MB
R3J 3T2
Phone: 1.800.665.1148
Fax: 1.800.0103
www.lb.ca

Foreign Rights
John Scott & Company
International Publisher's Agency
P.O. Box 878
Kimberton, PA 19442
USA
Tel: 610-827-1640
Fax: 610-827-1671

Japan
United Publishers Services Limited
1-32-5 Higashi-Shinagawa
Shinagawa-ku, Tokyo 140-0002
Japan
Tel: 03-5479-7251
Fax: 03-5479-7307
Email: kakimoto@ups.co.jp

United Kingdom, Europe,
Middle East, Africa
Eurospan Limited
3, Henrietta Street,
Covent Garden,
London WC2E 8LU, UK
Within the UK: 0800 526830
Outside the UK: +44 (0)20 7845 0868
http://www.eurospanbookstore.com

Singapore, Thailand, Philippines,
Indonesia, Vietnam, Pacific Rim, Korea
McGraw-Hill Education
60 Tuas Basin Link
Singapore 638775
Tel: 65-6863-1580
Fax: 65-6862-3354
www.mcgraw-hill.com.sg

Australia, New Zealand
Elsevier Australia
Locked Bag 7500
Chatswood DC NSW 2067
Australia
Tel: 161 (2) 9422-8500
Fax: 161 (2) 9422-8562
www.elsevier.com.au

Brazil
SuperPedido Tecmedd
Beatriz Alves, Foreign Trade Department
R. Sansao Alves dos Santos, 102 | 7th floor
Brooklin Novo
Sao Pãolo 04571-090
Brazil
Tel: 55-16-3512-5539
www.superpedidotecmedd.com.br

India, Bangladesh, Pakistan, Sri Lanka, Malaysia
CBS Publishers
4819/X1 Prahlad Street 24
Ansari Road, Darya Ganj, New Delhi-110002
India
Tel: 91-11-23266861/67
Fax: 91-11-23266818
Email:cbspubs@vsnl.com

People's Republic of China
People's Medical Publishing House
International Trade Department
No. 19, Pan Jia Yuan Nan Li
Chaoyang District
Beijing 100021
P.R. China
Tel: 8610-67653342
Fax: 8610-67691034
www.pmph.com/en/

CONTENTS

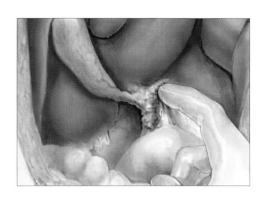

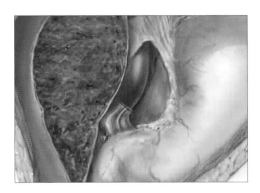

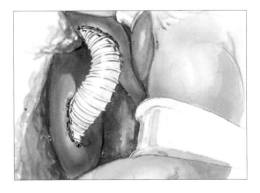

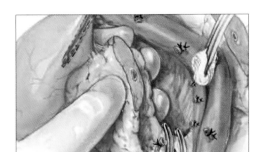

The Pancreas

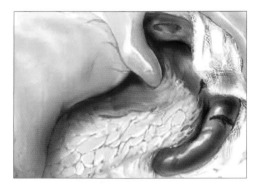

The Spleen

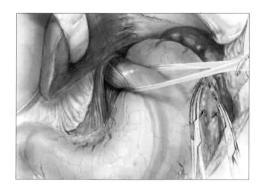

The Esophagus

CONTRIBUTORS

John L. Cameron, MD
Michael A. Choti, MD
Keith D. Lillemoe, MD
Mark A. Talamini, MD
Stephen C. Yang, MD
Charles J. Yeo, MD

The Department of Surgery
The Johns Hopkins Medical Institutions
Baltimore, Maryland

Corinne Sandone, MA, CMI

Department of Art as Applied to Medicine
Johns Hopkins University School of Medicine
Baltimore, Maryland

EDITOR'S PREFACE

This is the first of a two-volume atlas that represents the 2nd edition of our work published fourteen years ago. The distinguishing characteristic of the second edition is the same as for the first edition — the artist Corinne Sandone. She has established herself as one of the outstanding surgical illustrators of her era in this country. Her combining of accurate anatomical renderings, with unique angles and perspectives, via her magnificent watercolor technique, make her work unique. Because of her superb contribution, she is not only listed as the illustrator, but also as a coeditor of the atlas.

The first chief of surgery at the Johns Hopkins Hospital, Dr. William Stewart Halsted, was one of the pioneers of gastrointestinal surgery in this country. In the 1880s, when the great surgeons of Europe were attempting to anastomose intestine, with a high failure rate, Halsted was the first to demonstrate that intestinal sutures should include the sub-mucosal layer, and not just the muscular layer of the intestine. This contribution led to the development of the field of gastrointestinal surgery. Halsted also made unique contributions to the area of biliary tract and gall bladder surgery, and was the first surgeon in the world to successfully resect a periampullary tumor. After Halsted's death, the next great era at Hopkins involved the emergence of cardiac surgery. Dr. Alfred Blalock and his brilliant trainees were important players in the development and emergence of this field.

In the 1970s and 1980s, with new leadership at Hopkins, gastrointestinal surgery again emerged as an important focus for the department. Beginning in the 1970s and extending up until the present, a school of gastrointestinal surgery emerged at Hopkins, which has produced many young surgeons who currently hold important chairs of surgery throughout the country. This atlas includes the techniques, operations, and procedures favored and performed, and in some instances initiated, by these gastrointestinal surgeons. Thus, the operations included in this atlas are not all inclusive in scope. In many instances there are other operations and procedures that are used by others, with equally good results.

Successful gastrointestinal surgical outcomes depend upon the surgeon, however, favorable outcomes depend upon having outstanding and supportive gastroenterologists, radiological interventionists, anesthesiologists, intensivists, nurses, house staff, and another group that is becoming more and more important to the care of patients with gastrointestinal diseases — nurse practitioners and physicians' assistants.

John L. Cameron
October 2006

ILLUSTRATOR'S PREFACE

The illustrations in this atlas are the result of a 20-year collaboration with many outstanding surgeons, including and especially Dr. John Cameron. Their willingness to have me observe and sketch and, more importantly, their descriptions of steps which could not be observed directly, contributed to the clarity, accuracy and didactic strength of these images. The surgeons' narratives through the operative steps, including pitfalls and technical details for success, were crucial to my understanding and subsequent depictions of their operative techniques.

Medical illustration began at Johns Hopkins in 1894 with the arrival of Max Brödel to the newly founded School of Medicine. Working with the early Hopkins faculty, Brödel skillfully illustrated the research publications that documented the groundbreaking work of William S. Halsted, Harvey Cushing, William H. Welch, William Osler, Howard A. Kelly and Thomas Cullen. In 1911, the Department of Art as Applied to Medicine was created, formalizing Max Brödel's training of exceptional young artists to become capable medical illustrators. Currently in its 10th decade, the program grants a Master of Arts degree to medical illustrators who train alongside medical students and collaborate with Hopkins clinicians and researchers as their fields evolve.

Technology has provided new tools for the surgeon and the illustrator in the past two decades. These tools, however, do not replace or substitute for the talent, knowledge, experience and decision-making ability required for success in both fields. Since work was begun on the first edition of this atlas, new equipment in the operative suite - laparoscopic devices, intraoperative ultrasound - has been paralleled by developments in the studio equipment - scanners, digitized drawing tools. These change the way we work, but not the essence of what we do.

The challenge of my work is to provide the clarity, that a camera could never capture, to the operative steps while maintaining the realism of peering into the operative field. Less relevant is whether I achieve this by pushing wet pigment around with a traditional paintbrush or by moving pixels with a digitized pen tool. Many of the paintings in the volume are reprints of the original watercolors, a significant portion have been revised and updated, and many more are new - created using a combination of traditional and new media.

It has been my pleasure to work with the surgical teams at Hopkins. The second edition of this atlas will further disseminate their knowledge and techniques, allowing the reader to learn and see what I have had the privilege to observe, understand and illustrate.

Corinne Sandone
October 2006

DEDICATION

To all who participate in the care of the patient with a surgical gastrointestinal disease, particularly those surgeons who trained or spent time here, and are now building their own schools of gastrointestinal surgery, this atlas is dedicated.

JLC

For Dan, Carlene and Claudia - smart, funny and kind.

CS

GALL BLADDER

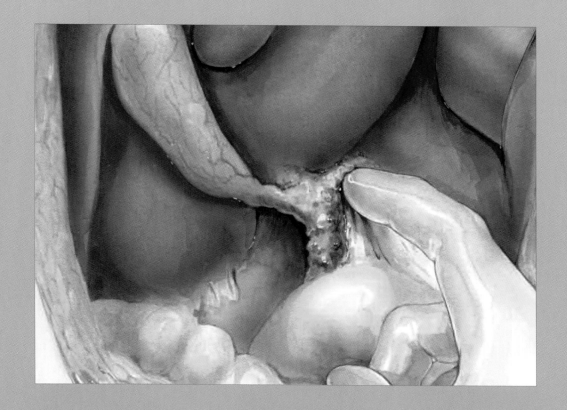

Laparoscopic Cholecystectomy

Operative Indications

Laparoscopic cholecystectomy has become the procedure of choice for nearly all patients undergoing cholecystectomy regardless of the indication. The most common indication for cholecystectomy is symptomatic gallstones. In the past many patients with asymptomatic gallstones were also thought to benefit from cholecystectomy. However, natural history data demonstrated that most patients with asymptomatic gallstones do not require cholecystectomy. The ease and reduced pain of laparoscopic cholecystectomy have not changed that recommendation. When the procedure was introduced in 1989, a number of relative contraindications for laparoscopic cholecystectomy existed, including previous upper abdominal surgery, acute cholecystitis, common bile duct stones, and pregnancy. However, as experience with the procedure has increased, there currently are few contraindications to the procedure. Patients with acute cholecystitis can often successfully undergo laparoscopic cholecystectomy, although the technical difficulties and chance for conversion to open cholecystectomy are greater. In addition, experienced laparoscopic surgeons have extended the procedure to include laparoscopic management of common bile duct stones. Whenever significant technical difficulties arise or the anatomy becomes unclear, the laparoscopic technique should be abandoned and a laparotomy performed.

Operative Technique

The procedure is performed under general anesthesia with a standard abdominal preparation. A Foley catheter and orogastric tube are placed. Four laparoscopic trocars are necessary for almost all patients. An initial trocar, 10 to 11 mm, is placed in the supraumbilical position and serves as the primary location for the laparoscopic telescope and attached camera. A second 5 mm trocar is placed in the subxiphoid area in the midline. Two 5 mm trocars are placed laterally in the right subcostal area, one near the midclavicular line and one near the anterior axillary line.

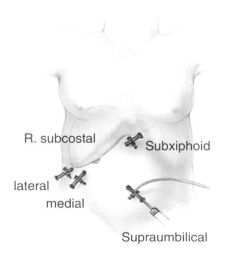

R. subcostal

Subxiphoid

lateral

medial

Supraumbilical

①

Umbilicus

The placement of the final three trocars varies somewhat from patient to patient, based on body habitus and the location of the gall bladder within the right upper quadrant. Proper trocar placement is essential; care must be taken to avoid placing the most medial of the 5 mm trocars in the direct view of the laparoscopic camera or in the way of the operating port.

The placement of trocars begins with a small, transverse supraumbilical incision about 1½ cm in length (1). The incision is carried through the skin and subcutaneous tissue, exposing the anterior fascia. In the absence of prior abdominal surgery, the patient is placed in the Trendelenburg position for placement of the Veress needle for insufflation. Two large towel clips are placed into the skin on both sides of the supraumbilical incision to provide countertraction for the passage of the Veress needle (2). In the obese patient, a somewhat longer transverse incision can be made, the dissection carried down through the subcutaneous tissue, and the towel clips placed directly on the fascia. In addition, the surgeon and an assistant can grasp the abdominal wall, laterally lifting it up further to minimize the chances of excessive advancement of the needle. The needle should be advanced with finger pressure only, with the hand resting on the abdomen to avoid a dangerous uncontrolled thrust. To avoid injury to the underlying aorta and vena cava, the needle is angled slightly toward the pelvis as it is advanced. Proper placement of the Veress needle should be ensured by aspirating with a syringe. Aspiration of blood, urine, or intestinal contents indicates improper placement of the needle. Before beginning insufflation, the "drop test" should be performed. A drop of saline is placed into the open lumen of the Veress needle. Normally, negative pressure in the peritoneal cavity causes the drop of saline to fall through the lumen of the Veress needle.

Insufflation with carbon dioxide is begun at a low rate, approximately 1.5 L/min. This is continued until reaching the desired intra-abdominal pressure, usually 12 to 14 mm Hg.

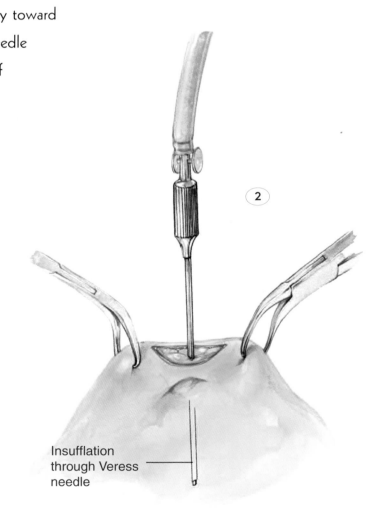

②

Insufflation through Veress needle

An alternative method of establishing a pneumoperitoneum, favored by many surgeons and essential for patients with previous abdominal surgery, involves the placement of the Hasson cannula (3). The fascia is exposed and is incised with Mayo scissors or the cautery. Sutures of 0 polypropylene are placed on both sides of the fascial defect, and free entry into the peritoneal cavity is obtained. The blunt tip of the Hasson cannula is inserted and the previously placed sutures are secured to its wings. Insufflation is begun at high flow. To inspect the peritoneal cavity, the scope is introduced and advanced early in the insufflation process.

The laparoscopic telescope is placed into the supraumbilical trocar, and the abdomen is inspected. A 30-degree side-viewing laparoscope is most useful for performing laparoscopic cholecystectomy and is recommended. After inspection of the pelvis and lower abdomen, the patient is repositioned in the reverse Trendelenburg position at about 30 degrees to allow the colon and omentum to fall away from the upper abdomen, providing better exposure of the gall bladder. Laparoscopic inspection of the surface of the stomach, liver, and upper abdominal viscera is completed.

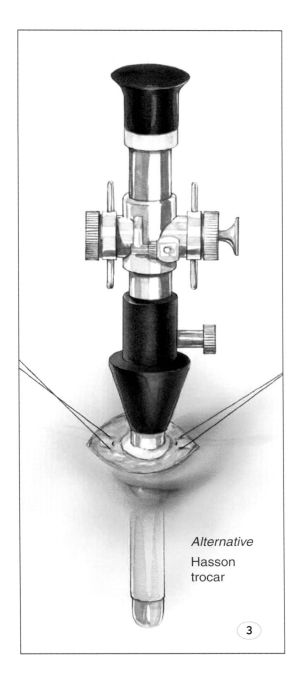

Alternative
Hasson
trocar

3

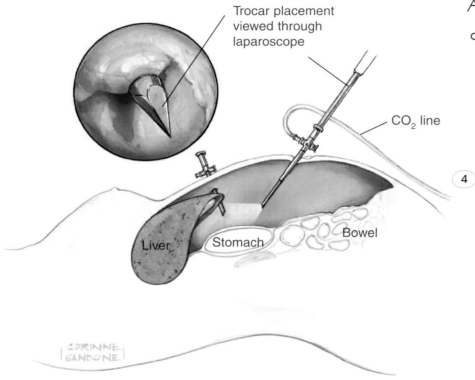

Trocar placement viewed through laparoscope

CO_2 line

Liver   Stomach   Bowel

④

Attention is turned to placement of the other trocars The position of the additional trocars has been previously discussed. The second trocar placed is a 5 mm trocar in the subxiphoid position. After the initial "blind" placement of the supraumbilical trocar, all remaining trocars are placed under direct vision. The surgeon is able to identify the safe site for entrance into the peritoneal cavity by first pressing on the abdominal wall in the desired area. The impression of the finger on the abdominal wall is viewed through the laparoscope and locates the safe site of entry and desired position in the peritoneal cavity. The trocar is advanced until its sharp point pierces through the peritoneum (4). The inner point of the trocar is then withdrawn, and the outer sheath can be advanced until it reaches the desired position.

After proper placement of the three remaining trocars, grasping instruments are passed through the two lateral 5 mm trocars. The grasping instruments can be either with or without teeth. In minimally inflamed gall bladders, graspers without teeth are usually preferred because they are less apt to tear the thin-walled gall bladder. However, if inflammation exists with thickening of the gall bladder wall, a grasper with teeth is usually a better instrument for grasping and retracting. The most lateral grasper is usually used to grasp the gall bladder close to the fundus. In some patients, when the gall bladder is not easily seen, a dissecting instrument placed through the subxiphoid trocar can lift up the edge of the liver to expose the fundus of the gall bladder. After a secure grasp on the fundus is obtained, the gall bladder is lifted superiorly toward the right shoulder. In many patients, there are filmy adhesions of the omentum, duodenum, or the transverse colon along the gall bladder's lower border. These adhesions are taken down bluntly, either using a dissecting grasper, a cautery hook, or scissors. After the entire peritoneal surface of the gall bladder has been exposed, the second grasper is applied to the gall bladder at the infundibulum near the neck. Retraction with this instrument is lateral and toward the abdominal wall. This maneuver exposes the cystic duct and places it on traction in the direction away from the common bile duct. Excessive force, however, must not be applied to avoid tearing the gall bladder and spilling bile and stones. If a hole is made, it is controlled with the grasping instrument or with the application of a clip or laparoscopic looped suture.

The filmy adhesions over the cystic duct are best taken down bluntly using a gently curved dissector from the subxiphoid position (5). These adhesions are usually avascular. However, a cautery attachment to the grasping instrument can be used for hemostasis if necessary. Dissection begins along the gall bladder and proceeds toward the cystic duct/common bile duct junction. Dissection continues circumferentially around the cystic duct until it is completely exposed.

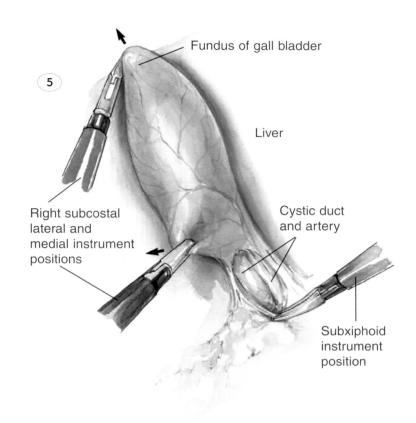

Fundus of gall bladder

Liver

Right subcostal lateral and medial instrument positions

Cystic duct and artery

Subxiphoid instrument position

The dissecting instrument is spread in both a parallel and perpendicular fashion to the cystic duct to clear an adequate space (6). It is usually helpful to place the dissecting instrument in and out of this space several times to ensure easy later passage of the clip applier.

The indications for cholangiography during a laparoscopic cholecystectomy are similar to those with open cholecystectomy. Some surgeons believe that routine cholangiography is essential in the performance of a laparoscopic cholecystectomy. This is in response to the increased incidence of bile duct injury with this procedure. However, it is my opinion that the indications for cholangiography during laparoscopic cholecystectomy are no different

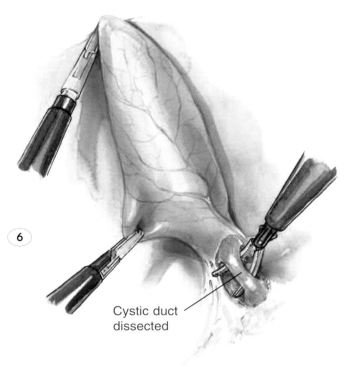

Cystic duct dissected

than those during open cholecystectomy and include suggestion of common bile duct stones, and uncertain anatomy. To perform an operative cholangiogram during laparoscopic cholecystectomy, the gall bladder neck is clipped with a single staple at its junction with the cystic duct (7) . This clip is applied to prevent leakage of gall bladder bile as the cystic duct is opened. A pair of small, fine scissors is then passed through the subxiphoid port, and a small nick is made in the anterior and superior surface of the cystic duct (8). Entrance into the duct lumen is demonstrated by leakage of a small amount of bile from the cystic duct. A cholangiocatheter is introduced, and in most cases can be passed easily through the cystic duct to the junction of the common bile duct for performance of cholangiography (9).

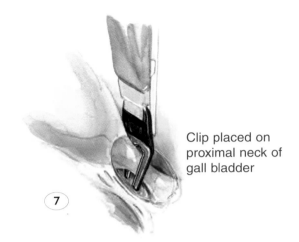

Clip placed on proximal neck of gall bladder

7

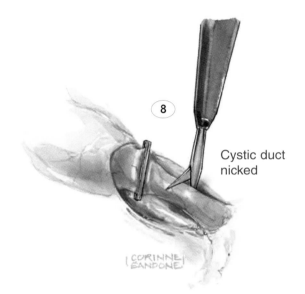

8

Cystic duct nicked

CORINNE SANDONE

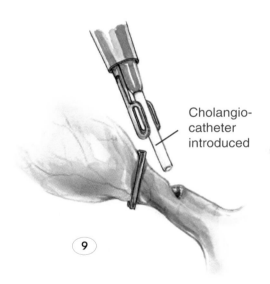

Cholangio-catheter introduced

9

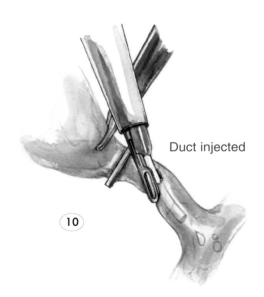

Duct injected

10

Fluoroscopy is essential for optimal performance of cholangiography during laparoscopic cholecystectomy because the position of many of the metallic instruments may impair the view of essential structures in the radiograph (10). A satisfactory cholangiogram should show not only filling of the common bile duct distally and the passage of contrast into the duodenum, but also essential filling of the proximal biliary tree. The most common error leading to major bile duct injury during laparoscopic cholecystectomy is mistaking the common bile or common hepatic duct for the cystic duct. At the point of cholangiography, a clip will have already been misplaced in most cases across the common bile duct or common hepatic duct, thus impairing the flow of bile into the proximal biliary tree. If during operative cholangiography the proximal biliary tree cannot be filled, substantial concern should be raised that the bile duct may be occluded by the applied clip.

If cholangiography demonstrates a normal biliary tree, the cholangiocatheter is removed. Two clips are placed distally on the cystic duct (11). Proper application of the clips is essential to avoid the complication of postoperative cystic duct leak. The clips must not be applied until the back jaw of the clip applier can be visualized completely around the cystic duct to ensure that the jaws of the clips completely cross the duct. The two clips should be placed parallel and should not cross over each other in any fashion that might impair the cystic duct closure.

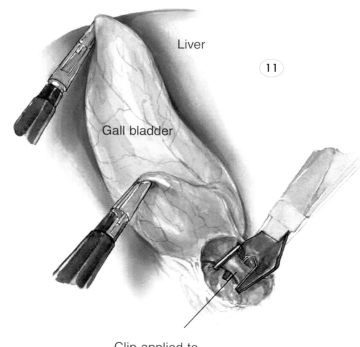

Clip applied to
distal cystic duct

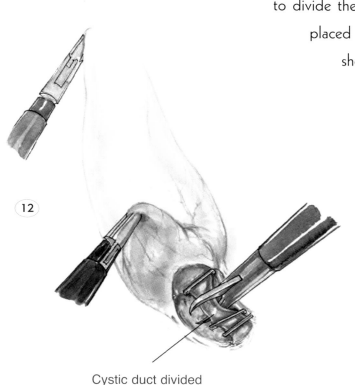

Cystic duct divided

After successful placement of the two distal clips, the hook scissors are used to divide the cystic duct (12). The back immobile jaw of the scissors is placed behind the cystic duct. After hooking the cystic duct, it should be elevated slightly away from other structures to avoid injury to any underlying tissues by the jaws of the scissors.

After dividing the cystic duct, blunt dissection is continued until the cystic artery is identified. The cystic artery is usually well visualized as a distinct structure located within millimeters of the cystic duct and running parallel to it. In some cases the cystic artery may divide into an anterior and posterior branch at variable locations near the gall bladder wall. Care should be taken to make sure that the path of the cystic artery is directly toward the gall bladder to avoid dividing a tortuous right hepatic artery. The dissection of the cystic artery must be gentle because the artery can tear, which may result in troublesome bleeding. If such bleeding does occur, it is essential to *not*

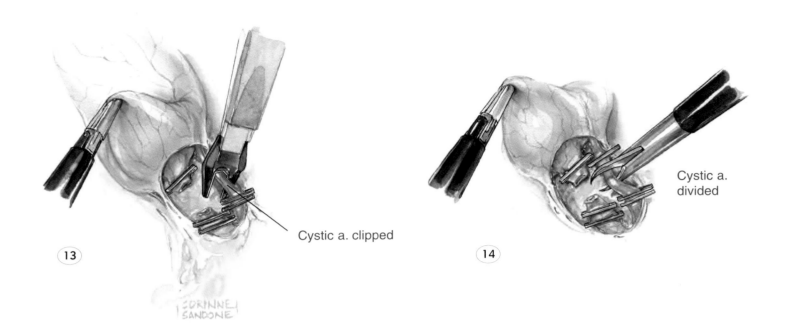

Cystic a. clipped

(13)

Cystic a. divided

(14)

place clips blindly into the area, because bile duct injury may result. If the bleeding artery can be seen, placement of the grasping instrument on the artery to retract it away from the portal structures will often allow placement of a clip across the artery to control the bleeding.

Once the cystic artery has been doubly clipped (13), the structure is divided with the hook scissors (14). Care again must be taken to avoid injury to underlying structures with the jaws of the scissors. The cystic duct and cystic artery clips should be reinspected, and the area should be irrigated to check for bleeding or bile leakage. It is essential that the clips be inspected at this point, because after the gall bladder has been mobilized from its bed, viewing these structures is sometimes difficult.

To facilitate dissection of the gall bladder from its bed, the two lateral graspers are used in concert to expose first the superior and then the inferior junction of the gall bladder's peritoneal surface with the liver. The grasper on the fundus of the gall bladder retracts medially, and the grasper near the cystic duct is pulled laterally. This exposes the superior surface of the junction of the gall bladder's peritoneal surface with the liver, which is divided from the neck toward the fundus (15). This dissection can be performed with either a hook or a spatula electrocautery. The hook cautery offers the

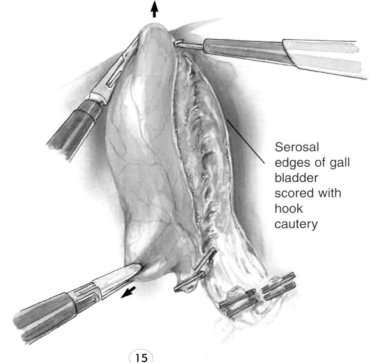

Serosal edges of gall bladder scored with hook cautery

(15)

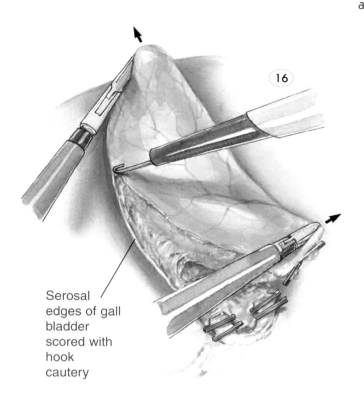

Serosal edges of gall bladder scored with hook cautery

advantage of pulling the tissue away from the gall bladder to avoid a cautery injury to the gall bladder wall, which may result in leakage of bile. The serosal edge of the gall bladder is incised as far as possible on the superior surface. The two lateral graspers are then repositioned with the fundus retracted toward the more lateral superior aspect, whereas the grasper on the cystic duct pushes the infundibulum medially. This exposes the inferior surface of the junction of the gall bladder peritoneum with the liver, which is also incised as far as possible (16).

After dividing the serosal surface on the superior and inferior aspects of the gall bladder, the infundibulum grasper is repositioned to the undersurface of the cystic duct, allowing the neck of the gall bladder to be lifted away from the gall bladder bed (17). Because tissue in this area is often avascular, traction of the gall bladder makes it easy for this plane to be dissected with either the hook or spatula cautery. As this dissection approaches the fundus, the gall bladder will be attached to the liver only at the fundus.

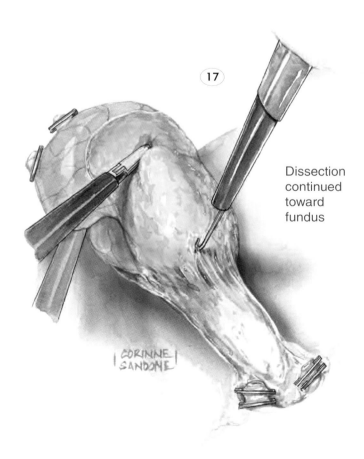

Dissection continued toward fundus

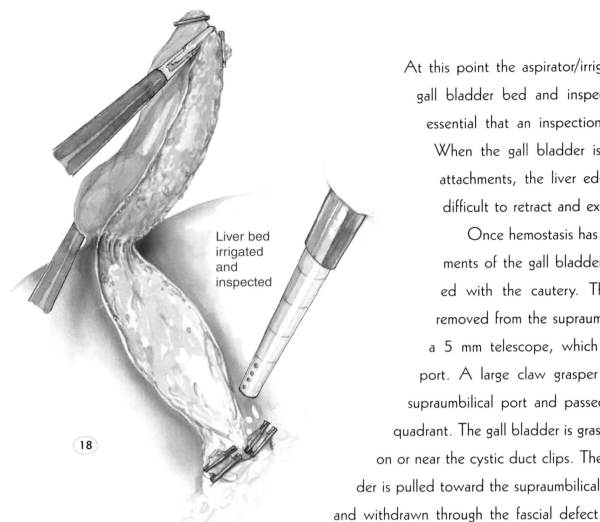

Liver bed irrigated and inspected

(18)

At this point the aspirator/irrigator is inserted to irrigate the gall bladder bed and inspect for hemostasis (18). It is essential that an inspection be performed at this point. When the gall bladder is separated from its final liver attachments, the liver edge will drop down, making it difficult to retract and expose the gall bladder bed.

Once hemostasis has been ensured, the final attachments of the gall bladder fundus to the liver are divided with the cautery. The telescope and camera are removed from the supraumbilical port and exchanged for a 5 mm telescope, which is inserted in the subxiphoid port. A large claw grasper is then placed through the supraumbilical port and passed into the right upper quadrant. The gall bladder is grasped at the neck, on or near the cystic duct clips. The gall bladder is pulled toward the supraumbilical port and withdrawn through the fascial defect as the trocar is withdrawn. When the gall bladder has been aspirated, or the bile has been spilled, the collapsed gall bladder can often be pulled directly through the fascia and removed. However, when the bile and stones are still present in the gall bladder, pulling the gall bladder through the small fascial hole is often impossible. The trocar should then be pulled out of the abdominal cavity with the gall bladder remaining tightly in the claws of the grasper (19). A Kelly clamp is used to grasp the gall bladder at its neck, and the grasping instrument is removed.

(19)

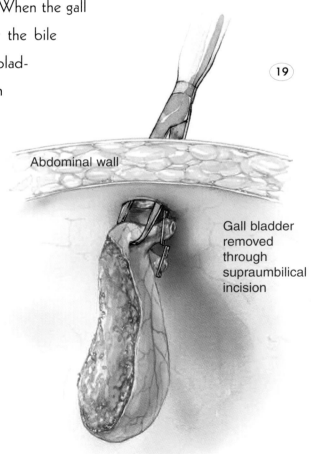

Abdominal wall

Gall bladder removed through supraumbilical incision

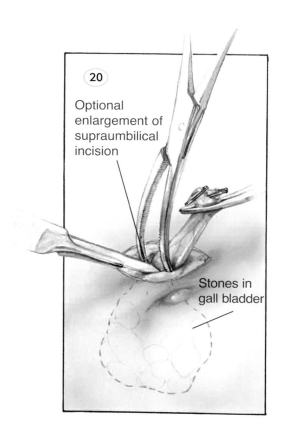

(20) Optional enlargement of supraumbilical incision

Stones in gall bladder

The supraumbilical fascial incision can be widened somewhat by either spreading a Kelly clamp or using a small knife blade to incise the fascia between the jaws of a clamp (20). The telescope monitors this process from its subxiphoid position (21). After the gall bladder is removed from the peritoneal cavity, the pneumoperitoneum will not be maintained because of the open fascial defect. The fascial defect is then closed by using simple interrupted sutures through both the superior and inferior fascial surface edges. After closure of the fascia, the abdomen is reinsufflated with carbon dioxide, and the supraumbilical closure is inspected. The area of the gall bladder bed is also reinspected, and irrigation over the dome of the liver and in the subhepatic space with an antibiotic solution is performed. At the completion of irrigation, as much fluid as possible should be aspirated. If there has been spillage of bile or stones, the irrigation should be continued until all traces of bile in the fluid have cleared. In many cases, the sucker or a grasping instrument can be used successfully to remove spilled stones.

After completion of irrigation, the pneumoperitoneum is evacuated, insufflation is stopped, and the trocars are removed. It is not necessary to close the remaining trocar fascial defects. The skin incisions should be closed with subcuticular absorbable sutures and Steri-Strips.

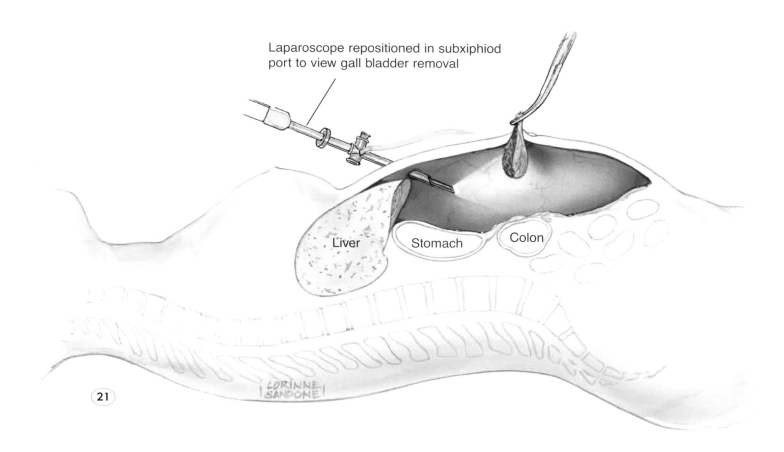

Laparoscope repositioned in subxiphiod port to view gall bladder removal

Liver   Stomach   Colon

(21)

Laparoscopic Bile Duct Exploration: Transcystic Approach

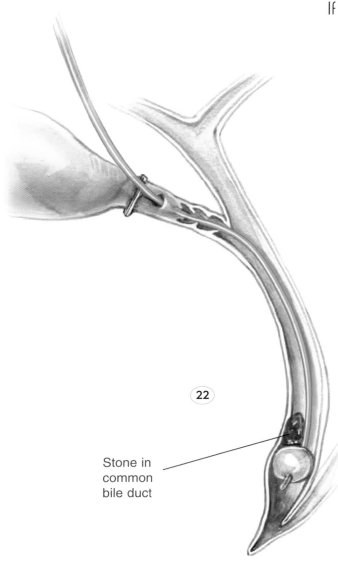

(22)

Stone in
common
bile duct

If a common bile duct exploration is indicated, the transcystic approach is usually attempted first. The cystic duct can be dilated using a 4 or 5 French balloon catheter. The position of the balloon should be confirmed by fluoroscopy (22). The balloon is then insufflated to the manufacturer's specification and held inflated for at least three minutes.

One can attempt to remove the stone by using the same balloon catheter or a Fogarty embolectomy catheter. Insert the balloon into the distal common duct or the duodenum. Confirm the position using fluoroscopy. Insufflate the balloon and pull the balloon out using minimal pulling force. After removing the stone(s), cholangiography is repeated.

Using a more proximal ductotomy, a flexible choledochoscope with a working port is advanced under direct vision using "picture-in-picture" technology on one monitor, or using two separate monitors. Irrigation through the scope's working channel should be started to allow clear visualization of the duct. The scope should ideally be no more than 3 mm in diameter.

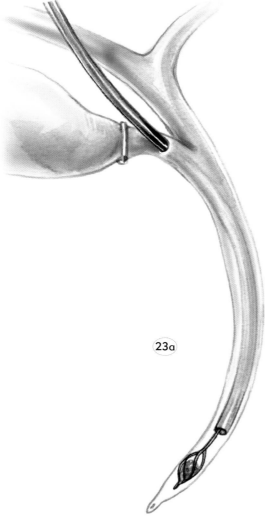

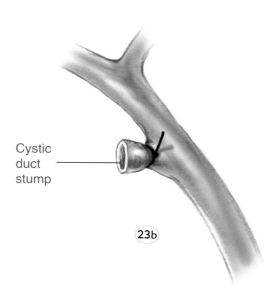

Cystic
duct
stump

Observing the direct view of the common bile duct, the scope is advanced by the surgeon. The scope may need laparoscopic instrument assistance, particularly once the common bile duct is entered. When stones are encountered, the irrigation is decreased to facilitate catching them. A wire basket catheter is advanced past the stone, so that the stone lies between the basket and the end of the scope. The basket is opened and the stone is grasped and pulled close to the scope (23a). The scope is then pulled back into the abdomen along with the basket and the stone. Repeat choledochoscopy is then performed, eventually down and through the ampulla, to make sure that all stones were completely removed.

The cystic duct stump is closed using clips or an endo-loop. Often the diameter of the duct is too big to close with just a large clip, making an endo-loop necessary (23b). Stones greater than 1cm are usually difficult to extract using this technique.

Laparoscopic CBD Exploration: Choledochotomy Approach

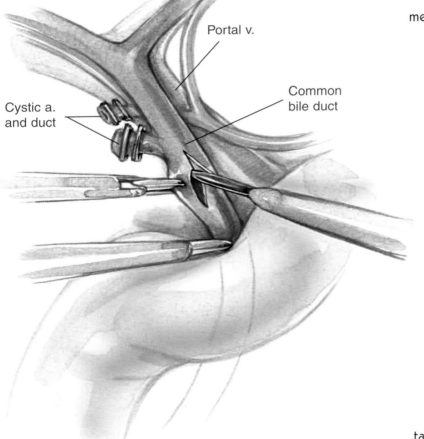

Portal v.

Common
bile duct

Cystic a.
and duct

(24)

The choledochotomy approach is indicated when there is a stone greater than 1 cm, or when the surgeon is unable to retrieve smaller stones using the transcystic approach. For ease in manipulation, retraction, and suturing, an additional 5 mm port is placed medially and slightly inferior to the medial right upper quadrant port. This port should be aligned with the common bile duct.

While retracting the gall bladder cephalad and medially, dissection of the cystic duct is accomplished using blunt dissection and carefully applied short bursts of an electrocautery. This dissection is continued to a point approximately 2 cm distal to the cystic duct junction on the anterior surface of the common bile duct. Stay stitches are placed on the anterior surface of the common bile duct to aid in the incision and retraction. A longitudinal choledochotomy is created on the anterior aspect of the common bile duct distal to the cystic duct junction (24). The incision should not be any longer than the diameter of the largest stone.

The stone is then milked proximally or removed using a biliary Fogarty catheter (25) or a vascular Fogarty catheter (which is longer). Once the stone has been retrieved, choledochoscopy or a cholangiogram should be carried out to ensure the integrity of the distal duct and to be certain that there are no residual stones. The choledochotomy is then closed over a T-tube. The 10–14 French T-tube is fashioned so that the short end is placed proximally and the long end distally (26). Additionally, a strip of the back wall of the T-tube is cut out longitudinally, and the ends are cut at an angle. The corner sutures are placed first (27, 28) because it makes the in-between sutures easier to place. 4-0 or 5-0 absorbable sutures are placed in an interrupted manner. The end of the T-tube is then brought out through one of the lateral 5 mm trocar sites. A cholangiogram is performed through the T-tube.

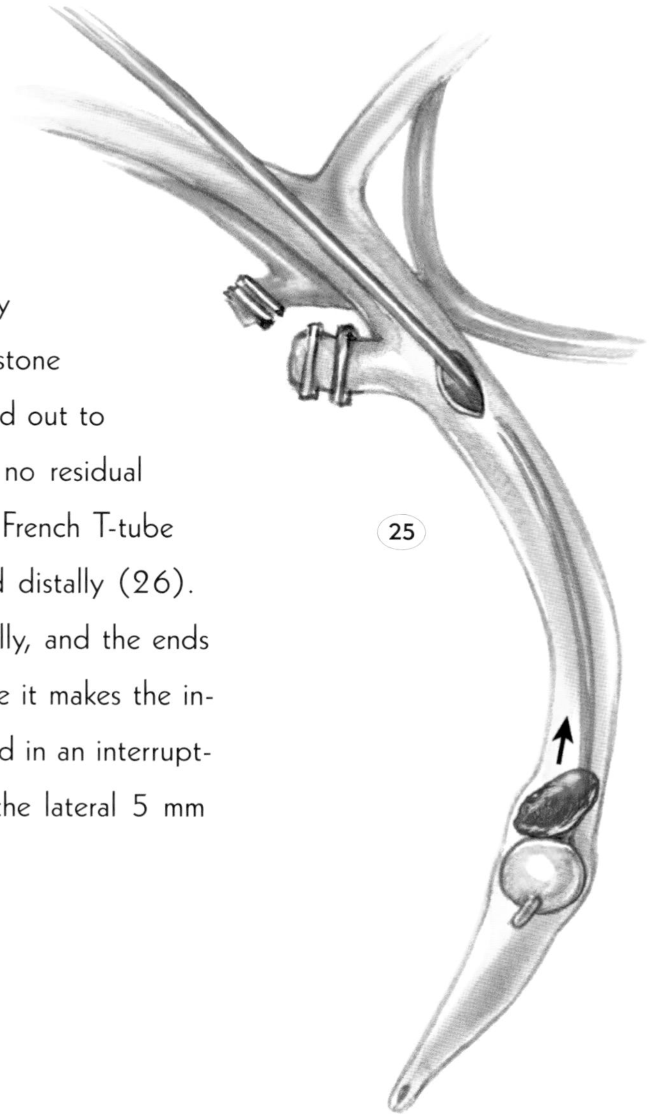

25

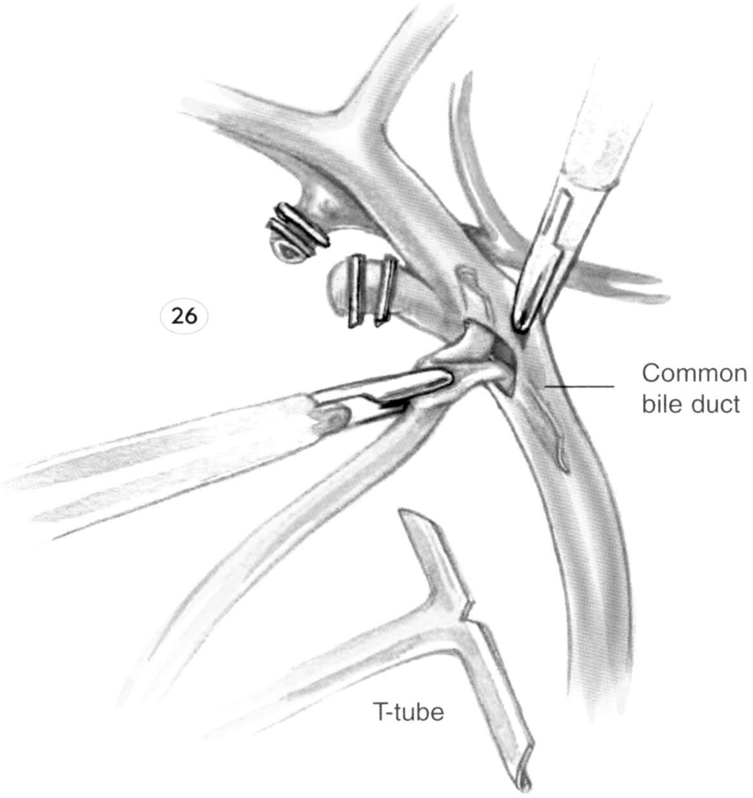

26

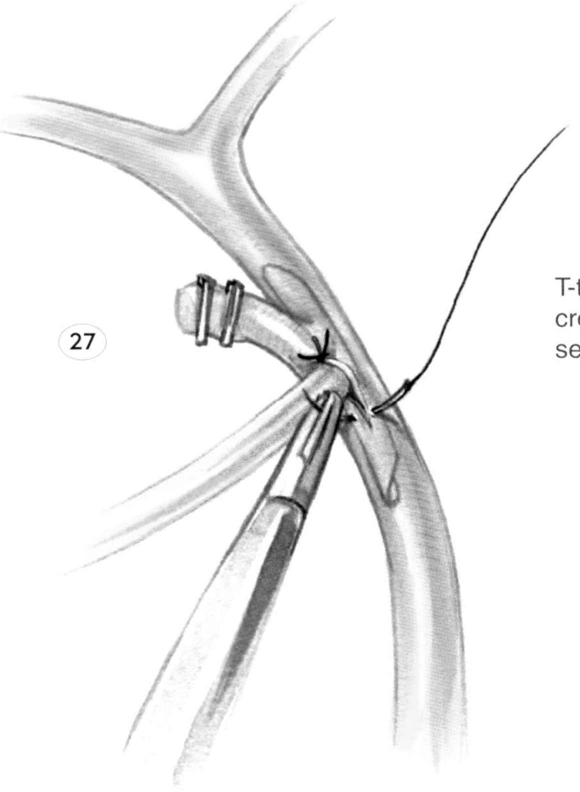

Common bile duct

T-tube

27

T-tube in cross section

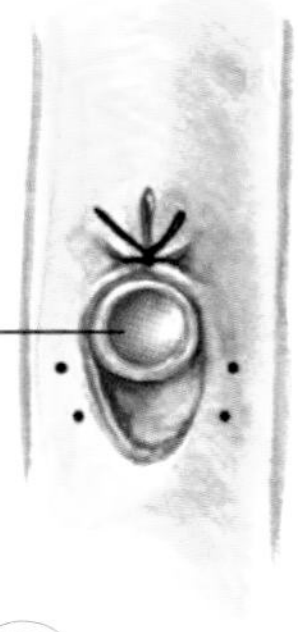

28

Open Cholecystectomy

Operative Indications:

Patients with symptomatic gallstones are candidates for cholecystectomy. In the past, even patients with asymptomatic gallstones were thought to require a cholecystectomy. Natural history data, however, suggest that unless patients with gallstones have symptoms referable to their biliary tract, the likelihood of developing significant morbidity is low enough to justify merely following the patient and performing cholecystectomy only if symptoms arise.

The introduction of laparoscopic cholecystectomy in 1989 has loosened somewhat the indications for cholecystectomy. For most physicians and surgeons, however, patients need to be symptomatic before a clear indication for cholecystectomy is considered.

There are exceptions, however, to the rule that gallstones have to be symptomatic before a cholecystectomy is indicated. An individual living in or traveling to remote areas where medical care is not readily available may be a candidate for prophylactic cholecystectomy if stones are present, particularly if there are multiple small stones. In addition, patients with calcified gall bladders, the so-called porcelain gall bladder, are felt to be at high risk to develop cancer of the gall bladder, and thus, that is considered an appropriate indication for cholecystectomy. Other factors such as diabetes or other systemic illnesses may modify the decision. Patients with gallstones who are asymptomatic, but who are to undergo a solid organ transplant and are immunosuppressed may also be considered for cholecystectomy if gallstones are present. Individuals who are having a hepatic artery pump inserted for the management of colorectal metastases to the liver routinely undergo cholecystectomy. Finally, patients with a single, very large gallstone occupying most of the lumen of the gall bladder are thought to be at very high risk for developing a complication, and thus may be considered for cholecystectomy even though they are asymptomatic.

Well over 90% of patients who undergo elective cholecystectomy, do so laparoscopically. There are still indications, however, for open cholecystectomy. If, during a laparoscopic procedure technical difficulties arise, such as too many adhesions to accurately expose the gall bladder, bleeding difficult to control, unclear anatomy, or a bile leak, one should convert to an open cholecystectomy. Furthermore, in some patients who have had multiple right upper quadrant operative procedures, laparoscopic cholecystectomy should probably not be attempted, and open cholecystectomy should be performed. Finally, if, during an open procedure for another indication, gallstones are found —whether or not the patient is symptomatic—the surgeon may decide to perform an open cholecystectomy.

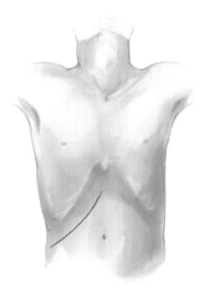

Operative Technique:

The operation is generally performed through a right subcostal incision, although an upper mid-line abdominal incision or even a right paramedian incision provides excellent exposure. It has been our feeling, however, that a right paramedian incision should rarely be used for any operative procedure.

Once the abdomen is entered, the peritoneal cavity is explored for evidence of other pathology. When none is found, the surgeon proceeds with the open cholecystectomy. Exposure is greatly facilitated if one of a variety of self-retaining retractors is used. Use of the upper hand retractor is an excellent way to retract the skin, subcutaneous tissues, and costal margin in the right upper quadrant. A Deaver retractor then easily exposes the under-surface of the liver (1). The hepatic flexure of the colon is mobilized by dividing the peritoneal attachments just cephalad to the hepatic flexure, that frequently extend up over the second portion of the duodenum and head of the pancreas. The colon is then retracted in a caudal direction, using a Mikulicz pad. The stomach is packed medially, also with a Mikulicz pad. A Kelly clamp is placed on the gall bladder infundibulum, and the gall bladder is retracted in a cephalad and lateral direction.

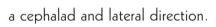

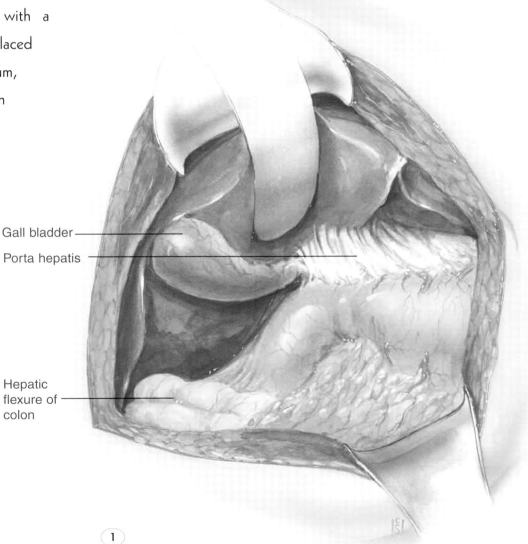

Gall bladder

Porta hepatis

Hepatic flexure of colon

1

The serosa overlying the porta hepatis is opened and the portal structures identified (2). The cystic duct is usually easily identified first and is looped with a 2-0 silk tie. If it is doubly looped, this will prevent gallstones from passing through the cystic duct into the common duct during manipulation of the gall bladder.

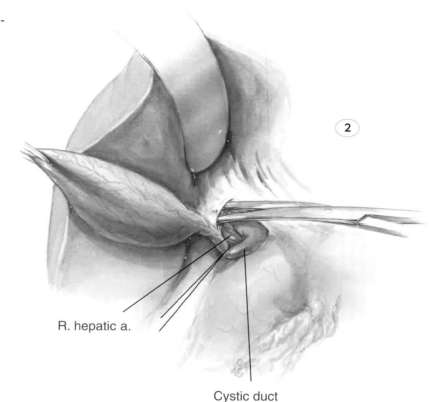

R. hepatic a.

Cystic duct

Dissection of Calot's triangle allows identification of the cystic artery, which may arise from the common hepatic artery, or more frequently from the right hepatic artery (3). This anatomy is extremely variable, and this area has to be dissected carefully and completely to clearly identify the cystic duct and cystic artery to avoid injuring anomalous structures. The right hepatic artery frequently follows the cystic duct and/or gall bladder very closely before curving back up into the liver parenchyma, and for a 1 cm or 2 cm course, it can easily be confused with the cystic artery. The arterial anatomy has to be dissected such that the cystic artery is clearly seen joining the gall bladder before one can be certain of its identification. The cystic artery often approaches the gall bladder just above the cystic duct, from a perpendicular direction. Again, an arterial structure running parallel to the cystic duct is more apt to be the right hepatic artery.

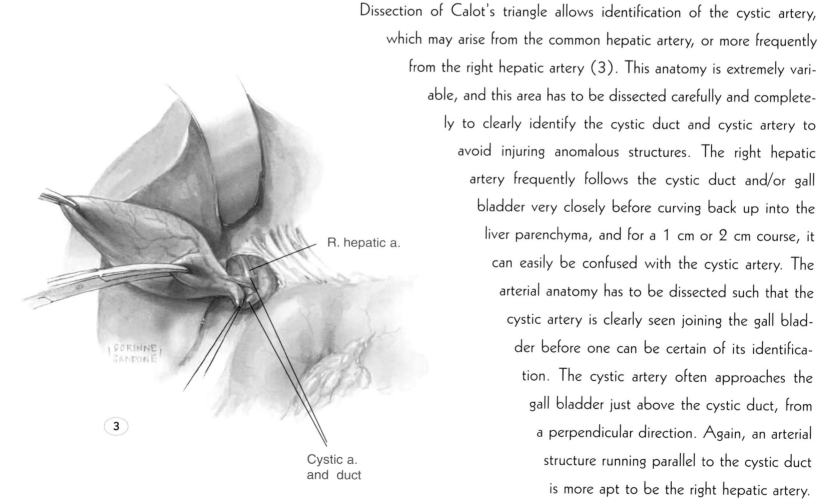

R. hepatic a.

Cystic a.
and duct

The cystic duct can also present confusing anatomy. The cystic duct usually arises from the common hepatic duct, but it may arise from the right hepatic duct or from one of the two segmental ducts to the right lobe of the liver. It also may arise very low posterior to the duodenum and course up parallel to the common hepatic duct up into the hilum of the liver before coursing to the right to enter the gall bladder. This area has to be very carefully and completely dissected to be certain of the anatomy, so that important structures are not injured. If the anatomy of the cystic duct/hepatic duct junction cannot clearly be delineated, one should stop further dissection in this area and proceed to mobilize the gall bladder from above downward. When the gall bladder has been mobilized out of the liver bed, the anatomy of this area will become clear. Early cholangiography, performed by injecting contrast directly into the gall bladder or ductal system may also be helpful. It remains controversial as to whether or not routine cholangiography should be performed with every cholecystectomy. With the introduction of laparoscopic cholecystectomy, where routine cholangiography is more difficult and time consuming, this argument has lessened somewhat and now there are many more surgeons who feel that only selective cholangiography should be performed. Everyone is in agreement, however, that if the anatomy is unclear, cholangiography is indicated.

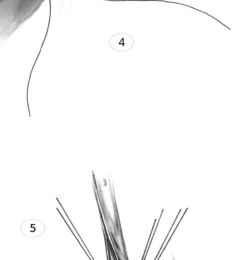

R. hepatic a.

Cystic duct

4

Cystic a.

5

Cystic a. and duct

Once the anatomy of the cystic artery is clear, it should be triply ligated with 2-0 silks and divided (4, 5). We would like to emphasize, once again, that the cystic artery should not be ligated and divided until one is certain of the anatomy. Mobilizing the fundus of the gall bladder and taking it from above downward prior to dividing the cystic artery can usually accomplish this.

Once the cystic artery has been divided, the gall bladder is mobilized out of the liver bed (6). I prefer to mobilize it from above downward. The serosa is opened three or four millimeters from the liver, and then elevated with a fine clamp. Using the electrocautery, the serosa is divided from above downward circumferentially around the entire gall bladder. The gall bladder is then dissected out of the liver bed utilizing the electrocautery, sharp dissection using scissors (7), or by blunt dissection. One needs to be aware that small anomalous ducts may enter the gall bladder directly from the liver, and these should be clamped and ligated, or suture ligated. If the cystic artery has been divided prior to mobilization of the gall bladder, very little bleeding occurs. Any bleeding that is present is easily controlled with the electrocautery or an argon beam coagulator.

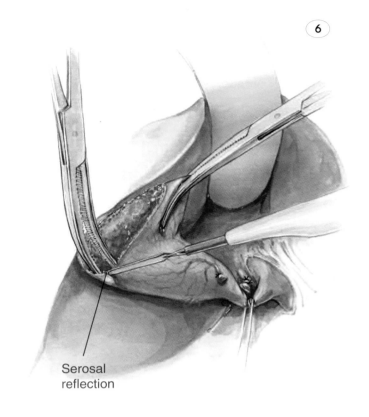

Serosal reflection

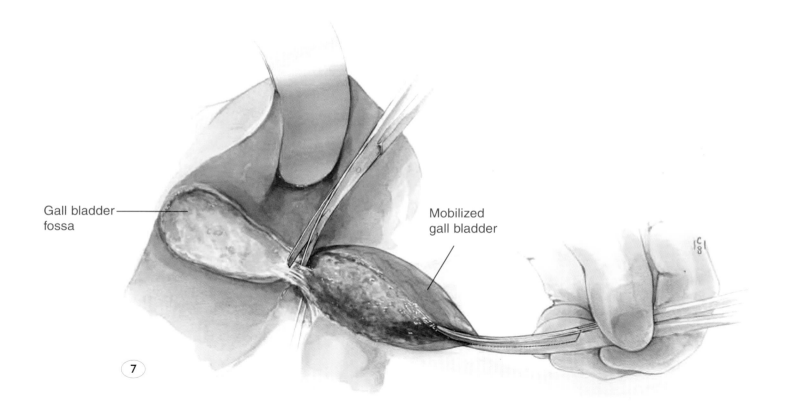

Gall bladder fossa

Mobilized gall bladder

Once the gall bladder has been completely mobilized out of the liver bed, the anatomy is generally clear, and if the cystic artery has not been previously identified, control of that vessel can now be accomplished. If one has decided to perform operative cholangiography, once the gall bladder mobilization has been completed, it is time to perform the procedure (8).

In most patients with normal liver function, and no other clear indications for cholangiography, it will not be necessary. However, in some patients operative cholangiography will be required. In patients who have a history of cholangitis or pancreatitis and with multiple small stones in the gall bladder, many feel cholangiography is indicated. If the common duct is dilated, and if there has been a clear history of common duct stones, cholangiography should be performed. After placing a tie at the cystic–duct–gall bladder junction, a small opening is made distally in the cystic duct, approximately 1 cm from its junction with the common hepatic duct. A cholangiocatheter is inserted and secured with a 2-0 silk that is tied around the distal cystic duct containing the catheter (8). After adequate cholangiography has been obtained, the cholangiocatheter is removed, the cystic duct is doubly clamped and divided (9), and the gall bladder is removed from the operative field.

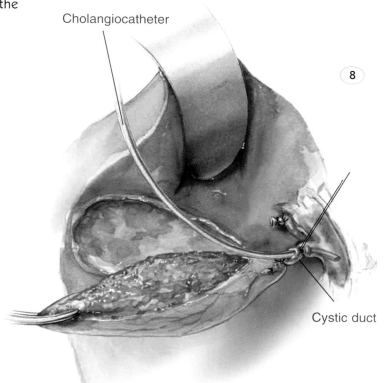

Cholangiocatheter

8

Cystic duct

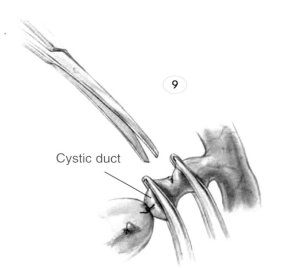

9

Cystic duct

The cystic duct stump is then ligated with a 2-0 silk (10). Most surgeons continue to use silk, as we do. Others are concerned that silk may act as a nidus for gallstone formation and thus use a synthetic absorbable material. Clips may also be used. Clips are used routinely during laparoscopic cholecystectomy. The right upper quadrant is copiously irrigated with an antibiotic-containing saline solution, hemostasis in the bed of the liver is achieved with the electrocautery or argon beam coagulator, and the abdomen is closed (11). Most surgeons do not leave a drain following a routine cholecystectomy. However, if the cholecystectomy was for acute cholecystitis, or if there has been bile leakage from the gall bladder bed in the liver, leaving a closed suction Silastic drain is appropriate.

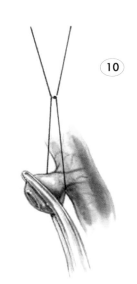

Many studies have shown drains to be unnecessary following cholecystectomy.

The only reason for leaving a drain behind is if an unexpected bile leak occurs from a small unrecognized bile ductule in the bed of the liver. Leaving a drain in place obviates the need for percutaneous drainage if a biloma or abscess occurs. Even though rare, it seems to us that the discomfort of a drain is worth the avoidance of a potential biloma or subhepatic abscess, in the face of acute cholecystitis, or bile seeping from the gall bladder bed in the liver. If biliary drainage does not occur within 48 hours, it can be removed, often on an outpatient basis. There are virtually no significant liabilities from draining the operative site following elective cholecystectomy.

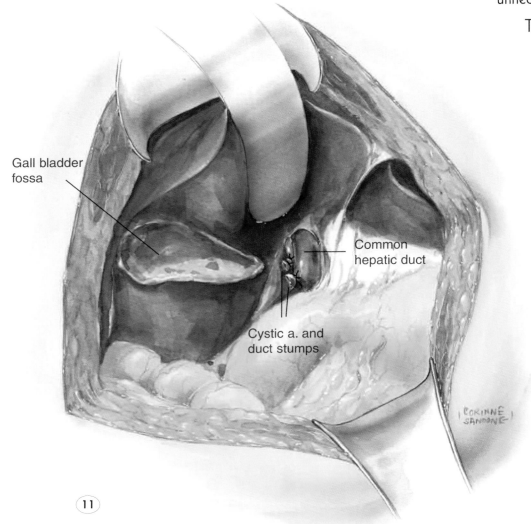

Gall bladder fossa

Common hepatic duct

Cystic a. and duct stumps

Common Duct Exploration

Operative Indications:

In the past, common duct exploration was a common procedure performed by general surgeons. Today it is only infrequently indicated. Most patients with common duct stones can be managed by endoscopic techniques. Endoscopic retrograde cholangiography can delineate the anatomy, and following papillotomy, most stones can be endoscopically extracted from the duct using balloons or baskets. Those that cannot be easily extracted generally pass spontaneously within the next few days. Some patients are not candidates for endoscopic papillotomy. Patients who have had gastric resections with a Billroth II reconstruction, generally are not candidates for endoscopic retrograde procedures on the biliary tree. Many of those patients can be managed percutaneously and transhepatically with catheters, either pushing the stone forward through the ampulla into the duodenum, or extracting them out a mature percutaneous tract. Occasionally, there will be patients who are not candidates for either endoscopic or percutaneous procedures—who, at the time of open cholecystectomy, will have indications for common duct exploration.

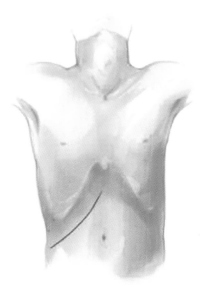

Operative Technique

The operation is generally performed through a right subcostal incision.

Prior to performing a choledochotomy the duodenum is kocherized extensively (1). This allows one to palpate the distal common duct as it passes behind the first portion of the duodenum and the head of the pancreas, prior to entering the distal second portion of the duodenum through the ampulla. The common duct itself is cleaned for a 2 cm or 3 cm length, generally between the cystic duct stump and the duodenum. Stay sutures of 5-O synthetic nonabsorbable material are placed in the common duct, and a choledochotomy is performed (2). The choledochotomy should be of ample length, at least 1½ cm, to allow for easy instrumentation of the duct without traumatic extension. Stones are often spontaneously evacuated as bile issues forth from the common duct opening. At the same time, any stones that are palpated in the distal common duct can be milked up toward the choledochotomy and removed (3).

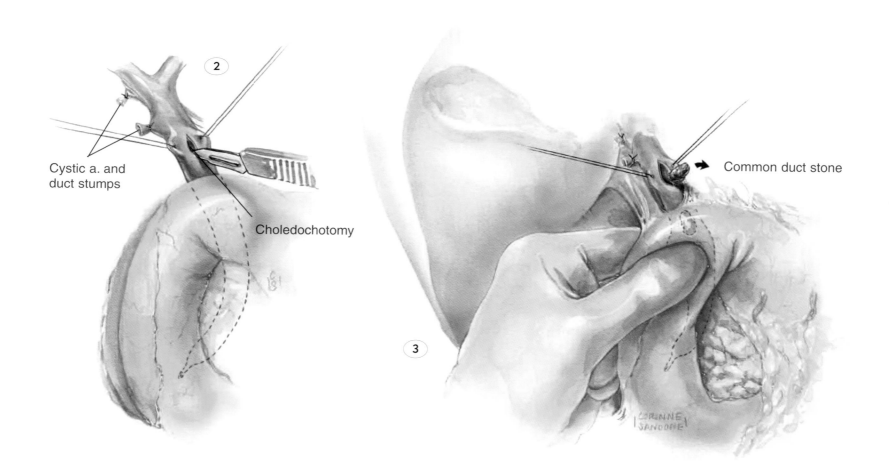

There are a variety of instruments that one can utilize to explore the biliary tree. Generally, we utilize all of these instruments in an effort to completely rid the biliary tree of calculi. It is important that the choledochotomy be made adequate in length, so that the instruments used to extract biliary calculi do not traumatically extend the incision. A variety of scoops with malleable handles can be used to pass distally down to the ampulla (4) and proximally up into the intrahepatic biliary tree via both the right and left hepatic ducts. These scoops come in a variety of sizes and can be extremely effective in removing small stones or biliary sludge.

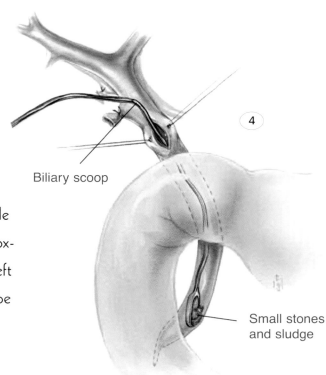

Biliary scoop

4

Small stones and sludge

Randall stone forceps are also utilized (5), and many surgeons use these instruments initially in the duct exploration. These forceps come with a variety of curves that range from almost straight, to right-angled and even acutely angled. These instruments are very effective in grasping larger well-formed stones. The biliary balloon catheter is particularly useful. It can be passed down distally through the ampulla and then inflated to document patency of the distal biliary tree into the duodenum. This is perhaps the safest way to demonstrate an open ampulla. In using the balloon catheter, one has to be careful that it is not overdistended. Experimental studies have demonstrated intrahepatic ductal disruptions and liver abscesses from overinflation of the balloon. If one constantly moves the catheter back and forth as the balloon is inflated, being certain that the balloon catheter remains mobile within the ductal system, overinflation is unlikely.

Intrahepatic stone

5

Randall stone forceps

The balloon catheter is particularly effective in retrieving intra-hepatic stones (6).

One of the most effective maneuvers in ridding the biliary tree of small stones and biliary sludge is irrigation using a small catheter. A 12 French catheter placed intrahepatically into the right and left hepatic ducts, together with large volume irrigation with saline, is extremely effective in ridding the entire biliary tree of small stones (7).

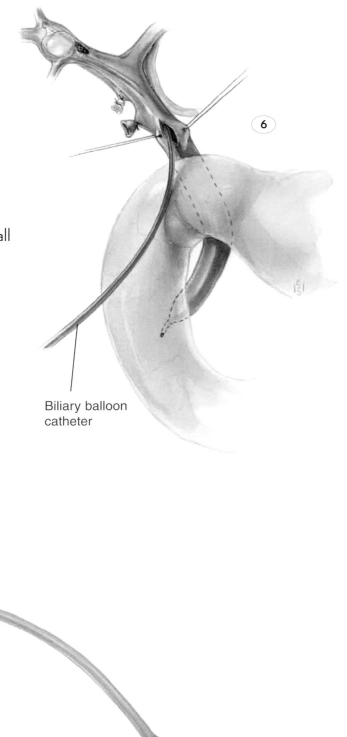

Biliary balloon catheter

Irrigation catheter

Operative Technique:

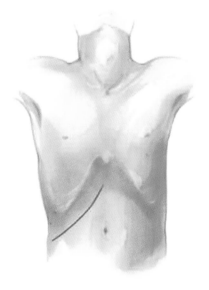

The abdomen is usually entered through a right subcostal incision. If the gall bladder is in place, a cholecystectomy is performed. After the gall bladder has been mobilized, cholangiography is often carried out. After the decision has been made to perform a sphincteroplasty, a small opening is made in the cystic duct, and a balloon catheter is inserted into the common duct, distally through the ampulla, and into the duodenum. The duodenum is kocherized and, following balloon inflation, the area of the ampulla can be identified by palpation. A longitudinal duodenotomy is made over the point where the surgeon palpates the balloon. If the gall bladder is not in place, an effort is made to palpate the ampulla through the duodenum to locate the correct position for the duodenotomy. If the ampulla cannot be palpated, a small choledochotomy can be performed and a Bakes dilator inserted down through the distal biliary tree and through the ampulla into the duodenum.

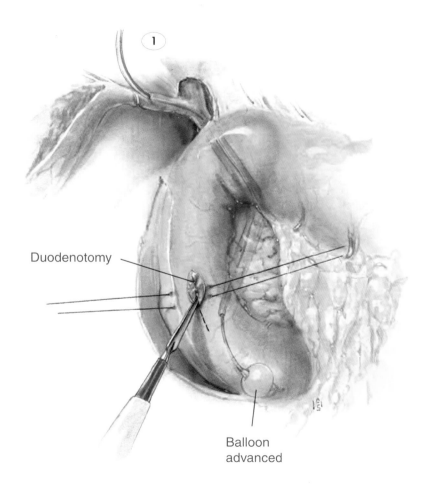

Duodenotomy

Balloon
advanced

Stay sutures of 3-0 silk are placed in the duodenum over the ampulla. The balloon catheter is then advanced beyond the ampulla so as not to perforate the balloon when the duodenotomy is performed. The duodenotomy is performed with the electrocautery (1). After the duodenotomy is completed, the ampulla can easily be seen by identifying the balloon catheter emanating from the biliary tree.

Once the location of the ampulla has been clearly identified, the duodenotomy can be extended in either or both directions for adequate exposure. Stay sutures of 5-0 synthetic absorbable material are placed at 3 o'clock and 9 o'clock into the muscular fibrous tissue of the ampulla. Using the balloon catheter as a guide, a sphincterotomy is performed at 11 o'clock or 12 o'clock with the electrocautery (2).

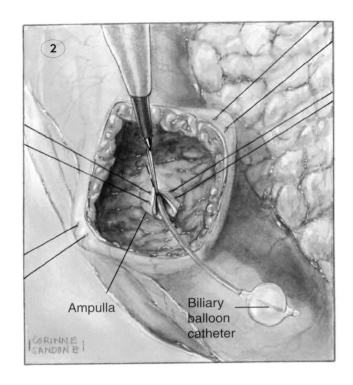

Ampulla

Biliary balloon catheter

The opening is extended three or four millimeters at a time. Once the ampulla has been opened, the ductal mucosa is sutured to the duodenum mucosa with a series of interrupted 5-0 synthetic absorbable sutures (3). These sutures are gathered in a hemostat. The retraction provides further exposure of the area.

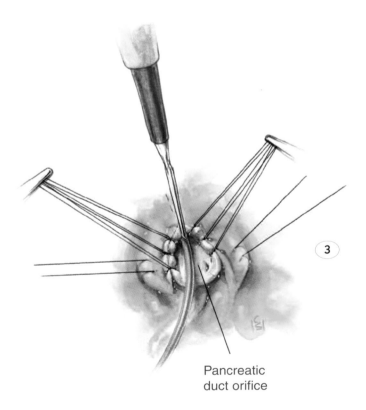

Pancreatic duct orifice

After the initial sphincterotomy incision, the pancreatic duct orifice can be identified with a silver probe (4). The sphincterotomy is generally extended for 1 cm or 2 cm with further 5-0 synthetic absorbable sutures being placed to approximate the duodenal and ductal mucosa. Finally, an apex suture is placed when the length of the sphincterotomy is deemed sufficient. There is little sense in making a sphincterotomy incision that is larger than the diameter of the common duct.

The length of the sphincteroplasty incision will vary depending upon the reason for its use. If one is performing a sphincteroplasty merely to dislodge an impacted common duct stone, a larger incision is unnecessary once the incision is large enough to dislodge the stone. On the other hand, if one is performing a sphincteroplasty incision in a markedly dilated common duct because of the concern of leaving behind retained stones, or if one is performing the sphincteroplasty because of recurrent primary common duct stones, a sphincteroplasty incision 2 cm to 3 cm in length may be carried out. One should be careful not to extend the sphincteroplasty incision beyond the point where the biliary tract and duodenum have a common wall. With careful approximation of the ductal and duodenal mucosa, however, risk of retroperitoneal or intraperitoneal leakage is virtually eliminated.

Apex suture

(4)

Probe in pancreatic duct

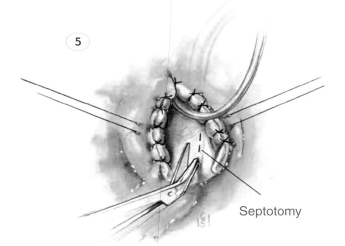

(5)

Septotomy

If the sphincteroplasty has been carried out for what are believed to be symptoms related to the pancreas, from a stenotic pancreatic duct orifice, a septotomy can be performed with Pott's scissors (5). This incision can usually be extended for four or five millimeters, at which point the septum thickens as the course of the pancreatic and biliary tree diverge. Some feel that the pancreatic and ductal mucosa should also be approximated with 5-0 or 6-0 synthetic absorbable material.

Following the completion of the sphincteroplasty, the balloon catheter is removed, the cystic duct is doubly clamped and divided, and the gall bladder is removed from the operative field. The cystic duct stump is ligated with a 2-0 silk. If it has been necessary to perform a choledochotomy for insertion of a Bakes dilator, a small T-tube should be left.

If the sphincteroplasty has been performed because of cholangiographic evidence of biliary calculi in a normal or small common duct, to avoid the technical and mechanical problems of exploring a small duct through a choledochotomy, we have utilized transampullary exploration. The common duct can be explored with the same variety of instruments as one utilizes with a traditional common duct explo- ration through a choledochotomy. Biliary scoops, Randall stone forceps (6), flushing through a French catheter, and a balloon catheter can all be utilized (7). At the end of the procedure, one does not have to be concerned about placing a small T-tube in a very small common duct. In addition, a sphinctero- plasty has been performed, so if one does not retrieve all the stones in the bil- iary tree, the stones have a free course to pass spontaneously.

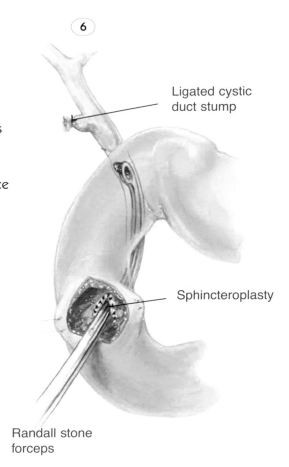

6

Ligated cystic duct stump

Sphincteroplasty

Randall stone forceps

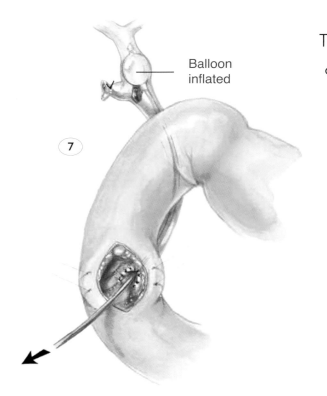

7

Balloon inflated

The lateral stay sutures are removed from the duodenum, and stay sutures of 3-0 silk are placed at each end of the duodenotomy. The duodeno- tomy can be closed longitudinally or transversely. We generally will close the duodenum longitudinally. It is closed in two layers; the inner layer is a continuous suture of 3-0 synthetic absorbable material placed in a Connell fashion. Sutures are started at each end and are tied in the middle. The outer layer is a row of inter- rupted, 3-0 silk, Lembert sutures. The duodenotomy may be drained with a Silastic closed suction drain. This is more for pro- tection in case the sphincteroplasty extends beyond the point where the biliary tree and duodenum share a common wall, rather than protection against leakage from the duodenotomy.

This suture is gathered in a similar fashion by holding both ends and the mid-portion of the suture in a hemostat. Again, this nicely aligns the duodenotomy and choledochotomy so that the anastomosis can be completed. The anastomosis is completed with a series of through-and-through, interrupted 3-0 silk sutures. The final three or four sutures of the side-to-side choledochoduodenostomy are held until all sutures are in place and then they are secured (6).

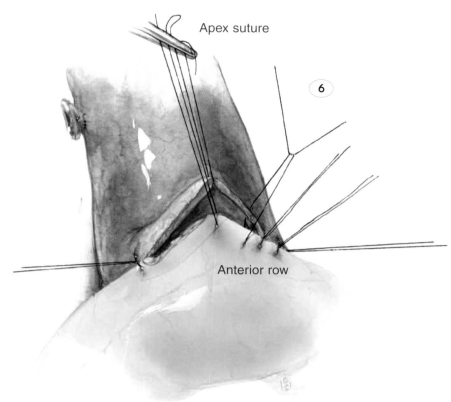

This is a side-to-side anastomosis, which is performed by pulling the first and second portions of the duodenum on top of the common duct, and then carrying out the anastomosis. The anastomosis can easily be palpated through the duodenum when the procedure is completed and should be widely patent. The anastomosis is demonstrated diagrammatically in (7). The theoretical shortcomings of the procedure are also nicely depicted. There is a segment of biliary tree that extends from the choledochoduodenostomy down to the ampulla. It has been reported that vegetable material from the duodenum can pass into the biliary tree through the side-to-side anastomosis and can become impacted distally, producing non-specific right upper quadrant symptoms referred to as "the sump syndrome." This is a theoretical disadvantage of the operative procedure, but we have never seen this complication. The area of the choledochoduodenostomy can be drained with a closed suction Silastic drain.

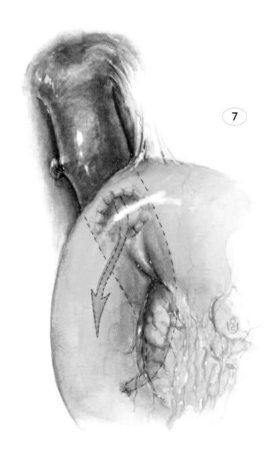

Resection of a Benign Bile Duct Stricture with Reconstruction Utilizing a Hepaticojejunostomy

Operative Indications:

Benign bile duct strictures can follow a variety of clinical situations. Scarring and fibrosis of the head of the pancreas from chronic pancreatitis can result in a distal biliary stricture. Mirizzi's syndrome, with impaction of a cystic duct stone obstructing the common hepatic duct, can also result in a benign biliary stricture. The majority of benign strictures, however, follow operative trauma, usually occurring during a laparoscopic cholecystectomy. Occasionally during a gastrectomy, operative trauma can also result in a biliary stricture. Prior to the introduction of laparoscopic cholecystectomy in 1989, the incidence of injury to the biliary tree during a cholecystectomy had fallen to approximately 1 in 1,000. Immediately following the introduction of laparoscopic cholecystectomy, the incidence increased to 1 in 100. Today, it has stabilized in the range of 2 to 5 in 1,000 cholecystectomies.

The total number of benign biliary strictures secondary to cholecystectomy is actually greater now than it was a decade or two ago, because of the introduction of laparoscopic cholecystectomy, and the higher incidence of injury. In addition, the injuries tend to be higher up in the hilum, presumably because of the easier access to this area laparoscopically, compared to an open procedure. If the biliary stricture involves the mid- or distal portion of the extrahepatic biliary tree, the repair is straightforward. The proximal biliary segment is dissected free, and a mucosal-to-mucosal anastomosis is performed between the common hepatic duct and a Roux-en-Y jejunal loop. Long-term stenting is not necessary. A T-tube may be used at the time of surgery to decompress the anastomosis, or if preoperatively inserted, a percutaneous transhepatic biliary catheter can be used. The T-tube or percutaneous biliary catheter can be removed 6 weeks after the repair. Today, however, most biliary tract surgeons would use no stent.

Many, if not most, extrahepatic injuries that occur during laparoscopic cholecystectomy, however, involve the common hepatic duct proximally, near or even involving the bifurcation. These high strictures are more difficult to manage. In recent years, the majority of patients referred to our institution with post-cholecystectomy strictures have had multiple ligaclips in the porta hepatis, and these often are found to be responsible for the stricture (1). It is our practice to perform preoperative percutaneous transhepatic cholangiography on all patients with a suspected stricture with the insertion of a percutaneous biliary catheter. If the injury is acute, and there are bilomas or subhepatic abscesses, these are drained percutaneously. At the time of percutaneous transhepatic cholangiography, the anatomy can be clearly delineated and external biliary drainage established. If biliary continuity has not been totally disrupted, passing the percutaneous biliary catheter through the area of injury into the duodenum will be important. In these patients, internal biliary drainage can be established. Once the bilomas and abscesses have been successfully drained and biliary drainage established (either externally or internally), the actual repair is often delayed for 6 weeks to 3 months, to allow the right upper quadrant inflammation to subside. If the injury is more chronic, however, and there is no evidence of biloma or intra-abdominal abscess formation, the repair can be carried out electively at any time. If there has been no intra-abdominal leakage, at the time of laparotomy for biliary stricture repair the amount of inflammation and adhesions can be minimal, compared to the era when most injuries were produced during open cholecystectomy.

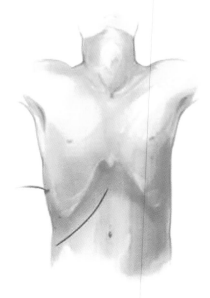

Cystic duct stump

Clip

Catheter in duodenum

Operative Technique:

Most patients today with benign biliary strictures will have undergone a cholecystectomy laparoscopically. However, some of these patients will have been converted to an open procedure. The patient is prepped and draped so that the percutaneous transhepatic biliary catheter is accessible in the prepped area during the procedure. The abdomen is entered through a right subcostal incision. Upon entering the abdomen, adhesions are encountered. These, however, are less severe following a laparoscopic cholecystectomy, compared to an open cholecystectomy. The adhesions are dissected both sharply and bluntly. By palpating in the porta hepatis for the previously placed percutaneous transhepatic biliary catheter, identification of the biliary tree is greatly facilitated. In the past, particularly if the patient had been operated upon several times, and no catheter was present within the biliary tree, dissection to identify the proximal biliary segment took hours. However, with a catheter in place, the dissection proceeds rapidly, and within a relatively short time, the proximal biliary segment can be identified.

Once the extrahepatic biliary tree has been identified, it is mobilized and encircled with a vessel loop (2). Dissection then proceeds proximally towards the bifurcation. The proximal biliary segment is frequently surrounded by a dense inflammatory reaction with fibrosis. Ligaclips often add to the difficulty of the dissection.

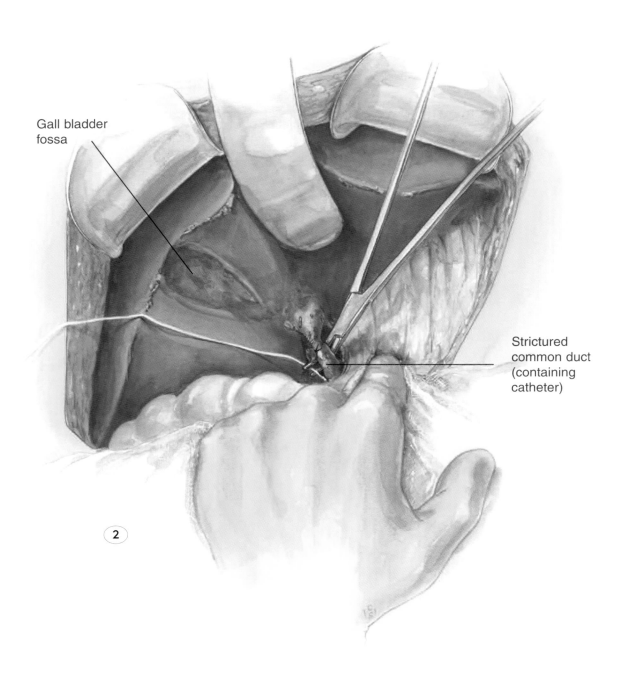

Gall bladder fossa

Strictured common duct (containing catheter)

2

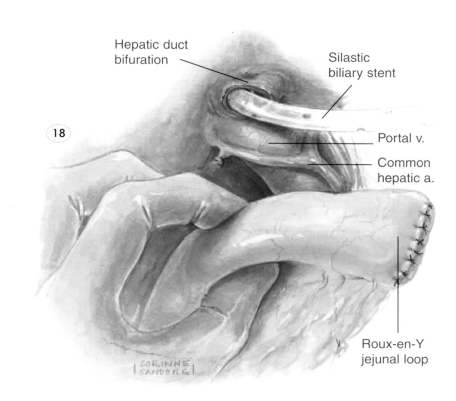

Hepatic duct bifuration

Silastic biliary stent

Portal v.

Common hepatic a.

Roux-en-Y jejunal loop

18

If the Roux-en-Y loop is 60 cm in length and the division in the small bowel mesentery is long enough, the Roux-en-Y loop will rest comfortably in the right upper quadrant without tension (18). The hepaticojejunostomy is performed in one layer. Interrupted 4-0 synthetic absorbable material is used.

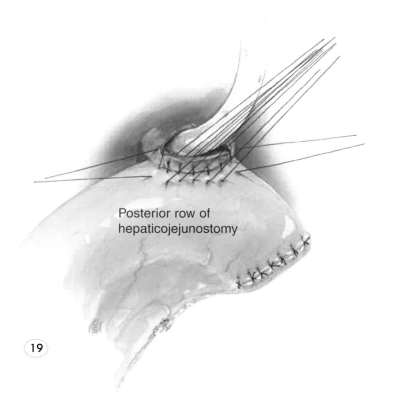

Posterior row of hepaticojejunostomy

19

The posterior row is placed first between the proximal biliary segment and the Roux-en-Y jejunal loop, prior to performing an enterotomy (19). The sutures pass into the submucosal layer of the jejunum and then through and through the proximal biliary segment. The proximal biliary segment may not be a complete rim of good mucosa, especially if the patient has had multiple attempts at prior repairs. This is the principal reason for using a transhepatic Silastic biliary stent, and leaving it for a prolonged period during healing and wound maturation.

Once the posterior row has been positioned, the sutures are secured and an enterotomy is performed with the electrocautery (20). The sutures are divided and the Silastic transhepatic biliary stent is passed through the enterotomy into the Roux-en-Y loop (21). The anterior row of sutures is completed with a single layer of interrupted through-and-through 4-0 synthetic absorbable sutures (22). This anastomosis is not, strictly speaking, a mucosal-to-mucosal anastomosis, because the posterior row was placed before the enterotomy. However, it functions as a mucosal-to-mucosal anastomosis and is easier to perform than if an enterotomy is made first.

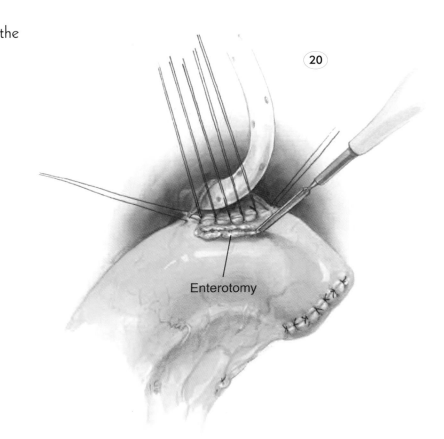

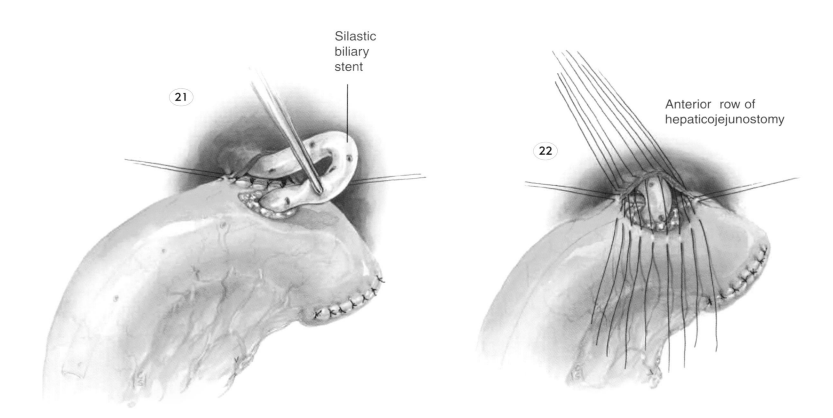

The Roux-en-Y loop may be tacked to periportal material on the undersurface of the liver to ensure that there is no tension on the anastomosis. We have found, however, that if the Roux-en-Y loop rests comfortably in the right upper quadrant, this step is not necessary. The Roux-en-Y loop is tacked to the opening in the transverse mesocolon to prevent small bowel herniation (23). The end of the Silastic biliary stent that emanates from the superior surface of the liver is brought out through a stab wound in the right upper quadrant. It is sutured in place to the skin using 5-0 stainless steel wire.

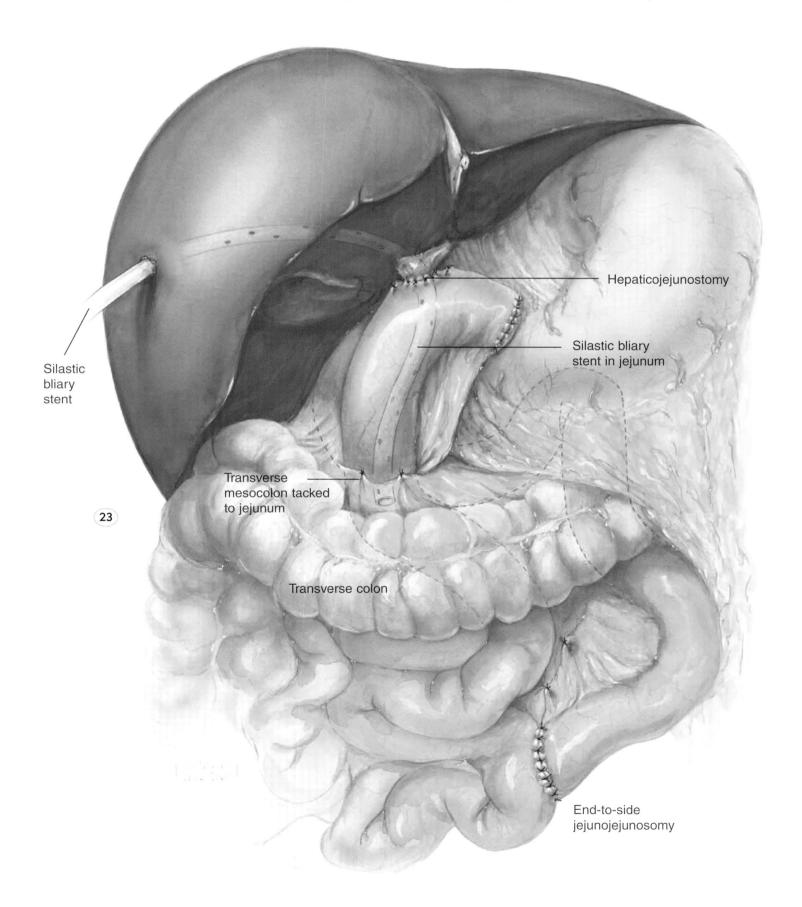

Silastic
bliary
stent

Hepaticojejunostomy

Silastic bliary
stent in jejunum

Transverse
mesocolon tacked
to jejunum

23

Transverse colon

End-to-side
jejunojejunosomy

It is placed to bile bag gravity drainage. A closed suction Silastic drain is left near the top of the liver at the egress site of the transhepatic biliary stent. The drain is brought out through a stab wound in the right upper quadrant. The hepaticojejunostomy is also drained with a closed suction Silastic drain.

At five days post-repair, cholangiography is performed through the Silastic stent, and if no leaks are evident at the anastomosis or at the superior surface of the liver, the stent is internalized. This can be accomplished by placing a three-way stopcock at the end of the biliary stent as it emanates out of the right upper quadrant, or by utilizing a heparin lock. The patient is taught to irrigate the tube twice a day with 20ml of saline. If an excellent mucosal-to-mucosal anastomosis has been performed, it is not necessary to leave the Silastic stent in for a prolonged period. Generally, 2 months after cholangiography, and after a clinical trial of leaving the stent in the liver but above the anastomosis for 2 weeks, and after performing a flow study, the stent is removed. However, if a good proximal biliary segment has not been present, and a good mucosal-to-mucosal anastomosis has not been performed, the stent is left in for a 12-month period to allow wound healing and contracture to proceed, in the face of a relatively non-reactive, large-bore, thick-walled Silastic stent. Even though the biliary stents are made of Silastic and are relatively non-reactive, biliary sludge can collect and occlude side holes. For this reason, the stents are changed every 3 or 4 months as an outpatient procedure. Under fluoroscopy, a guidewire is placed into the Roux-en-Y loop through the lumen of the old stent. The old stent is removed and a new one easily slipped in place. At the end of 1 year, the stent can be removed with virtual certainty that a stable anastomosis between the proximal biliary segment and jejunum has been created that will function obstruction-free indefinitely.

Prior to removing the stent, however, a good cholangiogram is performed with the stent pulled back into the liver to visualize the anastomosis. In addition, a clinical trial is carried out leaving the stent in the liver but above the anastomosis for a 2-week period. If cholangitis has not developed within that 2-week period, a flow study is performed. If the flow study using saline infused into the biliary stent above the anastomosis is normal, the stent is then removed.

If the benign stricture involves the hepatic duct bifurcation, it is necessary to resect the bifurcation and to perform bilateral hepaticojejunostomies. Preoperatively, transhepatic biliary catheters can be placed in both the right and left hepatic ducts. Following bifurcation resection, Silastic stents are placed in both the right and left hepatic ducts and bilateral hepaticojejunostomies are performed.

Resection of a Proximal Cholangiocarcinoma (Klatskin tumor) with Reconstruction via Bilateral Hepaticojejunostomies

Operative Indications:

With the frequent use of endoscopic and percutaneous cholangiography, as well as MR cholangiopancreatography, an increasing number of patients
with proximal biliary tumors have been identified.
These small adenocarcinomas, often referred to as
Klatskin tumors, are located at or near the hepatic duct
bifurcation. Today, any individual presenting with jaundice, who on computed tomography (CT) scan or ultrasonography is found to have dilated intrahepatic ducts with a
collapsed extrahepatic biliary tree and gall bladder, is highly suspected of having a proximal cholangiocarcinoma. We feel that such
patients should undergo percutaneous cholangiography, with insertion of percutaneous transhepatic biliary catheters into the right
and left hepatic ducts, through the tumor, and distally into the
duodenum (1). In our experience, virtually all patients can
have these catheters placed bilaterally through the tumor and
into the duodenum, despite the initial cholangiogram demonstrating complete obstruction at the bifurcation. Patients with
proximal cholangiocarcinomas are staged preoperatively with
cholangiography, and thin section three-dimensional CT scans.

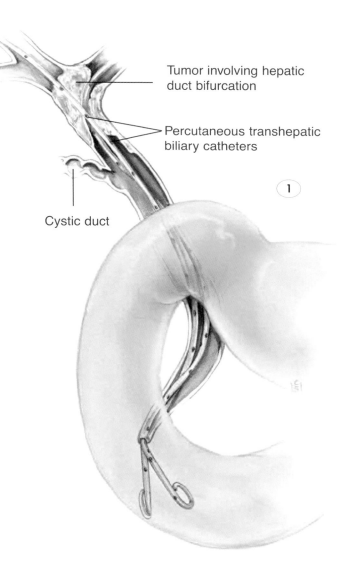

Tumor involving hepatic
duct bifurcation

Percutaneous transhepatic
biliary catheters

Cystic duct

1

Angiography was previously used for staging, but the accuracy of the three-dimensional CT scan, in most instances, has obviated its need. If, on cholangiography, the tumor clearly extends up into the hepatic parenchyma of both lobes, involving segmental branches on each side, the patient is palliated percutaneously with biliary catheters, and not explored. In addition, if a three-dimensional CT scan demonstrates encasement of the common hepatic artery or main portal vein, the patient is considered unresectable and is not explored. However, if only one branch of the hepatic artery or portal vein is involved, or if the tumor extends up into only one lobe, the patient still may be resectable if hepatic lobectomy is added (see next section, Resection of a Proximal Cholangiocarcinoma with Hepatic Lobectomy and Reconstruction with a Hepaticojejunostomy). After preoperative staging, approximately 60% of patients presenting with cholangiocarcinomas are candidates for resection.

In recent years, direct communication between the biliary tree bifurcation and the small ducts of the caudate lobe has been identified by several investigators. Thus, when the bifurcation is resected, inclusion of the caudate lobe, if possible, is preferable. However, because the portal vein and hepatic artery are interposed between the biliary tree and the caudate lobe, unless a hepatic lobectomy is performed, it can be exceedingly difficult to resect the caudate lobe.

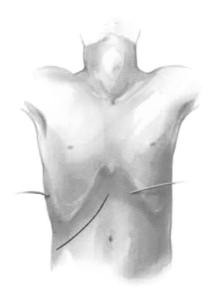

Operative Technique:

The patient is prepped and draped so that the surgeon has access to both percutaneous transhepatic biliary catheters in the operative field. A right subcostal incision is used. At the time of laparotomy the abdomen is explored for evidence of tumor dissemination. In our experience, liver metastases or peritoneal implants are uncommon. In addition, lymph node involvement is unusual. If a patient is unresectable, generally it is because of local involvement of parenchyma of both the right and left lobes, or involvement of the common hepatic artery or main portal vein.

Initially, at the time of laparotomy, the tumor generally cannot be seen or even felt. The gall bladder and extrahepatic biliary tree often appear normal. If one palpates high in the hilum of the liver, however, by feeling for the divergence of the biliary catheters, the area of the bifurcation and tumor can be identified (2). Two maneuvers greatly aid in exposing and dissecting the hepatic duct bifurcation. The first is mobilization of the gall bladder. If the gall bladder has not been removed previously, the cystic artery is identified, doubly clamped, divided, and ligated, and the gall bladder is mobilized out of the liver bed. This greatly improves access to the bifurcation. In addition, early in the dissection of the porta hepatis, the distal extrahepatic biliary tree is mobilized and looped with a vessel loop. Having the biliary catheters in place, particularly if the patient has been operated on previously, facilitates identification and dissection of the common duct.

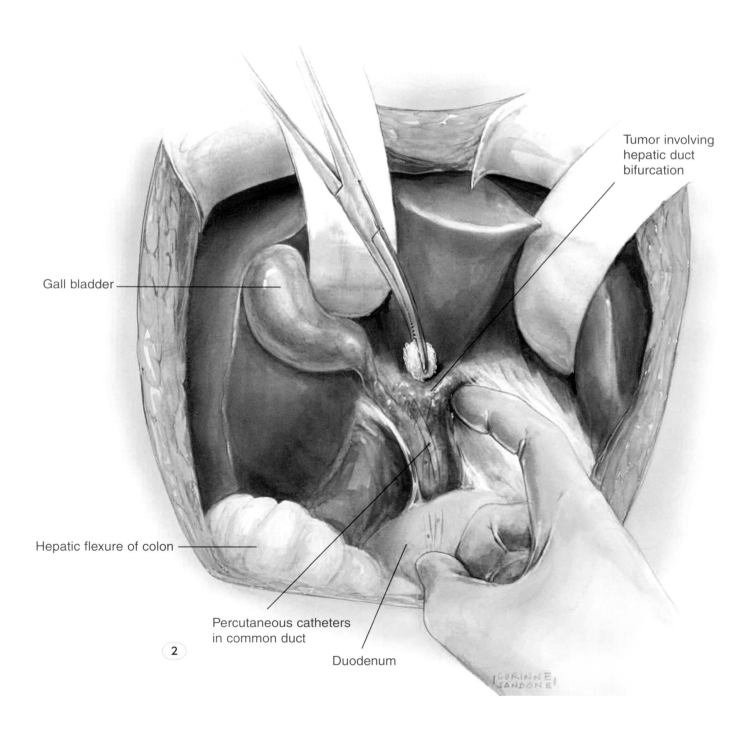

Tumor involving
hepatic duct
bifurcation

Gall bladder

Hepatic flexure of colon

Percutaneous catheters
in common duct

2

Duodenum

Once the duct has been mobilized, the anterior wall is opened, and the transhepatic biliary catheters extracted (3). The duct is then completely divided. The distal common duct can be ligated or closed with interrupted 3-0 silk sutures placed in a vertical mattress fashion. A distal margin of the biliary tree is sent for a frozen section to ensure that a distal negative margin has been obtained.

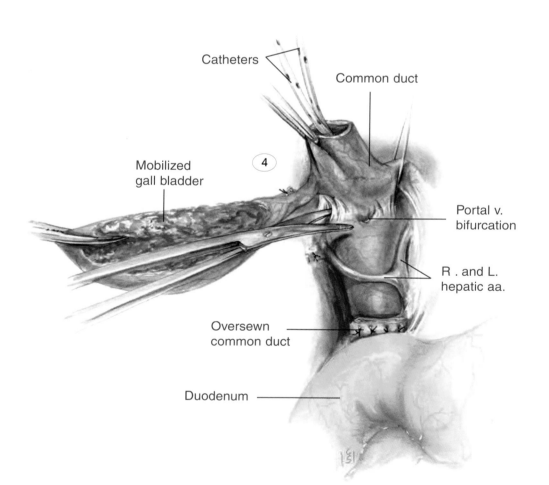

③ Tumor involving hepatic duct bifurcation

Catheters

Choledochotomy

④ Catheters

Common duct

Mobilized gall bladder

Portal v. bifurcation

R. and L. hepatic aa.

Oversewn common duct

Duodenum

These two maneuvers (mobilization of the gall bladder and early division of the distal common duct) aid greatly in access to and dissection of the bifurcation. Early division of the common duct allows one to dissect the bifurcation both anteriorly and posteriorly as the proximal biliary segment is being retracted cephalad (4). Retraction is aided by having the biliary catheters in place. The bifurcation of the biliary tree and the tumor rest on the bifurcation of the portal vein and hepatic artery. Dissection of this area without dividing

Once the posterior row of each hepaticojejunostomy has been placed, the sutures are secured. Bilateral enterotomies are made adjacent to the posterior row of sutures using the electrocautery (13).

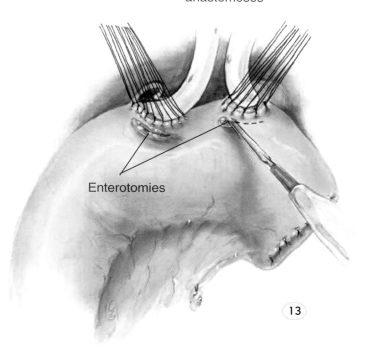

Posterior rows of anastomoses

Enterotomies

13

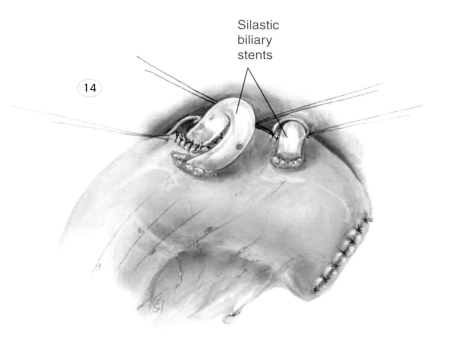

14

Silastic biliary stents

The posterior row of sutures, except for the two end sutures, is then divided, and the Silastic stents are placed in the Roux-en-Y loop via each enterotomy (14).

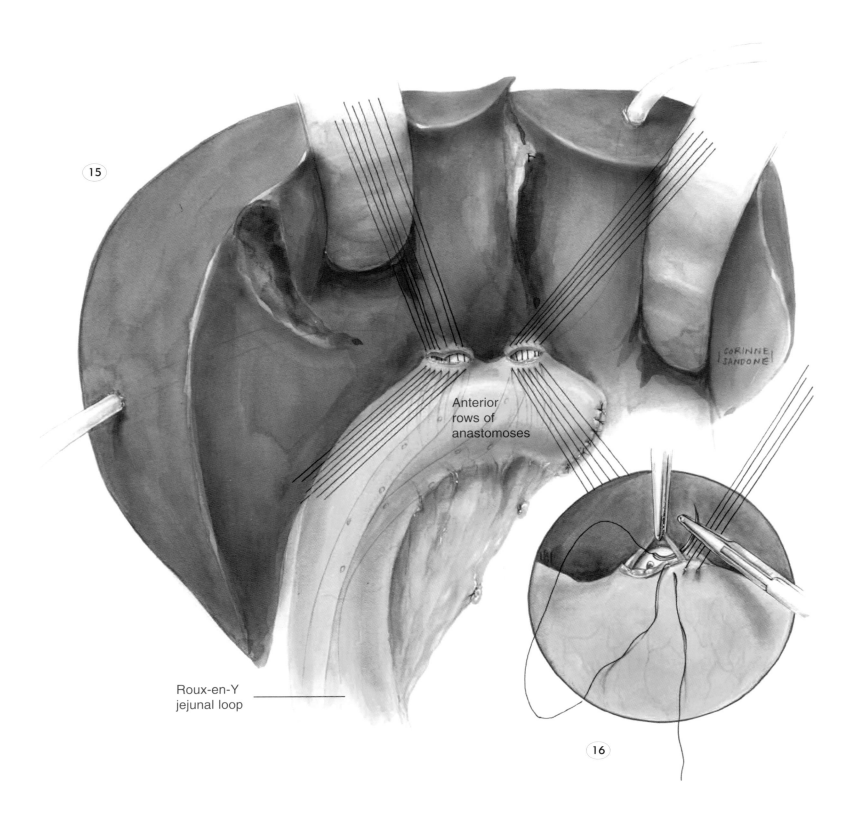

Each interrupted 4-0 synthetic absorbable suture is placed for the anterior layer of both hepaticojejunostomies, before securing the sutures (15). These sutures are simple sutures placed through and through the jejunum and then through and through the duct (16). Once all sutures of the anterior row of both hepaticojejunostomies have been placed, they are tied.

Once the anterior rows of both hepaticojejunostomies have been secured, the sutures are cut. The Roux-en-Y jejunal loop may be sutured to tissues on the undersurface of the liver with interrupted 3-0 silks to ensure that there is no tension on the anastomosis. With a Roux-en-Y loop 60 cm in length, however, it generally rests comfortably under the liver at the anastomosis, and fixation may not be necessary.

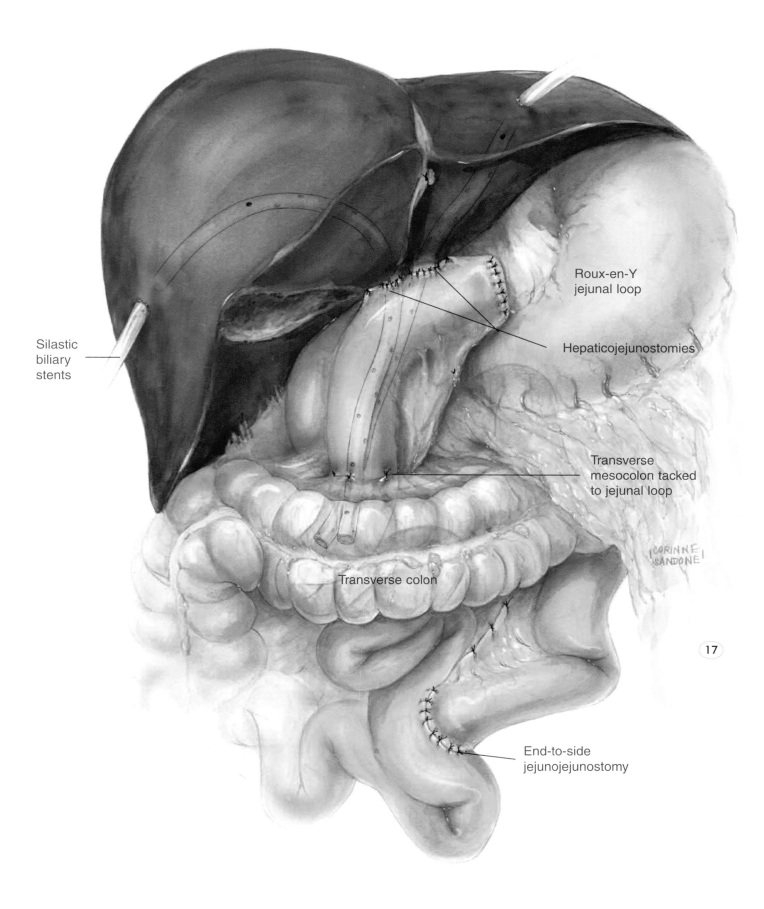

Silastic
biliary
stents

Roux-en-Y
jejunal loop

Hepaticojejunostomies

Transverse
mesocolon tacked
to jejunal loop

Transverse colon

End-to-side
jejunojejunostomy

(17)

The Roux-en-Y loop is sutured to the rent in the transverse mesocolon with interrupted 4-0 silks to prevent herniation of small bowel (17). Each Silastic transhepatic biliary stent is brought out through a separate stab wound in the right and left upper quadrants, and sutured to the skin with 5-0 stainless steel wire. The stents are connected to allow bile-bag drainage through gravity. The egress of each stent on the superior surface of the liver is drained with a closed suction Silastic drain brought out through separate stab wounds in the right and left upper quadrants. The bilateral hepaticojejunostomies are drained with a closed suction Silastic drain brought out through a stab wound in the mid-abdomen. The stents are left to allow gravity drainage for five days, at which time cholangiography is performed. If there are no leaks from the superior surface of the liver or at the anastomosis, the tubes are internalized by placing stopcocks or heparin locks on the ends of the stents.

The patients are taught to irrigate the stents twice a day with 20 mL of saline. Adjuvant therapy has not clearly been identified to be of benefit in these patients. However, we have had no long-term survivors who have not received radiotherapy. We thus generally deliver 5,000 rad of external beam radiotherapy to the tumor bed postoperatively. When this has been completed, the patients can be re-admitted and iridium 192 seeds lowered down through the bilateral transhepatic biliary stents and left in place for approximately 48 hours, to boost the radiation dosage an additional 2,000 rads. The transhepatic Silastic biliary stents are generally left in permanently. The stents are changed every 3 or 4 months as an outpatient procedure. This is carried out under fluoroscopy by placing a guidewire down through the old stent into the Roux-en-Y loop. The old stent is then removed, leaving the guidewire in place. A new stent is easily slipped in place over the guidewire and then the guidewire removed. The stents are left in long-term because, even though substantial prolongation of survival is achieved with this operative procedure, many patients are not cured and, eventually, the tumor will recur locally. If the Silastic stents are removed, biliary obstruction will recur. However, if a patient survives for three years, and there is no cholangiographic evidence of recurrent tumor, the Silastic stents may be removed.

Resection of a Proximal Cholangiocarcinoma with Hepatic Lobectomy and Reconstruction with a Hepaticojejunostomy

Operative Indications:

Patients with proximal cholangio-carcinomas will frequently have tumor extension up into one or the other lobe from the bifurcation (1). In most instances it will be on the right. In addition, it is not infrequent in such instances to have one branch of the portal vein or one branch of the hepatic artery on the involved side encased or occluded by tumor. Such patients may still be resectable if hepatic lobectomy is added to resection of the bifurcation and extrahepatic biliary tree. One is aware of this possibility prior to laparotomy because of preoperative cholangiographic and three-dimensional CT scan findings.

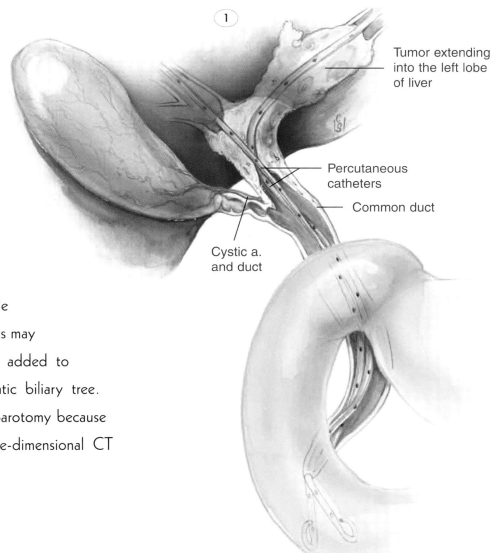

Tumor extending into the left lobe of liver

Percutaneous catheters

Common duct

Cystic a. and duct

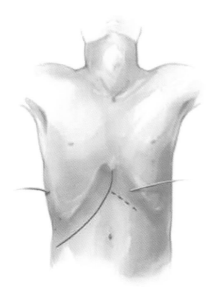

Operative Technique:

The patient is explored through a right subcostal incision, often extended up to the xiphoid in the midline, or over to the left side of the abdomen as a left subcostal extension. It is particularly important that these patients preoperatively have percutaneous transhepatic biliary catheters inserted bilaterally. The initial operative procedure is as described for resection of a proximal cholangiocarcinoma without hepatic lobectomy.

The gall bladder is mobilized to improve exposure of the bifurcation, and the distal common duct is divided (2) so that the proximal biliary segment can be reflected cephalad to facilitate bifurcation dissection.

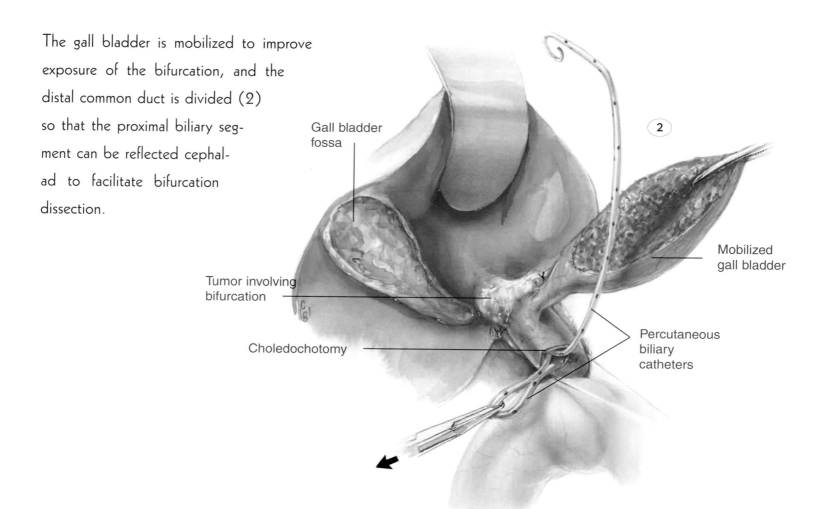

Gall bladder fossa

Tumor involving bifurcation

Choledochotomy

Mobilized gall bladder

Percutaneous biliary catheters

2

Once the hepatic duct bifurcation has been mobilized and dissected off the bifurcation of the portal vein and the hepatic artery (3), it is seen that the tumor extends well up into the left lobe of the liver, probably also involving the left branch of the hepatic artery and portal vein. On the right, however, normal hepatic duct can be identified by palpating the percutaneous biliary catheter above the tumor at the bifurcation.

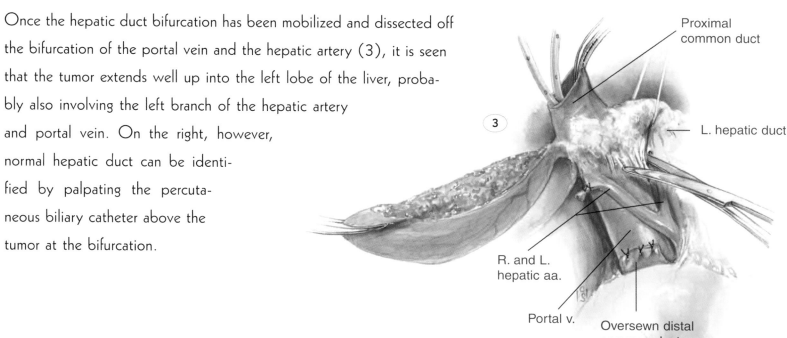

The right hepatic duct is divided (4) and the biliary catheter exposed and extracted. At this point, a frozen section should be taken of the right hepatic duct margin, and the distal common duct margin, to ensure that both of these margins are negative.

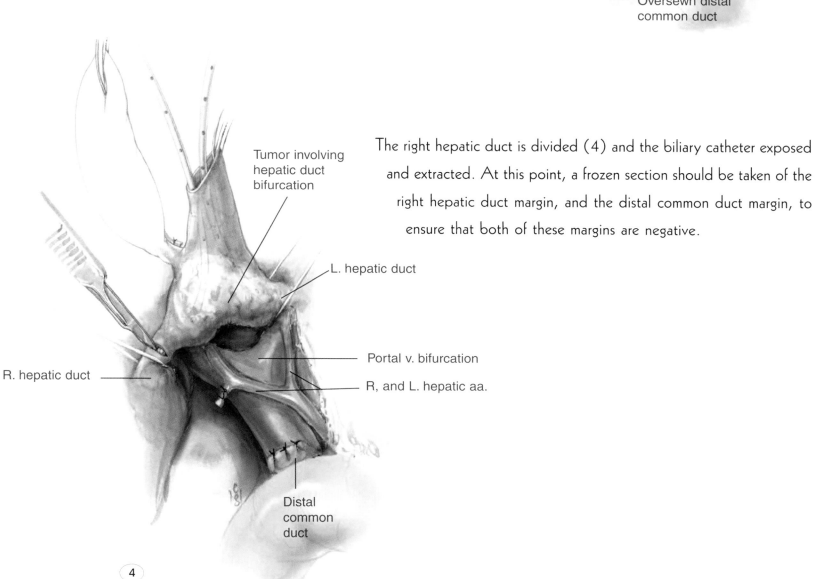

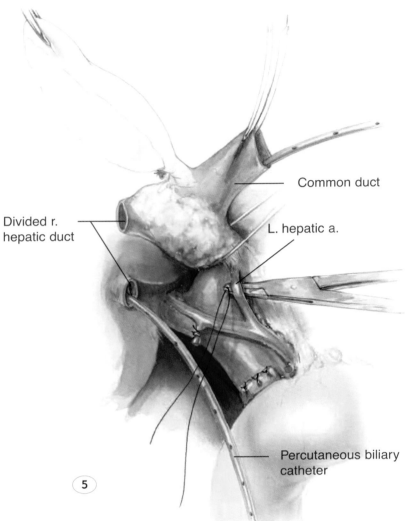

Common duct

Divided r.
hepatic duct

L. hepatic a.

Percutaneous biliary
catheter

5

The left branch of the hepatic artery is identified, dissected, doubly ligated and divided
(5). The left branch of the portal vein is dissected free, and doubly clamped with straight
Cooley clamps.

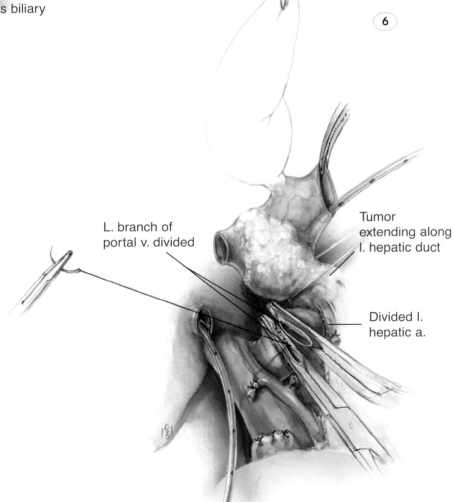

L. branch of
portal v. divided

Tumor
extending along
l. hepatic duct

Divided l.
hepatic a.

6

The left branch of the portal vein is then
divided and the proximal end oversewn
with a continuous 5-0 synthetic nonabsorbable suture (6). The distal end up
toward the left lobe of the liver, which is to
be resected, can be oversewn with a continuous 5-0 suture, or it can merely be ligated if
length permits.

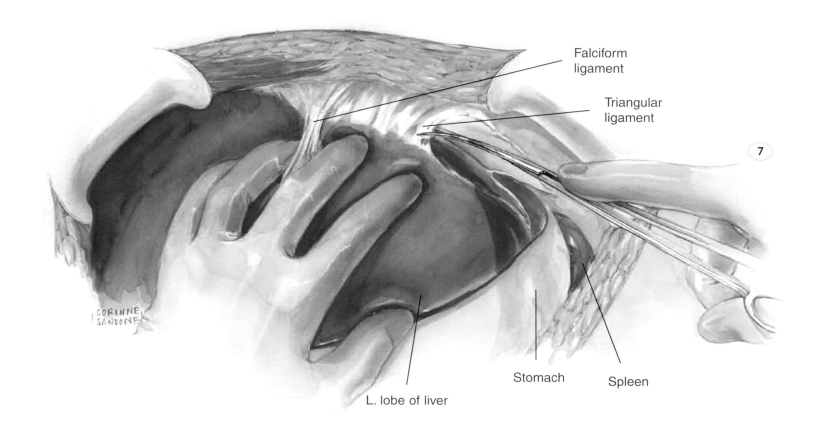

Falciform
ligament

Triangular
ligament

⑦

Stomach   Spleen

L. lobe of liver

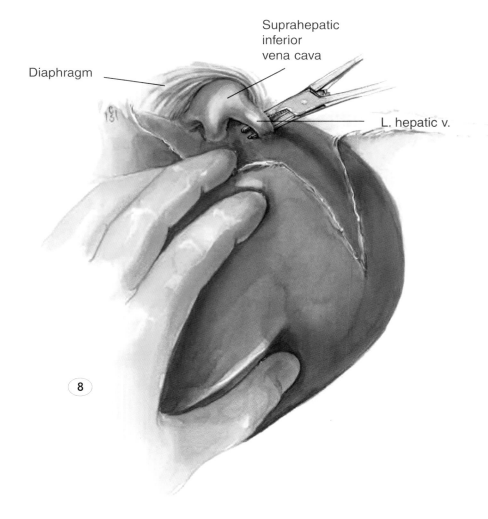

Suprahepatic
inferior
vena cava

Diaphragm

L. hepatic v.

⑧

Dividing the triangular and falciform ligaments allows mobilization of the left lobe of the liver (7). The hepatic veins are identified and the left hepatic vein is dissected free (8).

The left hepatic vein is doubly clamped with acutely curved Cooley clamps, divided, and each end oversewn with a continuous 5-0 synthetic non-absorbable suture (9).

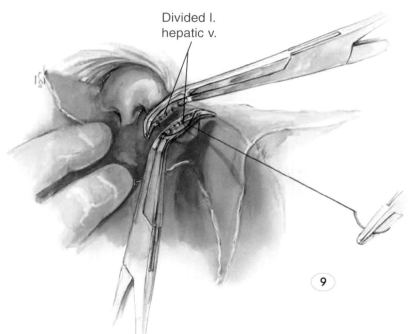

Divided l. hepatic v.

⑨

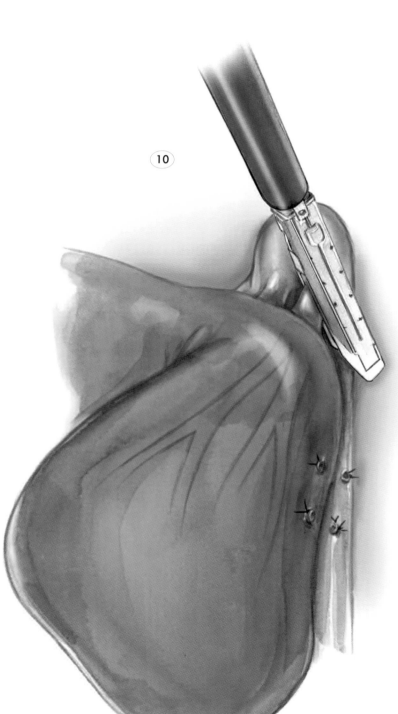

⑩

As an alternative, a stapling device can be used to divide and control the left hepatic vein (10). The left lobe of the liver has now been completely devascularized.

A variety of techniques are available for going through the hepatic parenchyma. In this example, parallel rows of No. 1 chromic catgut sutures are placed in a mattress fashion approximately 1 cm on either side of the plane that is to be divided between the right and left hepatic lobes. This plane generally extends from the gall bladder fossa to the hepatic veins as they enter the inferior vena cava. The liver parenchyma sutures should be snugged down to compress the liver, but not so tight as to cut through or necrose the liver. The line of division is first marked with the electrocautery (11). Two or three sutures are placed on each side, and then the hepatic parenchyma is divided with the electrocautery (12). Two or three more sutures are then placed, and more parenchyma divided with the cautery (13).

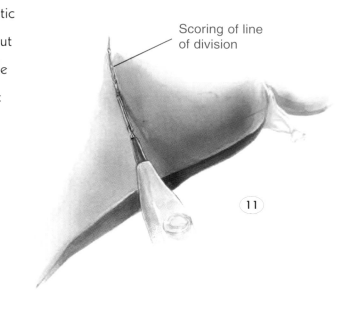

Scoring of line of division

11

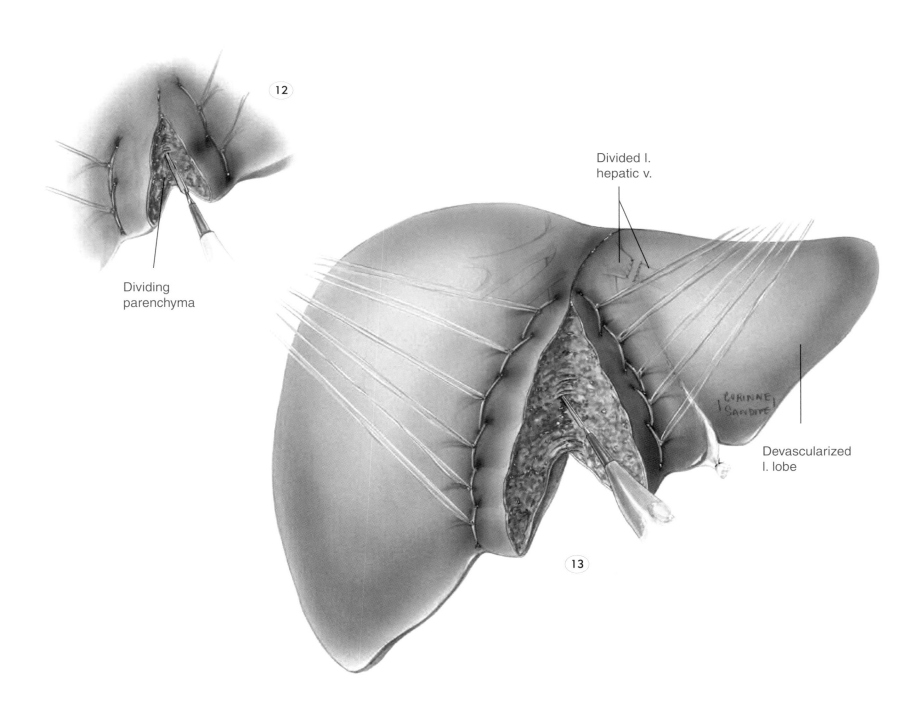

12

Dividing parenchyma

Divided l. hepatic v.

Devascularized l. lobe

13

This is perhaps the most bloodless way of dividing the hepatic parenchyma. The entire liver can generally be transected with virtually no loss of blood. The No. 1 chromic catgut sutures are wedged on large liver needles that can be controlled better if most of the curve is straightened. Other methods for dividing the hepatic parenchyma include using the Cavitron, and the TissueLink tools (see Liver).

When a hepatic lobectomy is performed, it is important that the caudate lobe be included with the resection. When only the bifurcation of the biliary tree is resected, it is difficult to access and remove the caudate lobe. However, when a hepatic lobectomy is included with bifurcation resection, the caudate lobe can be removed.

When division of the parenchyma has been completed, the specimen is removed from the operative field (14). The entire extrahepatic biliary tree, including the bifurcation, has been resected along with the left lobe of the liver. The tumor involves the bifurcation and clearly extends up into the left hepatic parenchyma.

Hemostasis is completed on the resected raw surface remaining on the right lobe of the liver using the electrocautery, figure-of-eight sutures of 3-0 synthetic absorbable material, and the argon beam coagulator (15). Because the stay sutures are compressing the hepatic parenchyma, very little hemostasis is generally required. Utilizing the preoperatively placed biliary catheter, a Silastic transhepatic biliary stent is placed. A guidewire is inserted through the biliary catheter so that the tract is not lost in case a catheter breaks or becomes dislodged during the exchange. A 16 French Silastic stent is threaded over the guidewire, and over the biliary catheter and sutured in place with two mattress sutures of 2-0 silk. The biliary stent is then extracted from the superior surface of the liver leaving the Silastic stent in position (16). That portion of the Silastic stent with side holes is left in the liver and in that portion of the stent that is placed in the Roux-en-Y loop. Obviously that portion of the Silastic stent that emanates out the top of the liver contains no side holes.

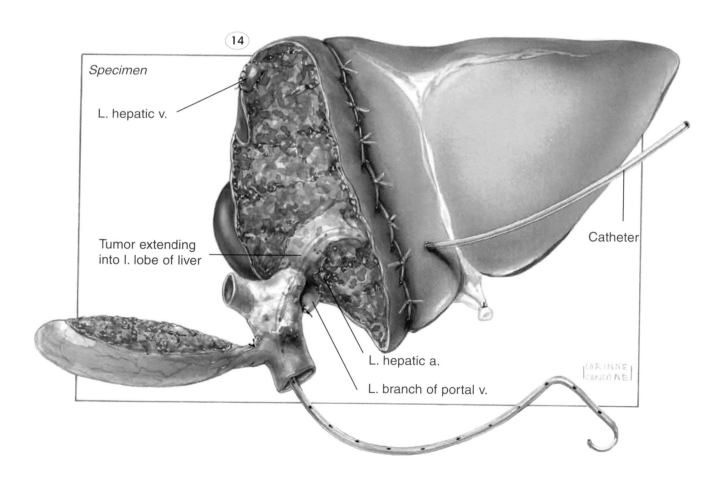

(14)

Specimen

L. hepatic v.

Tumor extending into l. lobe of liver

L. hepatic a.

L. branch of portal v.

Catheter

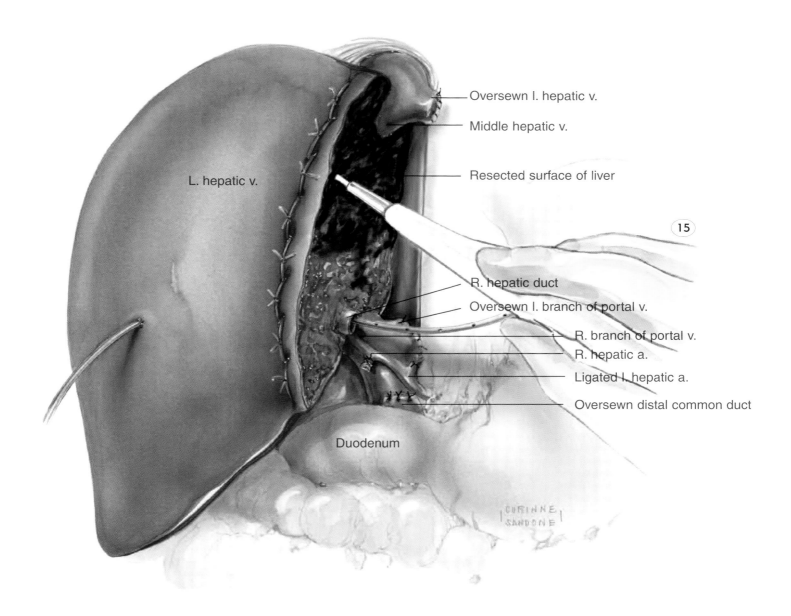

Oversewn l. hepatic v.

Middle hepatic v.

Resected surface of liver

L. hepatic v.

⑮

R. hepatic duct

Oversewn l. branch of portal v.

R. branch of portal v.

R. hepatic a.

Ligated l. hepatic a.

Oversewn distal common duct

Duodenum

A Roux-en-Y loop 60 cm in length is constructed, as previously demonstrated. It is brought up into the right upper quadrant in a retrocolic fashion on top of the second and third portions of the duodenum, through the bare area of the transverse mesocolon.

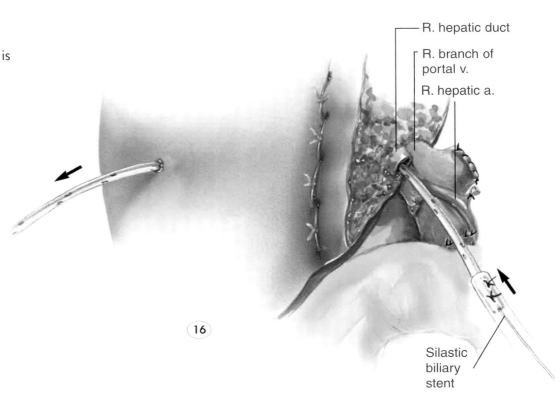

R. hepatic duct

R. branch of portal v.

R. hepatic a.

⑯

Silastic biliary stent

A hepaticojejunostomy is performed using one layer of interrupted 4-0 synthetic absorbable sutures (17). The technique of this anastomosis was demonstrated in the prior procedure. The end of the Silastic stent that emanates from the superior surface of the liver is brought out through a stab wound in the right upper quadrant, sutured to the skin with 5-0 stainless steel wire, and connected to dependent bile-bag drainage. The egress site of the biliary stent on the superior surface of the liver is drained with a closed suction Silastic drain brought out through a separate stab wound in the right upper quadrant. The resected surface of the liver and the hepaticojejunostomy are drained with two closed suction Silastic drains brought out through separate stab wounds in the mid-abdomen. The Roux-en-Y loop is sutured to the rent in the transverse mesocolon to prevent small bowel herniation (17). Postoperative cholangiography is performed at five days, and if no bile leaks are present, the stent is internalized by placing a three-way stopcock or heparin lock on the end of the stent. Patients are taught to irrigate the stents twice a day with 20 mL of saline. Postoperatively, patients are often treated with adjuvant radiotherapy, although no definitive proof of efficacy has been demonstrated. Five thousand rads of external beam radiotherapy are delivered to the area of the porta hepatis. When this is completed, patients may be readmitted to the hospital for approximately 48 hours so that iridium 192 seeds can be lowered down the biliary stent and positioned in the area of the anastomosis. An additional 2,000 rads of radiotherapy are delivered locally. The Silastic transhepatic biliary stent is left in permanently. Even though cures are possible, many patients will develop recurrent tumor. Thus, leaving the stent in place will prevent recurrent biliary obstruction and maximally prolong survival. The stents, however, are changed every three or four months prophylactically because of biliary sludge accumulation and obstruction of the side holes. This is easily and quickly carried out as an outpatient procedure under fluoroscopy in the catheterization laboratory. If the patient reaches 3 years post-resection, with no evidence of recurrent tumor, the Silastic stents may be removed.

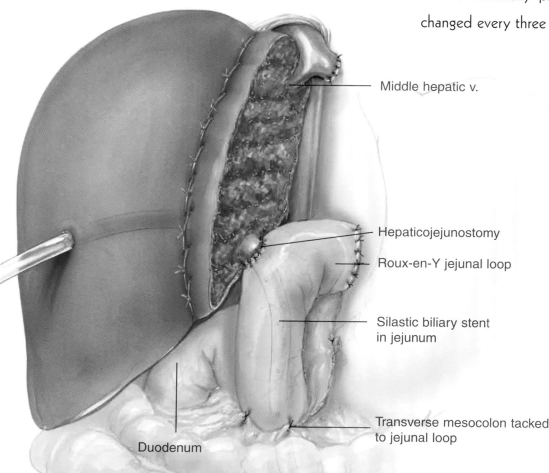

Middle hepatic v.

Hepaticojejunostomy

Roux-en-Y jejunal loop

Silastic biliary stent
in jejunum

Transverse mesocolon tacked
to jejunal loop

Duodenum

17

Proximal Cholangiocarcinoma: Palliation By Transhepatic Stenting and Hepaticojejunostomy

Operative Indications:

All patients with proximal cholangiocarcinomas are staged preoperatively by percutaneous cholangiography and thin section three-dimensional CT scans. Magnetic resonance angiography can also be utilized. If it appears that a patient is not potentially resectable for cure, palliation is achieved generally with percutaneous transhepatic biliary catheters. Occasionally, patients can be palliated endoscopically with endostents. Whichever approach is used, permanent, expandable metallic stents have become the treatment of choice. Such stents are more frequently placed successfully in an appropriate position transhepatically and percutaneously, than endoscopically. However, either approach can be used. These patients can then receive palliative irradiation following tissue confirmation of their disease. Again, there is no absolute proof that radiotherapy prolongs survival, but its utilization is common.

When patients who are thought to be potentially curable after staging are explored, at the time of surgery some will prove to be unresectable. These patients will have tumor extending up into both lobes of the liver (1), or tumor involving the portal vein and/or common hepatic artery. In such instances, we feel it is appropriate to replace the rigid percutaneous transhepatic biliary catheters with Silastic transhepatic biliary stents and to perform a hepaticojejunostomy. The thick-wall, large-bore Silastic transhepatic biliary stents provide better palliation than the rigid percutaneous catheters alone. They are more comfortable, are tolerated better by patients, and are less frequently associated with complications such as hematobilia and liver abscesses. Because of their large internal diameter, and thick wall, they are less likely to occlude with biliary sludge, or be compressed by tumor growth. Placing the Silastic stents is not worth a laparotomy in a patient who is clearly incurable by preoperative staging. However, if a patient has been explored with the hopes of a curative resection, and it is not possible, this procedure is appropriate and indicated. One needs to resect the biliary tree distal to the tumor and bifurcation, because otherwise, these large-bore Silastic stents will not be accommodated by a normal or small-sized common duct.

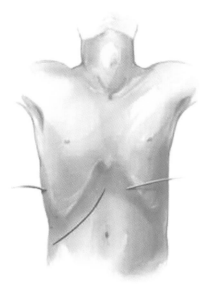

Operative Technique:

The patient is explored through a right subcostal incision. The two preoperatively placed percutaneous transhepatic biliary catheters are prepped into the field so they are accessible to the surgeon. When tumor extension is found into both lobes of the liver (1), or if the tumor is found to involve the main portal vein or common hepatic artery, it is important to confirm the diagnosis by tissue biopsy.

This may be difficult on frozen section because of the fibrotic sclerotic nature of the tumor. Nevertheless, the surgeon should persist so that the diagnosis is definitively confirmed. In preparation for removing the gall bladder, the cystic artery is identified, doubly clamped, divided, and ligated.

Tumor extending into
r. and l. lobes of liver

1

Percutaneous
catheters

Cystic duct

Duodenum

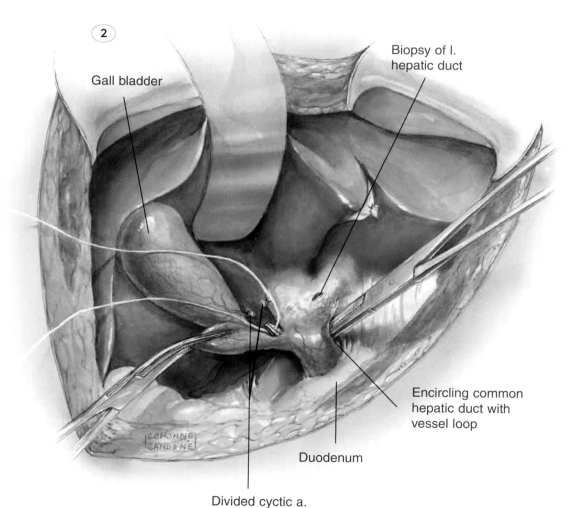

2

Gall bladder

Biopsy of l.
hepatic duct

Encircling common
hepatic duct with
vessel loop

Duodenum

Divided cyctic a.

At the same time, the common hepatic duct is mobilized and looped with a vessel loop (2).

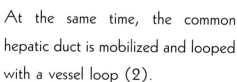

The gall bladder is mobilized, the common hepatic duct is divided, and the distal common duct is divided, removing the gall bladder and a segment of the extrahepatic biliary tree (3). The distal common duct is either ligated or oversewn with interrupted 3-0 silks. One is now left with a short segment of common hepatic duct, cholangiocarcinoma involving the common hepatic duct and bifurcation and extending up into both lobes, and percutaneous transhepatic biliary catheters in both the right and left hepatic ducts (4).

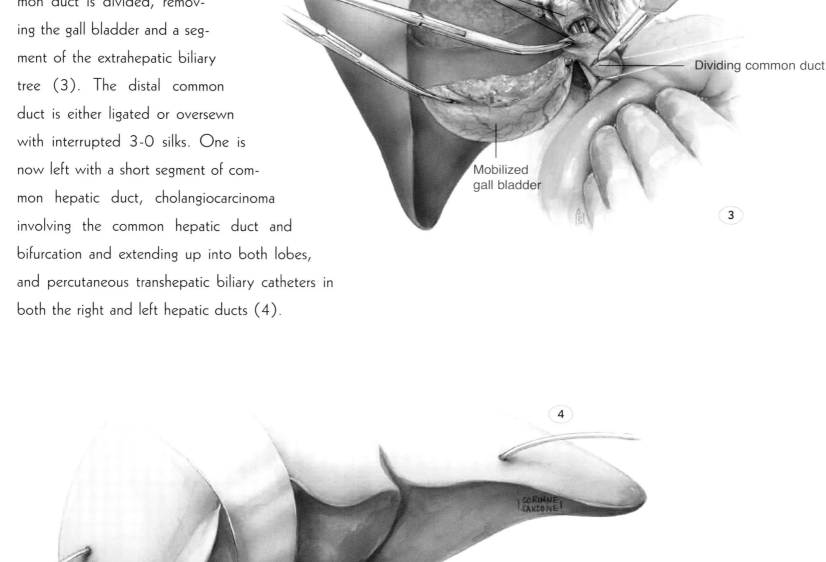

Divided common hepatic duct

Tumor extending into both lobes

Dividing common duct

Mobilized gall bladder

3

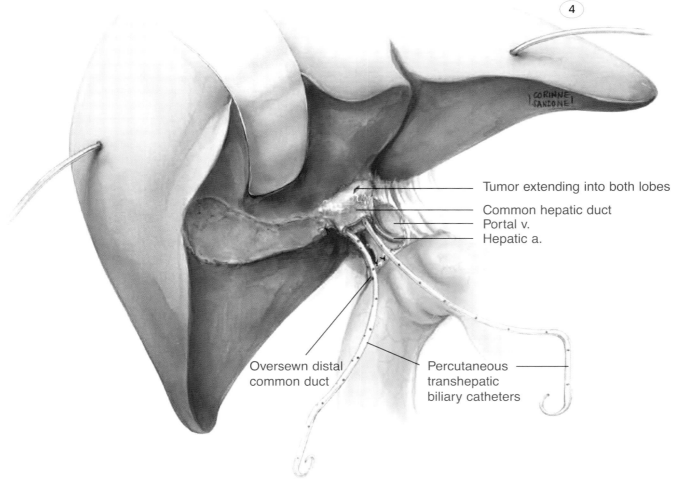

4

Tumor extending into both lobes
Common hepatic duct
Portal v.
Hepatic a.

Oversewn distal common duct

Percutaneous transhepatic biliary catheters

It is important that the gall bladder be removed, because with stents in place, the development of acute cholecystitis and an empyema of the gall bladder is common. This results from obstruction of the cystic duct by edema or by the stents themselves. Acute suppurative cholecystis is common in this setting. Since the distal biliary tree is of normal size, it cannot accommodate the two large Silastic stents, and it is necessary to construct a Roux-en-Y jejunal loop as a receptacle. The percutaneous transhepatic biliary catheters are then brought into the peritoneal cavity through the chest wall. A guidewire is inserted into each catheter to maintain the tract in case a catheter breaks or becomes dislodged during the following manipulation (5).

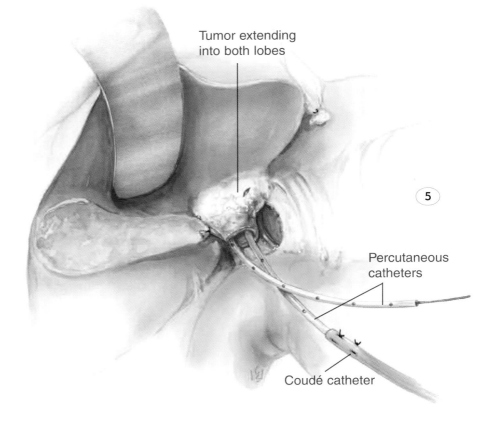

A 12 French red rubber Coude catheter with its tip cut off is then placed over the guidewire and biliary catheter and sutured in place. The Coude catheters are drawn up through the tumor, thereby dilating it and placing the Coude catheters in the right and left hepatic ducts. Often this is repeated with the next size Coude catheter—for instance a 14 French—before placing the 16 French Silastic transhepatic biliary stent (6). Without progressive dilatation, one may have difficulty in placing the Silastic transhepatic biliary stents. Using progressively larger Coude catheters, the tumor is dilated and the Silastic stents placed. Once both Silastic transhepatic biliary stents have been positioned, a Roux-en-Y loop 60 cm in length is constructed as previously demonstrated. The anastomosis is performed with a single layer of interrupted 4-0 synthetic absorbable material. The posterior row is placed prior to performing an enterotomy. The sutures pass into the submucosal layer of the bowel and through and through on the duct side (7). Thus the anastomosis is not actually mucosa-to-mucosa, but functionally it acts as one.

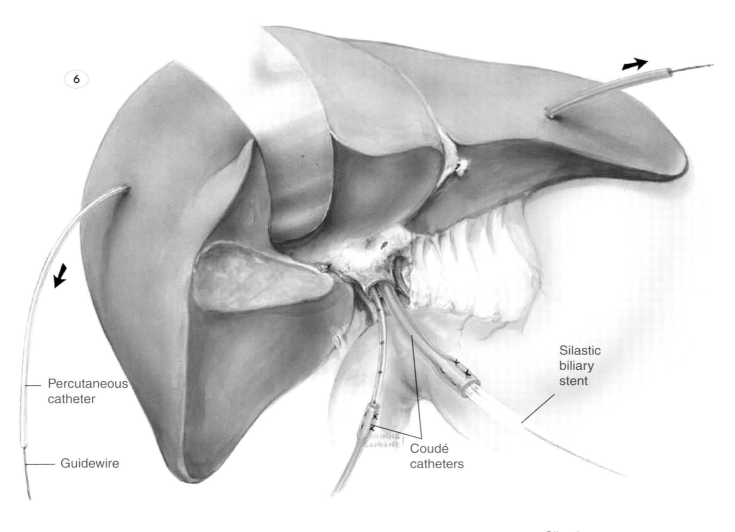

6

Percutaneous catheter

Guidewire

Silastic biliary stent

Coudé catheters

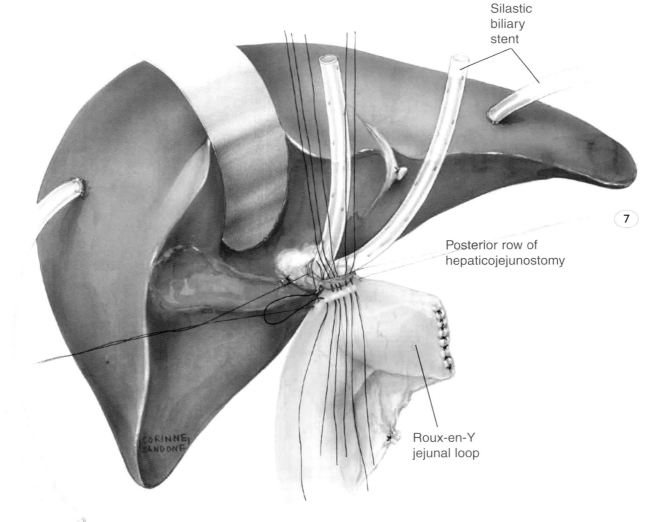

Silastic biliary stent

7

Posterior row of hepaticojejunostomy

Roux-en-Y jejunal loop

After the back row has been placed and the sutures secured, an enterotomy is made with the electrocautery (8). The posterior row of sutures is divided, and both stents are placed into the Roux-en-Y loop through the single enterotomy. The knots of the posterior layer are on the inside, but since the suture material is absorbable, this is of no consequence. The anterior row of the anastomosis is completed with a single interrupted layer of through and through sutures of 4-0 synthetic absorbable material (9). All such sutures are placed and then secured. Both Silastic transhepatic biliary stents are brought out through stab wounds in the right and left upper quadrants, and sutured to the skin with 5-0 stainless steel wire, and connected to gravity bile-bag drainage. Both egress sites on the superior surface of the liver are drained with closed-suction Silastic drains, brought out through separate stab wounds in the right and left upper quadrants. The anastomosis is drained with a third closed-suction Silastic drain brought out through a stab wound in the mid-abdomen. The Roux-en-Y loop may be sutured to the undersurface of the liver with interrupted 3-0 silks. With a 60 cm Roux-en-Y loop, however-er, it generally rests comfortably in the right upper quadrant, and this may not be necessary. The Roux-en-Y loop is sutured to the rent in the transverse mesocolon with interrupted 4-0 silks (10).

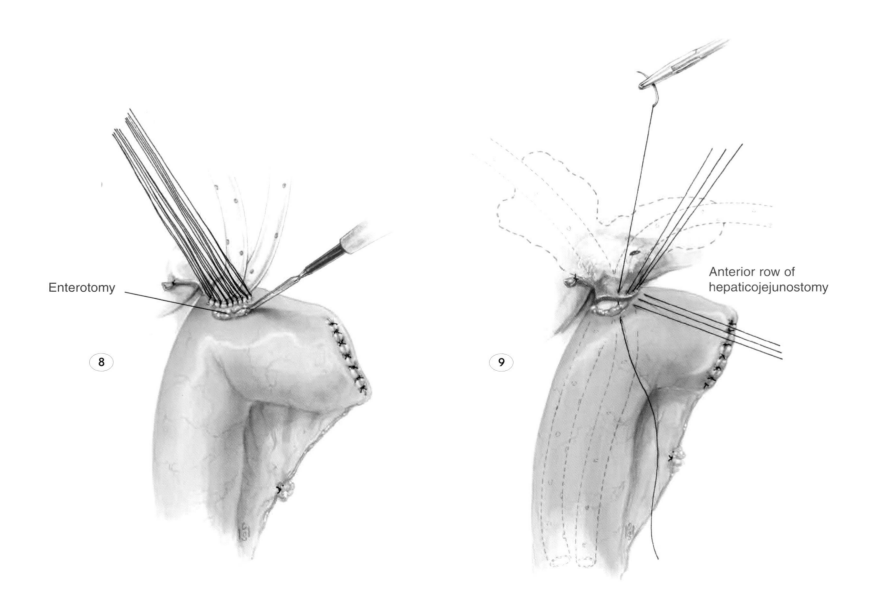

Enterotomy

8

Anterior row of
hepaticojejunostomy

9

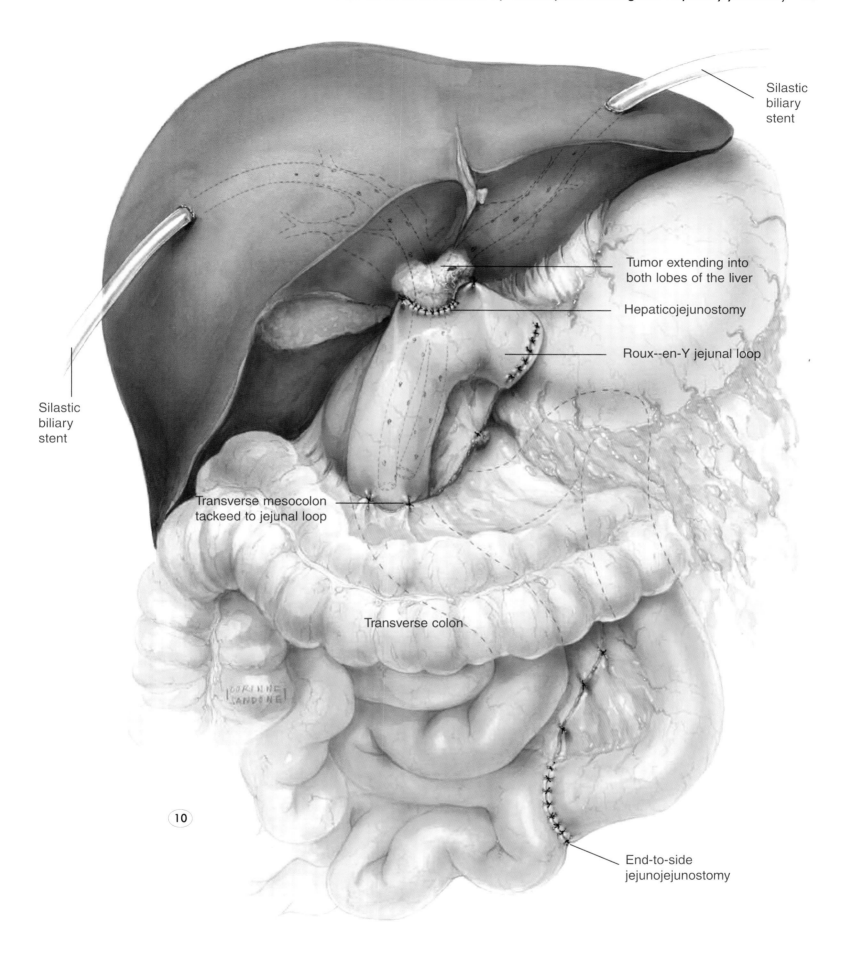

Silastic biliary stent

Tumor extending into both lobes of the liver

Hepaticojejunostomy

Roux--en-Y jejunal loop

Silastic biliary stent

Transverse mesocolon tackeed to jejunal loop

Transverse colon

End-to-side jejunojejunostomy

⑩

Postoperatively, the stents are placed to allow bile-bag drainage by gravity. In five days, cholangiography is performed and, if there are no bile leaks, the stents are internalized by placing three-way stopcocks or heparin locks on the ends. Patients are taught to irrigate the stents twice a day with 20 mL of saline. The Silastic transhepatic biliary stents are left in permanently to maintain patency of the biliary tree. The stents are changed every 3 or 4 months as an outpatient procedure, to prevent side-hole occlusion with biliary sludge. This is accomplished by passing a guidewire through the old stent into the jejunal loop and then removing the old stent, leaving the guidewire in place. A new stent is placed into the jejunal loop over the guidewire and the guidewire is removed.

Postoperative irradiation can be delivered in a fashion similar to irradiation after a curative resection. Five thousand rads are delivered to the hepatic duct bifurcation via external beam radiotherapy, and the patients may then be readmitted for the delivery of internal irradiation via iridium 192 seeds lowered down through the lumens of the Silastic biliary stents. The seeds are left in place for approximately 48 hours to deliver an additional 2,000 rads. This palliative procedure can prolong survival for an extended period following the initial presentation.

Proximal cholangiocarcinomas can be very slow growing. Long-term survival is possible. It is not clear whether postoperative irradiation is of benefit in prolonging survival, but it is commonly utilized.

Resection of Hepatic Duct Bifurcation, Dilatation of Intrahepatic Biliary Tree, and Prolonged Stenting with Transhepatic Biliary Stents for Sclerosing Cholangitis

Operative Indications:

Sclerosing cholangitis is an idiopathic disease that commonly affects middle-aged males and is often associated with inflammatory bowel disease. Autoimmune pancreatitis and Sjögren syndrome may also be associated with sclerosing cholangitis. Patients with sclerosing cholangitis often have diffuse involvement of both the intra- and extrahepatic biliary tree, with multiple benign inflammatory strictures. Even though the strictures involve the intra- and extrahepatic biliary tree diffusely, the area of most severe involvement is often at the hepatic duct bifurcation (1). Most patients present with intermittent painless jaundice, pruritus, and abnormalities of liver function, in particular a very high alkaline phosphatase. Patients with sclerosing cholangitis can have prolonged, variable, and episodic clinical courses.

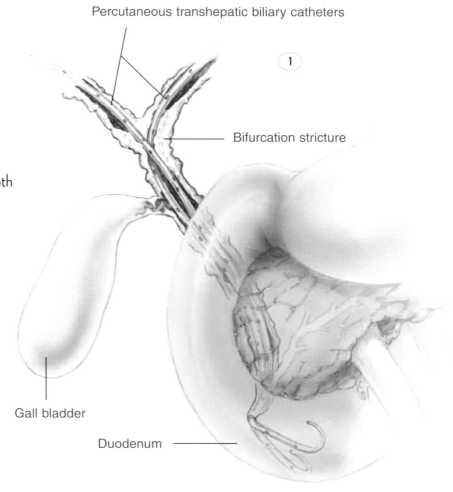

Percutaneous transhepatic biliary catheters

Bifurcation stricture

Gall bladder

Duodenum

When persistent jaundice develops, however, it is a sign of a poor prognosis. Such patients should undergo liver biopsy. If biliary cirrhosis is present, the patient is a candidate for liver transplantation.

But if biliary cirrhosis is not present, and there is a dominant bifurcation stricture, the patient should be considered for resection of the hepatic duct bifurcation, dilatation of the intrahepatic biliary tree, long-term stenting with transhepatic biliary stents, and bilateral hepaticojejunostomies. Patients with sclerosing cholangitis are also prone to developing cholangiocarcinoma, which is another reason to resect the bifurcation of the biliary tree if a dominant stricture is present.

This procedure is based on the premise that the bifurcation stricture and the proximal obstruction that results play a major role in the progressive parenchymal disease that eventually leads to hepatic failure. The functional significance of the bifurcation stricture is often difficult to detect because of the lack of proximal dilatation. In patients with sclerosing cholangitis, the entire biliary tree tends to be fibrotic and often does not dilate proximal to a stricture. Biliary tract surgeons have been slow to recognize the functional significance of these bifurcation lesions.

Thus, patients with sclerosing cholangitis who develop persistent jaundice over several months, who have a dominant stricture involving the hepatic duct bifurcation, and who on liver biopsy do not have biliary cirrhosis, are considered excellent candidates for bifurcation reconstruction and long-term stenting. Preoperative percutaneous cholangiography should be performed and percutaneous transhepatic biliary catheters should be inserted into both the right and left hepatic ducts, through the bifurcation stricture, and into the duodenum (1). These are placed preoperatively, not only to decompress the hyperbilirubinemia, but to aid the surgeon during the operative procedure.

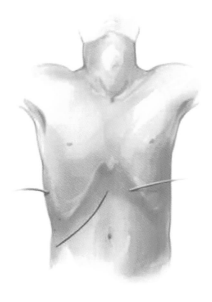

Operative Technique:

Patients are explored through a generous right subcostal incision. At the time of laparotomy, the abdomen is explored. The cholangiographic diagnosis of sclerosing cholangitis is highly accurate. But there is an increased incidence of cholangiocarcinoma developing in patients with sclerosing cholangitis; thus the liver and abdomen should be thoroughly explored for evidence of tumor. The entire extrahepatic biliary tree is usually sclerotic and fibrotic. The gall bladder, however, is often normal. The bifurcation of the biliary tree can usually be identified high in the porta hepatis by palpating for the point where the two percutaneous transhepatic biliary catheters diverge into the right and left hepatic ducts (2).

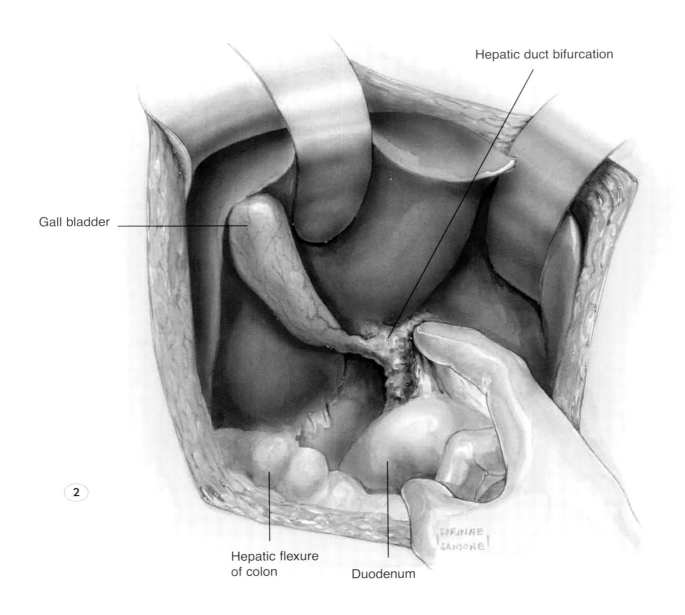

Hepatic duct bifurcation

Gall bladder

Hepatic flexure
of colon

Duodenum

2

After identifying, dividing, and ligating the cystic artery, the gall bladder is mobilized to improve access to the hepatic duct bifurcation. The extrahepatic biliary tree is dissected, and the common duct is encircled with a vessel loop. The distal common duct is divided (3), the two transhepatic biliary catheters are extracted, and the distal bile duct is either ligated or closed with a series of interrupted 3-0 silk sutures.

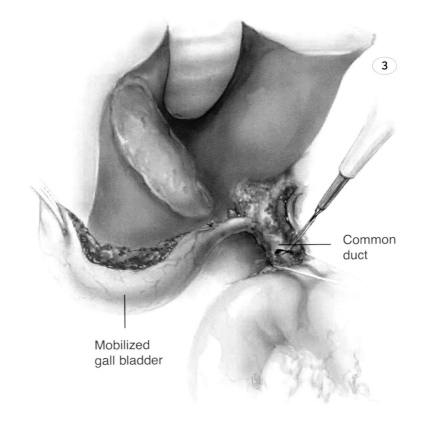

3

Common
duct

Mobilized
gall bladder

The proximal biliary segment is reflected cephalad, and the extrahepatic biliary tree is dissected off the hepatic artery and portal vein (4). The bifurcation of the hepatic duct rests on the bifurcation of the portal vein and the hepatic artery. Reflecting the proximal biliary segment so that the biliary tree can be dissected both anteriorly and posteriorly makes this a safe dissection. The right and left hepatic ducts are dissected free and looped with vessel loops. The right and left hepatic ducts are then divided (5) and the specimen removed from the operative field. The specimen should be sent for frozen sections of the distal biliary margin as well as the right and left hepatic duct margins, to be certain that a cholangiocarcinoma is not present and involving one of the margins of resection.

The next step involves dilatation of the fibrotic strictured intrahepatic biliary tree. Percutaneous transhepatic biliary catheters have previously been placed in the right and left hepatic ducts. The catheters are retrieved through the chest and the abdominal wall and brought into the peritoneal cavity. A guidewire is placed in the lumen of the biliary catheter to avoid losing the tract if a catheter breaks or becomes dislodged in the next series of manipulations. A 12 French Coude catheter is placed over the

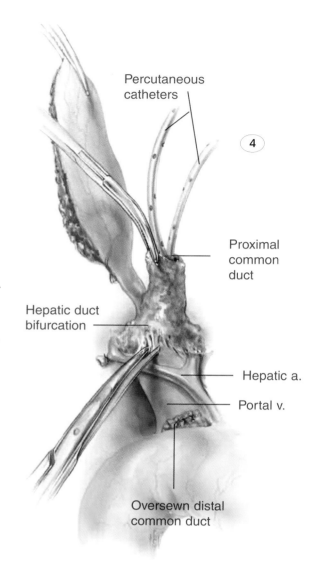

Percutaneous catheters

4

Proximal common duct

Hepatic duct bifurcation

Hepatic a.

Portal v.

Oversewn distal common duct

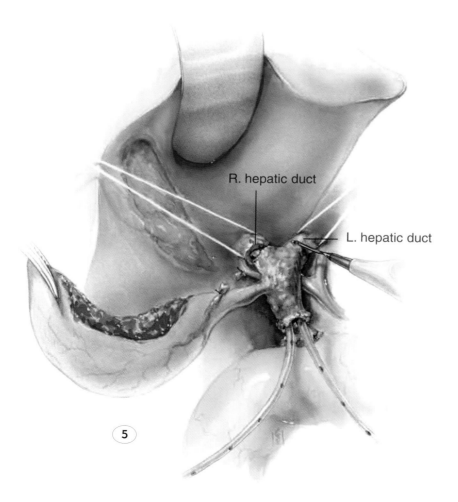

R. hepatic duct

L. hepatic duct

5

guidewire and onto the biliary catheter after cutting off the curved distal tip of the Coude catheter. The Coude catheter is sutured to the biliary catheter and then drawn up through the liver, thus dilating the intrahepatic biliary tree (6). A 14 French Coude catheter is then placed over the guidewire and sutured to the 12 French Coude catheter. Further dilatation is accomplished by pulling the 12 French Coude catheter through the top of the liver, thereby placing the 14 French Coude catheter. This can then be repeated with a 16 French Coude catheter. Gentle but very firm traction is usually required.

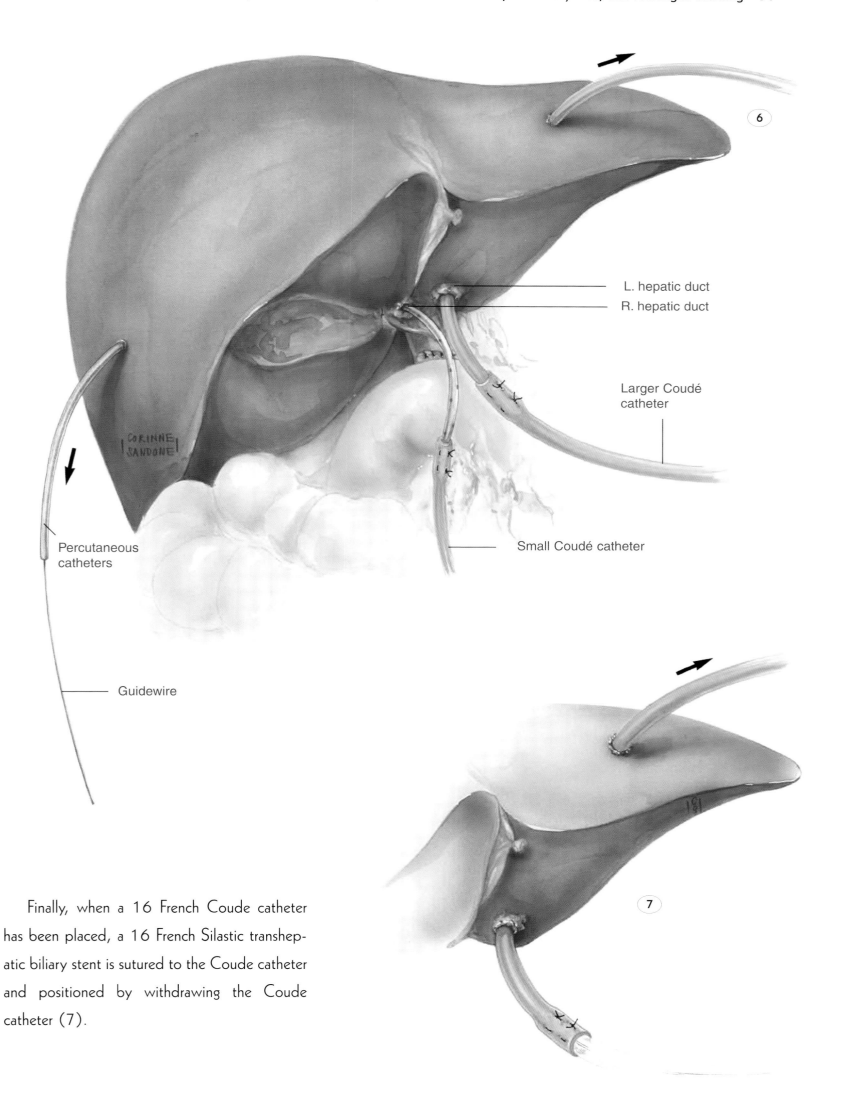

L. hepatic duct

R. hepatic duct

Larger Coudé catheter

Percutaneous catheters

Small Coudé catheter

Guidewire

Finally, when a 16 French Coude catheter has been placed, a 16 French Silastic transhepatic biliary stent is sutured to the Coude catheter and positioned by withdrawing the Coude catheter (7).

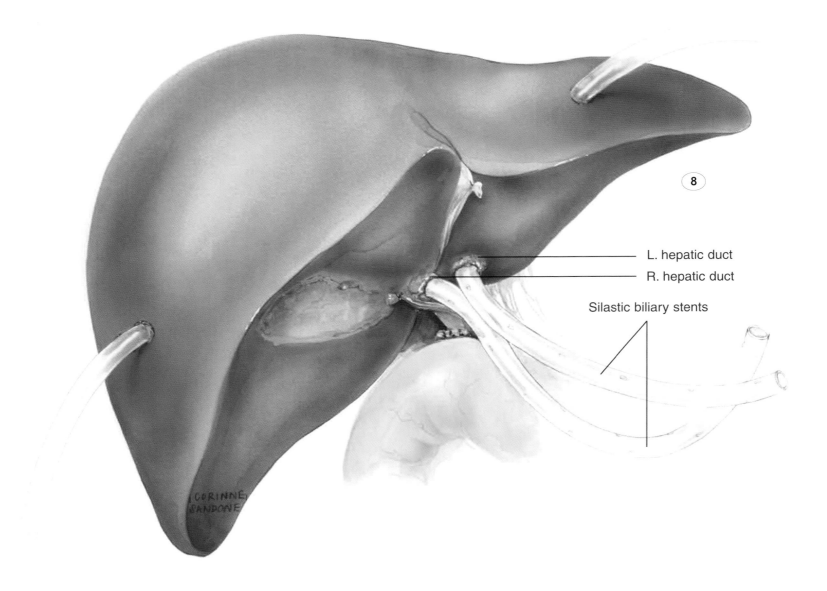

L. hepatic duct

R. hepatic duct

Silastic biliary stents

This series of manipulations not only dilates the strictured intrahepatic biliary tree, but also positions the Silastic transhepatic biliary stents used for the reconstruction (8).

The process of dilating the intrahepatic biliary tree is greatly simplified by having percutaneous transhepatic biliary catheters in place. If biliary catheters have not been inserted preoperatively, it is necessary to dilate the intrahepatic biliary tree after bifurcation resection with instruments such as Bakes dilator. This can be extremely tedious. One has to proceed cautiously to avoid making false passages. If a false passage is made, it is virtually impossible to get beyond the false passage to dilate the biliary tree up within the liver. By proceeding very cautiously, however, dilatation can eventually be performed. Once the intrahepatic biliary tree is dilated, the Bakes dilator can be pushed out the diaphragmatic surface of the liver and a Silastic stent sutured to it (9). The stent is positioned by withdrawing the Bakes dilator out the hilum of the liver. Securing the Silastic stent to the Bakes dilator is facilitated by having a hole drilled in the end of the olive tip.

A Roux-en-Y loop 60 cm in length is constructed as previously described. It is brought into the right upper quadrant in a retrocolic position on top of the second and third portions of the duodenum. Bilateral hepaticojejunostomies are then performed. These are constructed in one layer using interrupted 4-0 synthetic absorbable suture material. The sutures pass into the submucosal layer of the jejunum and through and through the duct. The entire posterior row is placed for each hepatico-

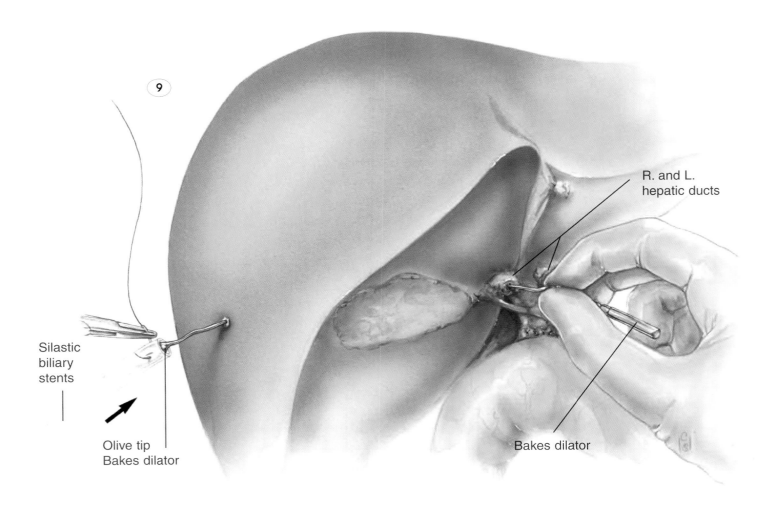

⑨

Silastic
biliary
stents

Olive tip
Bakes dilator

R. and L.
hepatic ducts

Bakes dilator

jejunostomy before the sutures are secured
(10). The intestinal sutures are placed in the
posterior row prior to performing an enterotomy; so, strictly speaking, it is not a
mucosa-to-mucosa anastomosis, although
functionally it acts as one. Each suture is
grasped in a separate hemostat and lined up
in order on a longer clamp. Once all the
sutures have been placed, they are secured. The
knots of the posterior row are on the inside, but
since the suture material is absorbable, this is of no
long-term consequence.

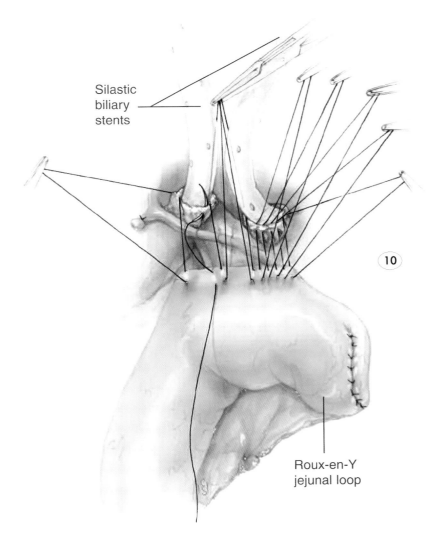

Silastic
biliary
stents

⑩

Roux-en-Y
jejunal loop

Bilateral enterotomies are performed with the electrocautery (11). The posterior row of sutures is divided, and the Silastic transhepatic biliary stents are placed through the enterotomies into the Roux-en-Y loop (12). The anterior rows of both hepaticojejunostomies are completed utilizing through-and-through simple sutures of 4-0 synthetic absorbable material (13). Both Silastic transhepatic biliary stents emanating from the top of the liver are brought out through separate stab wounds in the right and left upper quadrants, and sutured to the skin with 5-0 stainless steel wire sutures. The stents are then connected to gravity bilebag drainage. Both egress sites on the superior surface of the liver are drained with closed-suction Silastic drains brought out through separate stab wounds in the right and left upper quadrants.

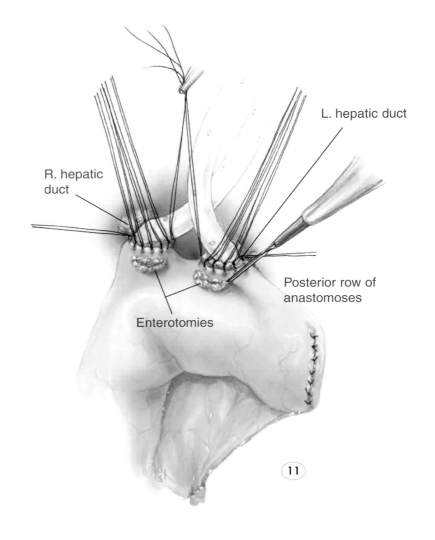

L. hepatic duct

R. hepatic duct

Posterior row of anastomoses

Enterotomies

11

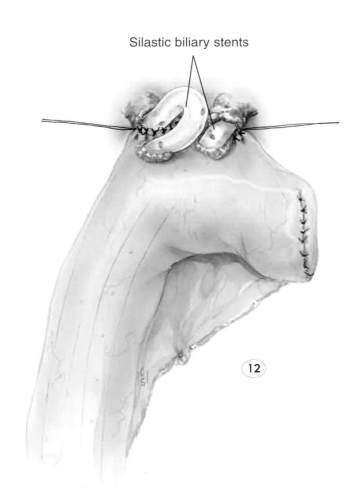

Silastic biliary stents

12

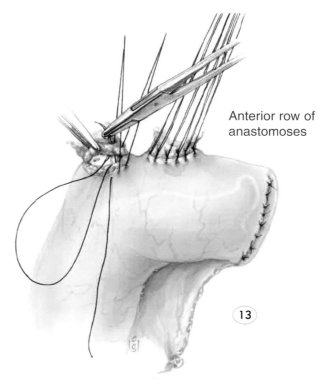

Anterior row of anastomoses

13

The Roux-en-Y loop is sutured to the undersurface of the liver with interrupted 3-0 silks, to prevent tension on the anastomosis. With a 60 cm Roux-en-Y loop, however, it generally rests comfortably under the liver and this step may not be necessary. The Roux-en-Y loop is sutured to the rent in the transverse mesocolon with interrupted 4-0 silks (14).

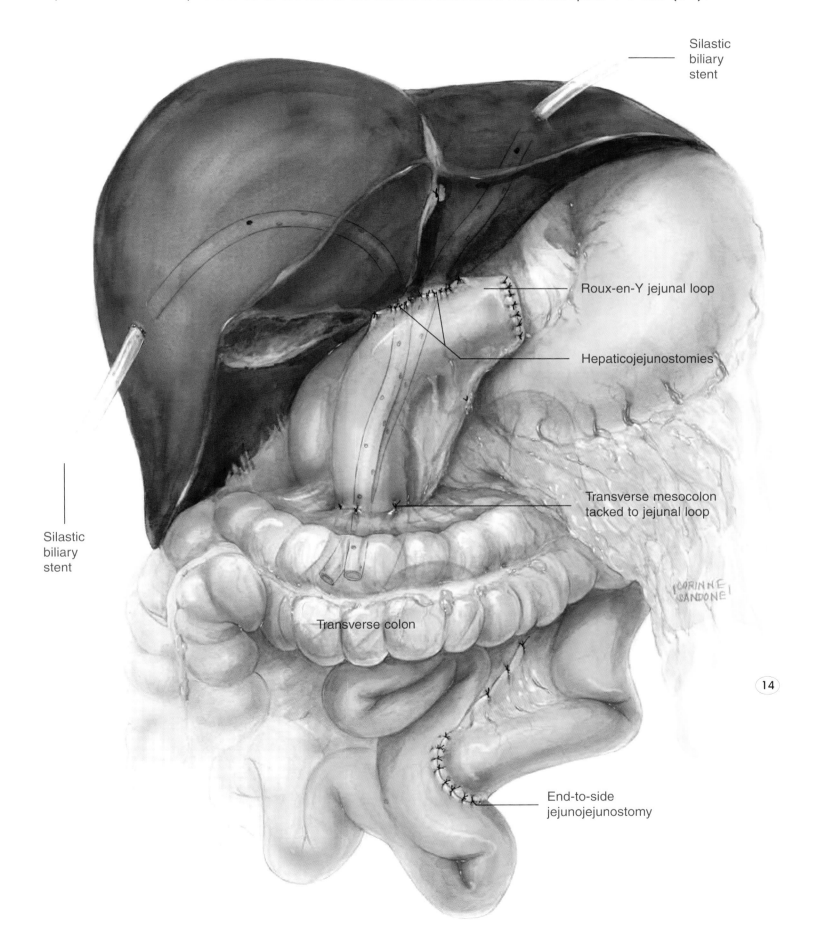

Silastic
biliary
stent

Silastic
biliary
stent

Roux-en-Y jejunal loop

Hepaticojejunostomies

Transverse mesocolon
tacked to jejunal loop

Transverse colon

End-to-side
jejunojejunostomy

14

The hepaticojejunostomies are drained with a closed-suction Silastic drain brought out through a stab wound in the mid-abdomen. Postoperatively, the stents are left to gravity drainage for five days. At five days, cholangiography is performed and, if no leaks are apparent, the stents are internalized by capping them with three-way stopcocks or heparin locks. The patients are taught to irrigate the stents twice a day with 20 mL of saline.

It has been our practice to leave the Silastic stents in permanently. The stents, however, are changed every 3 or 4 months as an outpatient procedure. Patients come in and, under fluoroscopy, a guidewire is placed through the old stent into the Roux-en-Y loop. The old stent is removed, leaving the guidewire in place. A new stent is then slipped in place over the guidewire and the guidewire is removed. Patients with sclerosing cholangitis tend to form biliary sludge more rapidly than patients with other disorders. Therefore, it is occasionally necessary to change the stents more frequently than every 3 or 4 months. Some patients who have done exceptionally well for several years, with no difficulty, have had their stents removed, assuming their disease is in a quiescent, arrested stage. But for many patients, the stents are left in permanently to prevent inevitable stricture. We have had several patients with stents in place for over 10 years. It is our feeling that, in many patients with sclerosing cholangitis this procedure prolongs survival, and in some instances, will put off—if not obviate—the need for eventual liver transplantation. In most instances, the hyperbilirubinemia will return to, or towards, normal after this procedure. If a patient's disease subsequently progresses, liver transplantation may be necessary. Many of our patients subsequently have undergone successful liver transplantation.

Resection of Choledochal Cyst

Operative Indications:

Choledochal cysts are thought to be congenital and, in the past, were recognized most frequently in infancy or early childhood. The triad of an abdominal mass, pain, and jaundice was associated with the diagnosis. In recent years, however, the entity has been diagnosed far more frequently in adulthood than in childhood. It often presents with mild abdominal pain, and occasionally, with hyperamylasemia. Many patients are felt to have gall bladder disease when they present with a choledochal cyst, and a laparoscopic cholecystectomy frequently leads to the diagnosis.

There are a variety of classifications of choledochal cyst. By far the most common type of cyst consists of a fusiform dilatation of the extrahepatic biliary tree that includes portions of both the common hepatic and common bile ducts (Type I). An anomalous high junction between the pancreatic duct and biliary tree has been recognized in virtually all patients with choledochal cysts. Many feel that reflux of pancreatic juice into the biliary tree results in destruction of the integrity of the bile duct wall, and subsequent dilatation.

Many patients are asymptomatic at the time of diagnosis of a choledochal cyst. But there is considerable risk of development of cholangiocarcinoma in a choledochal cyst, and therefore all choledochal cysts should be resected and biliary reconstruction carried out. In the past, choledochal cysts were drained into adjacent stomach, the duodenum, or into a Roux-en-Y loop. This is no longer acceptable management because of the risk of recurrent episodes of cholangitis, and the risk of cholangiocarcinoma. Thus, in each instance, the cyst should be resected.

The presentation today in adulthood is more frequently that of mild abdominal symptoms, occasionally associated with hyperamylasemia and/or with jaundice. Sonography or CT scan often suggests the diagnosis of a choledochal cyst in a patient being worked up for abdominal pain. The diagnosis can be confirmed by magnetic resonance cholangiopancreatography (MRCP), endoscopic retrograde cholangiopancreatography (ERCP), or by percutaneous transhepatic cholangiography.

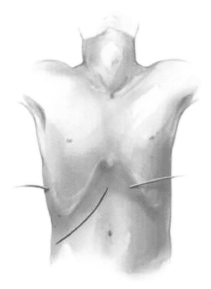

Operative Technique:

Prior to surgery, cholangiography is necessary to accurately define the anatomy of the choledochal cyst. If there is a long normal neck of common hepatic duct distal to the bifurcation, and no intrahepatic disease, it is not necessary to preoperatively insert percutaneous transhepatic biliary catheters. In many instances, however, the cyst extends to the bifurcation, and may at times involve the bifurcation. In these instances, prior to surgery percutaneous transhepatic biliary catheters are inserted into the intrahepatic biliary tree and then passed into the cyst. In the past, we used to pass the catheters distally through the ampulla into the duodenum. But because of the high insertion of the pancreatic duct into the biliary tree, pancreatitis can be initiated by passing the catheter into the duodenum, so now, generally they are left coiled in the cyst (1). If the cyst involves the hepatic duct bifurcation, and bifurcation resection is anticipated, percutaneous transhepatic biliary catheters are placed in both the right and left hepatic ducts and are left in the cyst.

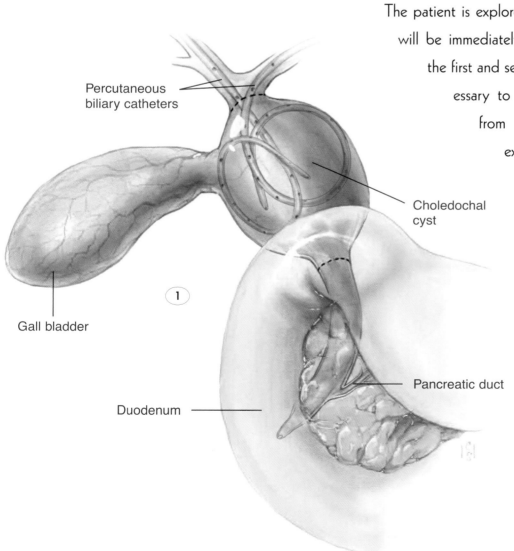

Percutaneous
biliary catheters

Choledochal
cyst

①

Gall bladder

Pancreatic duct

Duodenum

The patient is explored through a right subcostal incision. The cyst will be immediately evident. Frequently, it extends well behind the first and second portions of the duodenum, and it is necessary to divide the serosa and soft tissues extending from the duodenum onto the cyst to adequately expose the cyst (2).

The gall bladder usually rises from the mid portion of the cystic dilatation of the biliary tree. The cystic artery is identified, doubly clamped, divided and ligated. The gall bladder is mobilized out of the liver bed. The cyst is dissected free of overlying serosa (3). This generally requires mobilization of the duodenum off the anterior wall of the cyst and blunt and sharp dissection of the remaining cyst. There is

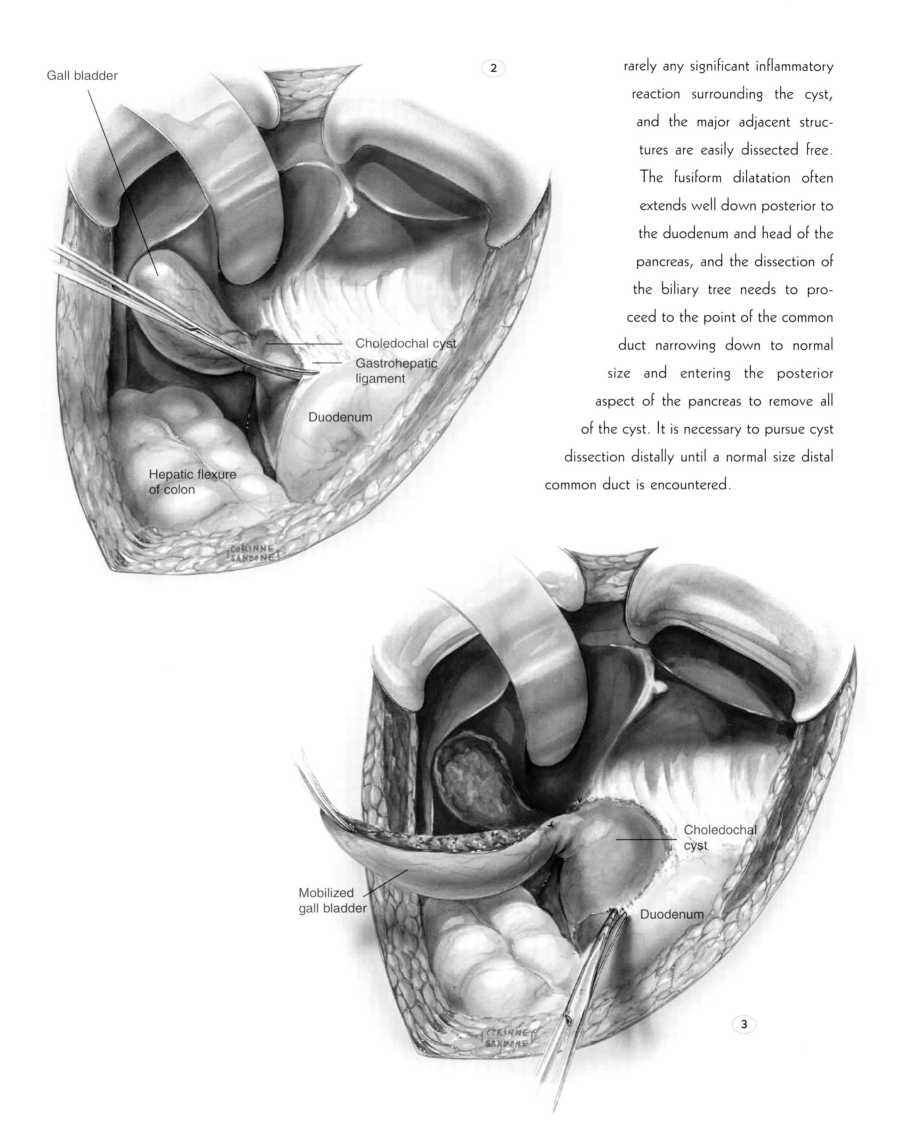

Gall bladder

Choledochal cyst

Gastrohepatic ligament

Duodenum

Hepatic flexure of colon

2

rarely any significant inflammatory reaction surrounding the cyst, and the major adjacent structures are easily dissected free. The fusiform dilatation often extends well down posterior to the duodenum and head of the pancreas, and the dissection of the biliary tree needs to proceed to the point of the common duct narrowing down to normal size and entering the posterior aspect of the pancreas to remove all of the cyst. It is necessary to pursue cyst dissection distally until a normal size distal common duct is encountered.

Choledochal cyst

Mobilized gall bladder

Duodenum

3

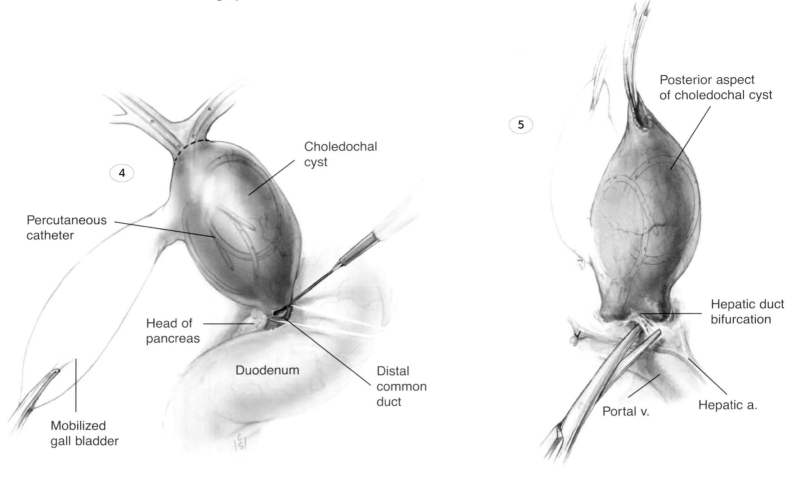

At this point, the distal normal-size common duct is divided (4). The distal common duct is oversewn with interrupted 3-0 silks. Once the choledochal cyst has been divided distally, it is reflected cephalad and easily dissected free from the hepatic artery and portal vein (5). These are generally fresh areolar planes that dissect bloodlessly and rapidly. The dissection is carried up to the bifurcation both anteriorly and posteriorly. In some instances, the cyst extends up to, and involves, the bifurcation, and there may be a stricture at the bifurcation where the right and left hepatic ducts join. If that is the case, the right and left hepatic ducts have to be dissected free and divided and the bifurcation resected. In this instance, the common hepatic duct appears to reconstitute fairly normally before the cystic dilatation of the choledochal cyst. Therefore, the common hepatic duct is divided just distal to the bifurcation, and the specimen is removed from the operative field (6).

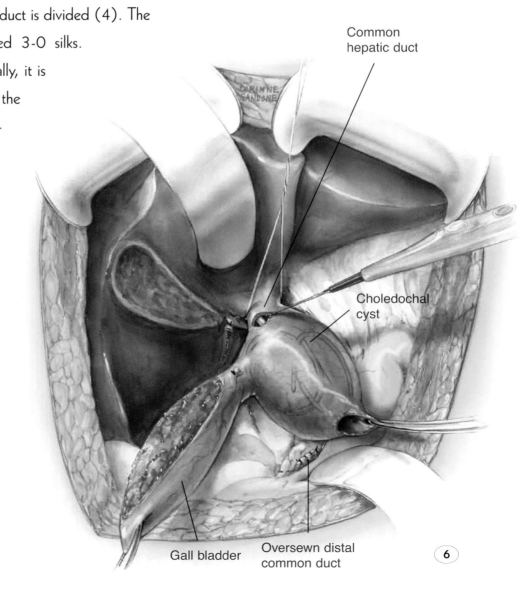

When the cyst has been resected, a Roux-en-Y jejunal loop 60 cm in length is constructed as previously described. The curved tips of the percutaneous transhepatic biliary catheters are amputated. In this instance, since the bifurcation was not resected, one biliary catheter insertion preoperatively could have sufficed. The Roux-en-Y loop is brought up into the right upper quadrant in a retrocolic position on top of the second and third portions of the duodenum (7). It easily rests without tension in the porta hepatis.

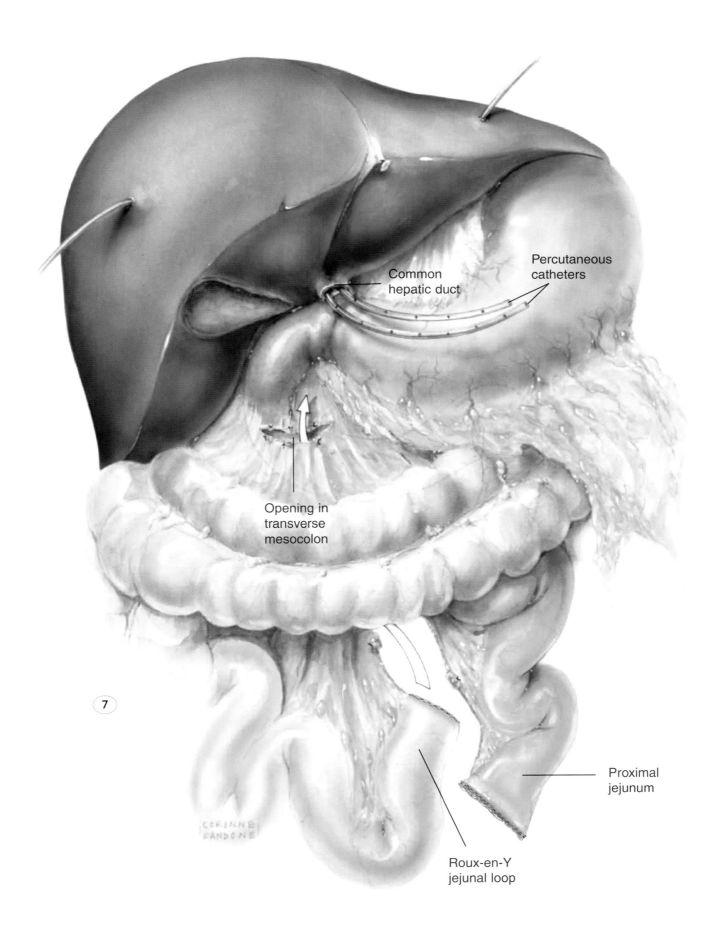

Common
hepatic duct

Percutaneous
catheters

Opening in
transverse
mesocolon

⑦

Proximal
jejunum

Roux-en-Y
jejunal loop

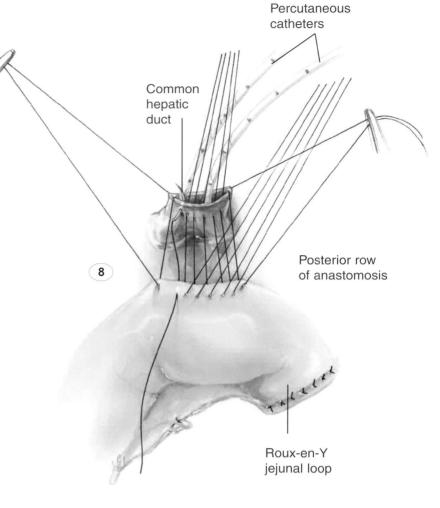

The hepaticojejunostomy is performed in a single layer using multiple interrupted 4-0 synthetic absorbable sutures. The posterior wall is placed in the jejunum prior to making an enterotomy. The sutures are placed into the submucosal layer of the jejunum and through and through the duct (8). All sutures are placed before they are tied.

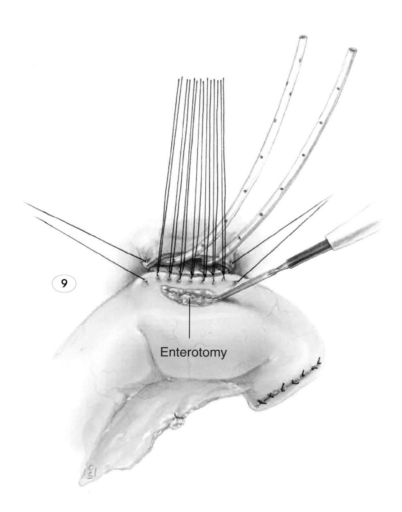

Once the sutures are secured, an enterotomy is carried out in the Roux-en-Y loop with the electrocautery (9).

The posterior layer of sutures is then divided and the two biliary catheters inserted into the Roux-en-Y loop (10). These are not exchanged for transhepatic Silastic biliary stents because the proximal biliary segment is normal, and a good mucosa-to-mucosa anastomosis can be performed. The two percutaneous transhepatic biliary catheters are not used as long-term stents, but will be left in for a month or 6 weeks merely to decompress the biliary anastomosis during healing. They are mostly used to help the surgeon identify the biliary structures at the time of surgery. The stents will be removed during an outpatient visit.

Percutaneous catheter

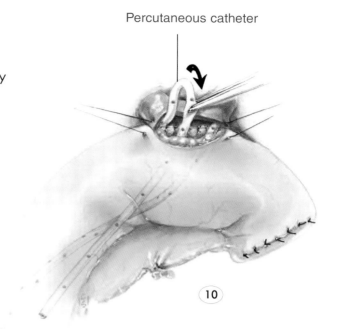

10

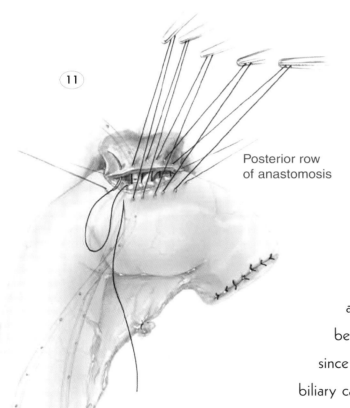

11

Posterior row
of anastomosis

The anterior row of sutures is placed using a single layer of interrupted 4-0 absorbable synthetic sutures placed through and through both duct and bowel (11). All sutures are placed before they are tied. As mentioned previously in this instance since the common hepatic duct was normal, only one percutaneous biliary catheter needs to be placed.

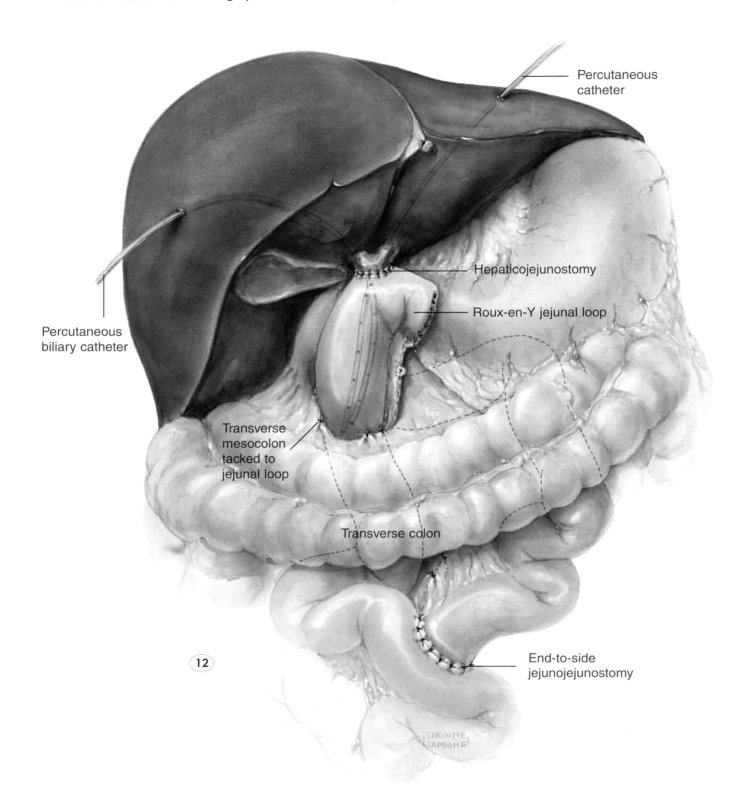

The Roux-en-Y loop is tacked to the rent in the transverse mesocolon with interrupted 4-0 silk sutures to prevent small bowel herniation (12). The two percutaneous biliary catheters were placed preoperatively and already have exit sites through the left upper quadrant and the right chest. The catheters are placed to allow bile-bag drainage by gravity. Five days after surgery cholangiography is performed. If no leaks are seen, the catheters are internalized by placing stopcocks or heparin locks on the ends. Patients are taught to irrigate the catheters twice a day with 20 mL of saline. The catheters are removed 4 to 6 weeks following surgery. The anastomosis is drained with a closed suction Silastic drain brought out through a stab wound in the right upper quadrant.

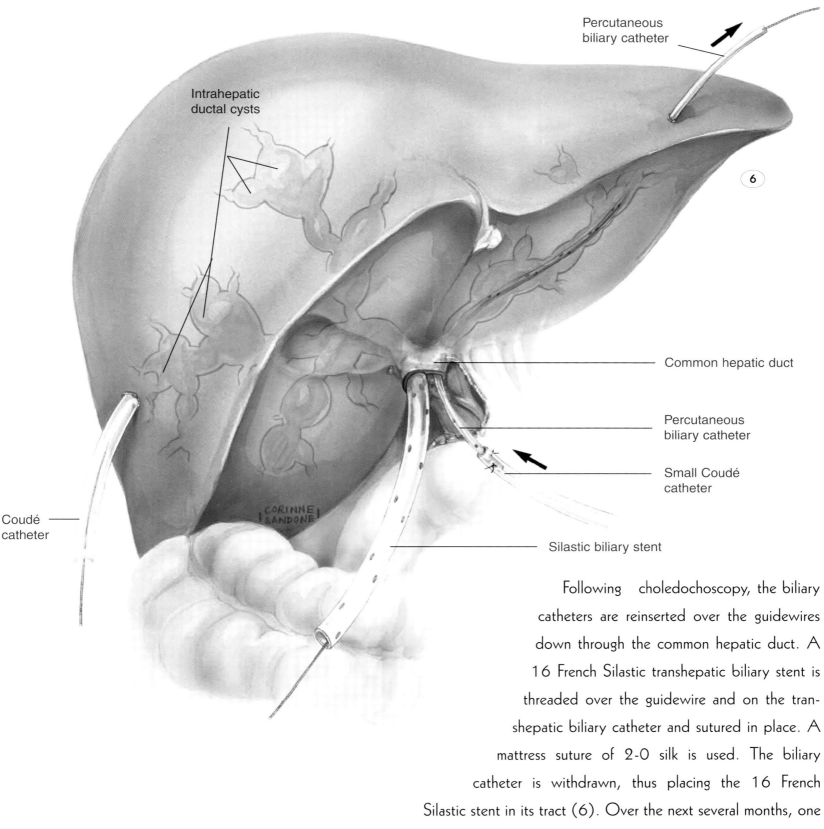

Percutaneous
biliary catheter

6

Intrahepatic
ductal cysts

Common hepatic duct

Percutaneous
biliary catheter

Small Coudé
catheter

Coudé
catheter

Silastic biliary stent

CORINNE
SANDONE

Following choledochoscopy, the biliary catheters are reinserted over the guidewires down through the common hepatic duct. A 16 French Silastic transhepatic biliary stent is threaded over the guidewire and on the transhepatic biliary catheter and sutured in place. A mattress suture of 2-0 silk is used. The biliary catheter is withdrawn, thus placing the 16 French Silastic stent in its tract (6). Over the next several months, one may decide to upsize the Silastic biliary stents to an 18 French or even a 20 French. This can easily be done in the catheterization laboratory following discharge from the hospital and when the tracts are secure. The side holes of the Silastic stents are positioned so they reside within the liver and in that portion of the stent that extends beyond the common hepatic duct and which will be placed in the Roux-en-Y loop. A Roux-en-Y jejunal loop 60 cm in length is constructed as previously described. It is brought up into the right upper quadrant in a retrocolic fashion, on top of the second and third portions of the duodenum, so that it rests without tension in the subhepatic space.

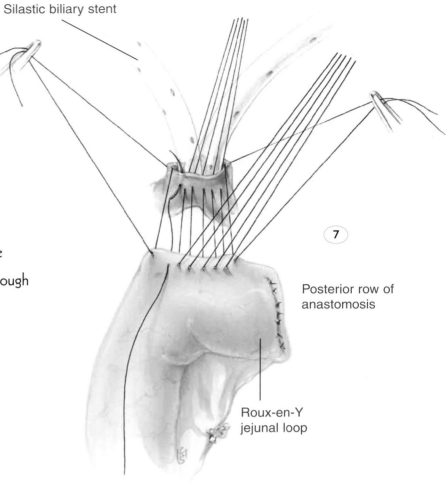

Silastic biliary stent

⑦

Posterior row of anastomosis

Roux-en-Y jejunal loop

A single-layer anastomosis is performed using interrupted 4-0 synthetic absorbable material. The posterior layer is placed prior to making an enterotomy. These sutures pass into the submucosal layer of the bowel and through and through the duct (7). Each is held with a hemostat.

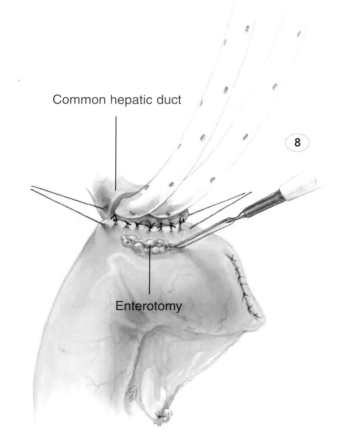

Common hepatic duct

⑧

Enterotomy

Once the sutures are all placed, they are secured, and an enterotomy is performed using the electrocautery (8).

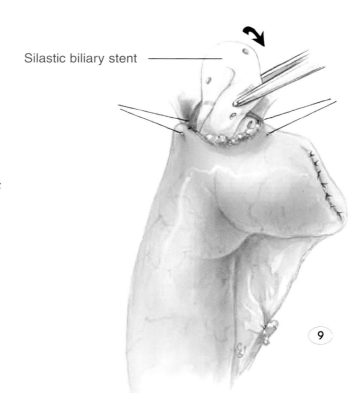

The back row of sutures is divided and the stents are placed in the Roux-en-Y loop (9).

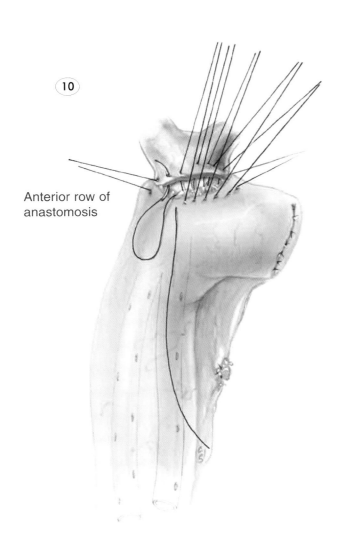

The anastomosis is completed with an anterior row of interrupted 4-0 synthetic absorbable sutures placed in a simple through-and-through fashion (10). All sutures are placed before they are secured.

The Roux-en-Y loop is tacked to the rent in the transverse mesocolon with interrupted 4-0 silks to prevent herniation of the small bowel (11). The Silastic transhepatic biliary stents are brought out through stab wounds in the right and left upper quadrants, sutured to the skin with 5-0 stainless steel wire, and connected to dependent bile-bag drainage. The egress sites of both stents on the superior surface of the liver are drained with closed-suction Silastic drains brought out through separate stab wounds in the right and left upper quadrants. A third closed-suction Silastic drain is used to drain the hepaticojejunostomy, and is brought out through a stab wound in the mid abdomen.

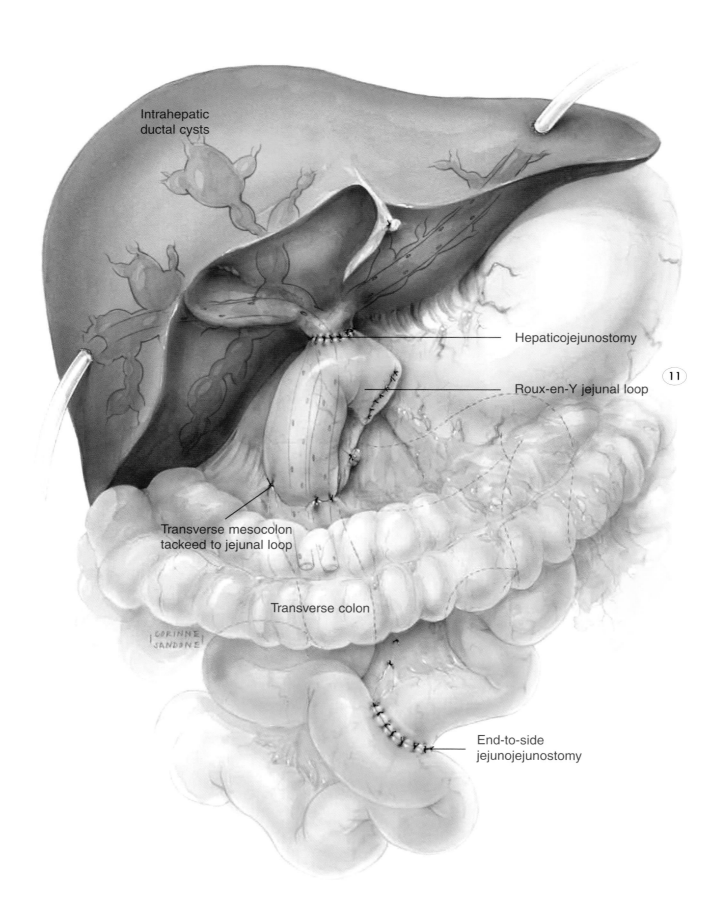

Intrahepatic
ductal cysts

Hepaticojejunostomy

Roux-en-Y jejunal loop

11

Transverse mesocolon
tackeed to jejunal loop

Transverse colon

CORINNE
SANDONE

End-to-side
jejunojejunostomy

current to performing the cholecystectomy. If the patient has already had a laparoscopic cholecystectomy and the diagnosis confirmed, one proceeds with a wedge resection of the gall bladder bed in the liver.

The hepatic flexure of the colon and omentum are dissected free and retracted inferiorly (3).

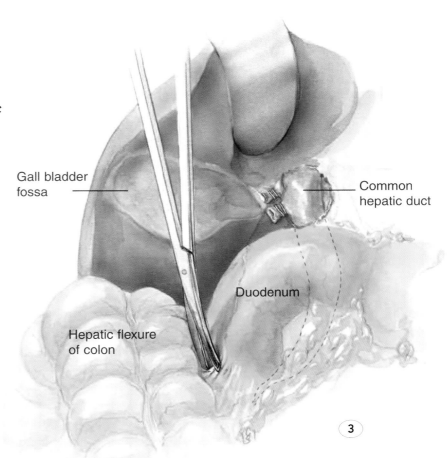

Gall bladder fossa

Common hepatic duct

Duodenum

Hepatic flexure of colon

3

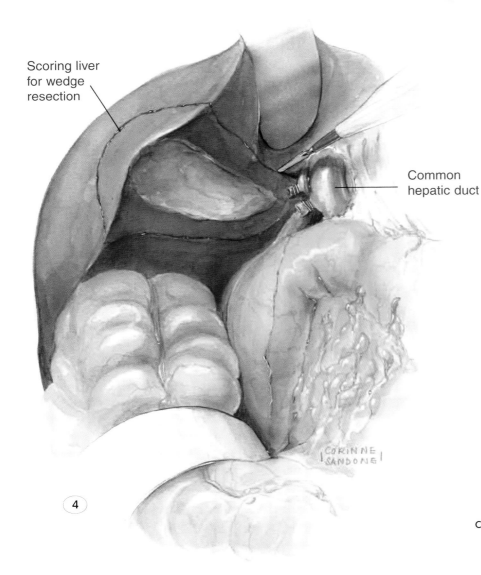

Scoring liver for wedge resection

Common hepatic duct

4

Since this patient has already undergone a laparoscopic cholecystectomy, using the electrocautery, the margins of the wedge resection can be outlined on the liver, surrounding the gall bladder bed (4). The wedge resection can be performed utilizing a variety of techniques. Many surgeons prefer to use the Cavitron or TissueLink for such nonanatomical liver resections. In this example, we demonstrate a technique of utilizing a series of overlapping No. 1 chromic catgut mattress sutures to compress surrounding hepatic parenchyma. The chromic catgut sutures compress the liver parenchyma, thus achieving hemostasis without compressing the liver to the point where necrosis occurs. The actual resection is then carried out with the electrocautery, using the ball tip (5). Generally, a 2 cm margin can easily be obtained using this technique. which results in a virtually bloodless resection. Small bleeding points or small bile ducts are further controlled with suture ligatures. Hemostasis can be achieved using the electrocautery and the argon beam coagulator.

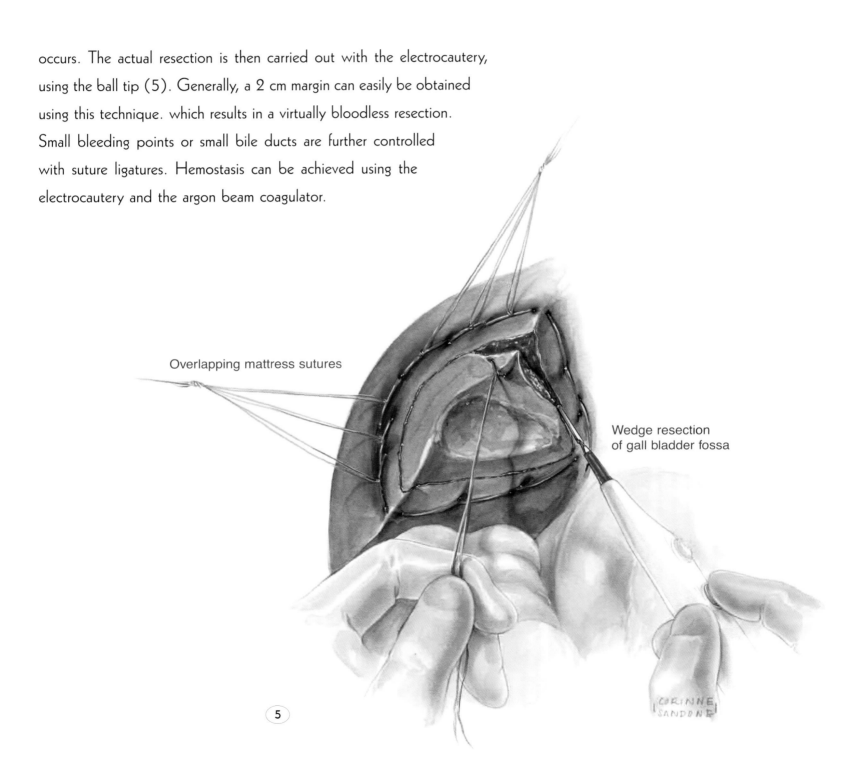

Overlapping mattress sutures

Wedge resection
of gall bladder fossa

5

Following the local wedge resection of the liver, a regional lymph node dissection is carried out removing all lymph nodes and surrounding areolar tissue from the bifurcation of the common hepatic duct down to the distal common duct and medially along the hepatic artery over to the celiac axis (6). Many nodes are actually posterior to the biliary tree. In the past, we have tried to perform this lymphadenectomy without removing the extrahepatic biliary tree. This is very difficult, and we now routinely divide the common hepatic duct just distal to the bifurcation, and include the entire extrahepatic biliary tree with the porta hepatis lymphadenectomy. This also gives a bigger margin on the gall bladder than just the cystic duct if only a cholecystectomy is performed. Following laparoscopic cholecystectomy, we have had instances when a normal-looking extrahepatic biliary tree has been removed in the course of the porta hepatis lymphadenectomy, and a histologically positive cystic duct margin has been found.

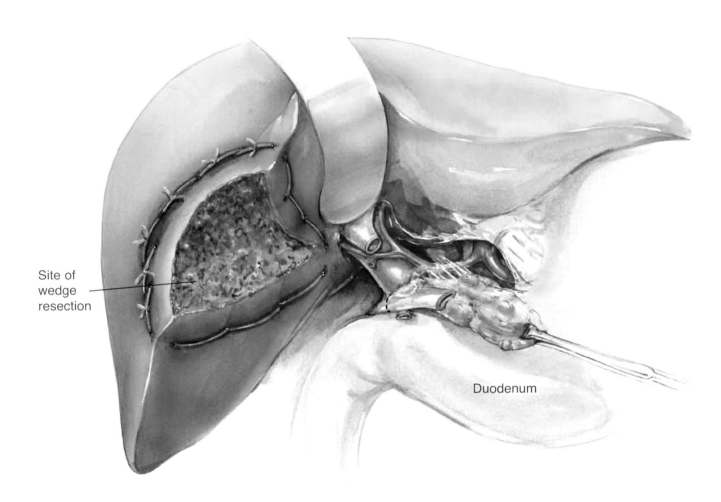

Site of
wedge
resection

Duodenum

6

Following the porta hepatis lymphadenectomy, a Roux-en-Y jejunal loop 60 cm in length is constructed in the fashion previously demonstrated (see "Insert Section Here"). It is brought up into the right upper quadrant through a rent in the transverse mesocolon on top of the second and third portions of the duodenum. A hepaticojejunostomy is performed with a single layer of interrupted 4-0 absorbable synthetic material (7) as previously described (see "Insert Section Here"). Stenting of the anastomosis is not necessary. We have generally followed the principle that, if tumor is present in the segment of liver removed with the wedge resection and/or positive lymph nodes or a positive cystic duct margin is present, post-operative adjuvant therapy is carried out using both radiotherapy and chemotherapy. If these three areas are negative, adjuvant therapy is not used.

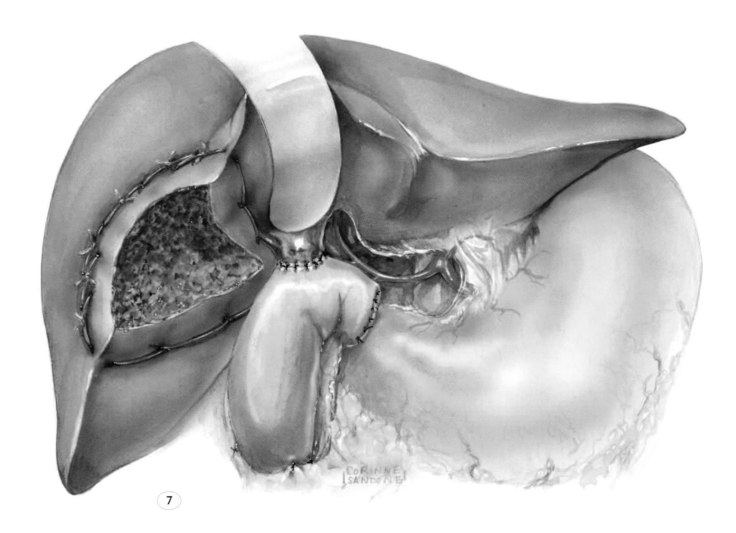

7

THE LIVER

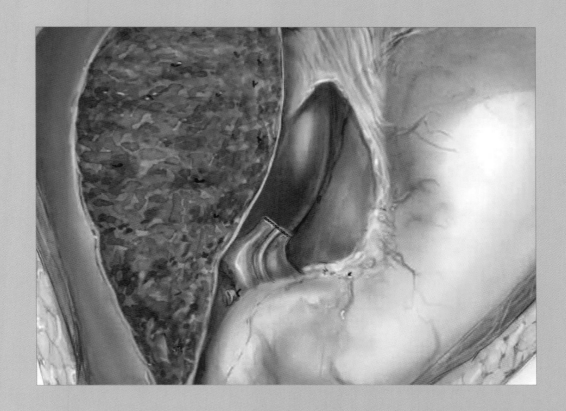

Anatomy of the Liver

Knowledge of the surgical anatomy of the liver and its blood supply has evolved in recent decades. Earlier classifications of liver anatomy, which were based on morphologic surface features, have evolved into one principally based on the functional vascular anatomy. First described by Cantlie in 1898 and expanded upon by Couinaud in 1957, the adoption of this functional anatomic classification has allowed for more clear descriptions of types of hepatic resection and helped to encourage anatomic resection techniques.

The liver occupies the entire right upper quadrant of the abdomen and extends well beyond the midline into the left abdomen. It ranges in weight from 1,200 to 1,600 g in the adult and is the single largest organ in the body. Most of its surfaces are covered with peritoneum, or Glisson's capsule. This layer extends to the hilum and encompasses the portal structures as they enter into the liver parenchyma, defining the portal pedicles. Superiorly, on either side of the inferior vena cava, and larger on the right, are the bare areas, which have no peritoneal covering. Suspensory ligaments or peritoneal attachments of the liver include the falciform ligament and the round ligament at the umbilical fissure. Additional attachments include the hepatoduodenal, gastro-heptic (lesser omentum), hepato-colic, hepatorenal, and left and right triangular ligaments.

According to the modi-fied Couinaud classifica-tion, the liver is divided into two hemilivers (or lobes), four sectors (or sections) and eight seg-ments, defined by the branching of the portal pedicles (1). The anatomic

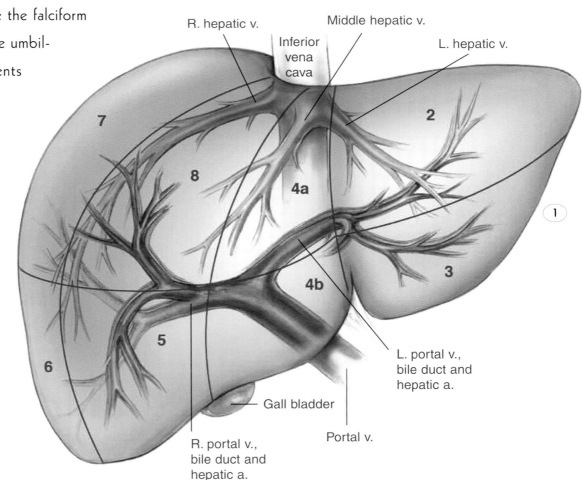

division between the left and right hemilivers follows a plane from the medial margin of the gall bladder bed to the vena cava posteriorly (Cantlie's plane). The left hemiliver is divided into the left medial and left lateral sectors, and three segments (segments 2 to 4). The right liver is divided into the right anterior and right posterior sectors and four segments (segments 5 to 8). The caudate lobe (segment 1) is located posteriorly between the right and left hemilivers with separate vasculature (2).

There are typically three main hepatic veins draining the liver, although considerable anatomic variability can be seen. The three veins enter the inferior vena cava at the superior aspect of the liver, just below the diaphragm (1). Occasionally, the middle vein will join the left vein before entering the inferior vena cava. In addition, there may also be additional smaller accessory veins that enter the inferior vena cava below the main hepatic venous confluence. The major hepatic veins, while not defining the segmental anatomy, are often found in the watershed areas between segments and can be used to identify the anatomy on imaging studies. The right hepatic vein runs between the right posterior and anterior hepatic sectors; and the middle vein often courses in the plane between the right and left hemiliver. In contrast, the left hepatic vein does not divide the sectors of the left liver (which is instead divided by the falciform ligament) but travels within the left lateral sector.

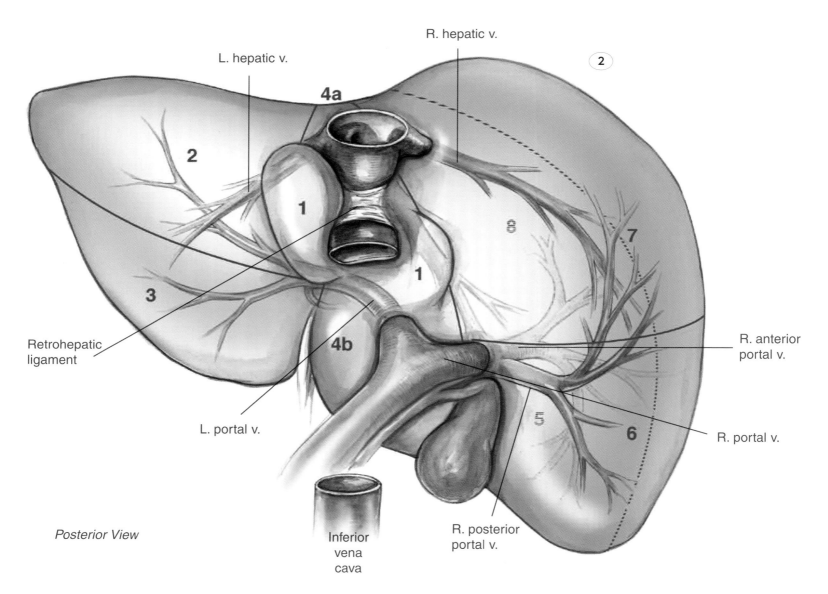

Structures within the Liver Hilum or Porta Hepatis

The confluence of the right and left bile ducts overlie the portal venous bifurcation (3). The hepatic arteries have a more variable anatomy, but most typically lie anterior and medial to the biliary and portal structures. The right hepatic artery often crosses the portal vein immediately posterior to the biliary confluence (3). The extrahepatic portion of the right portal pedicle is short. In contrast, the left pedicle has a longer extrahepatic segment, coursing below segment 4B and included in the hilar plate.

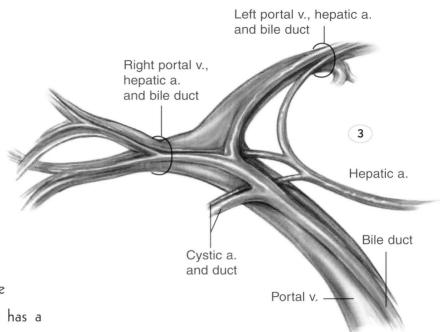

A useful way to assess the segmental anatomy of the liver is in the context of transverse planes as would be visualized on cross-sectional imaging (4, 5). Here, a high "slice" through the liver (A) visualizes the hepatic venous confluence and superior segments of the liver. Slice B distinguishes the umbilical fissure and left portal pedicle. Slice C is at the level of the main right portal vein and demarcates the approximate level between the superior and inferior segments of the liver. Finally, the lower slice (D) identifies the lowest portion of the liver and gall bladder.

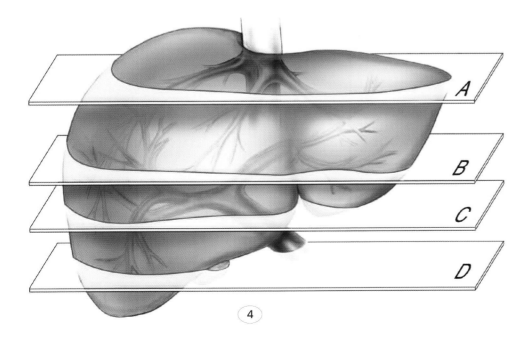

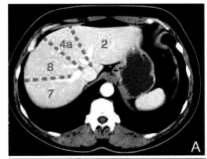

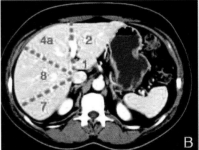

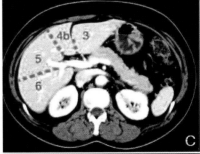

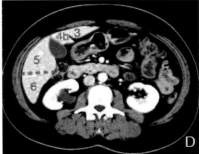

Hepatic Ultrasonography: Open and Laparoscopic

Intraoperative ultrasonography (IOUS) is used frequently by surgeons performing major hepatobiliary surgery. IOUS not only improves the ability to image and detect liver tumors at operation, but provides detailed visualization of intrahepatic structures which results in more precise hepatic resection. Ultrasonic imaging of the liver is performed using a relatively low frequency transducer ranging from 5 to 7.5 MHz. The range allows for the penetration necessary to image deeply within the hepatic parenchyma. Probe configurations can be either in linear or curvilinear array and can be either handheld or used through a laparoscope. Probes are gas-sterilized or placed within a disposable sterile plastic cover and applied directly on the surface of the liver.

When used prior to liver resection, IOUS is typically performed with the open abdomen and after partial or complete mobilization of the liver. Saline is used on the surface of the liver for improved acoustic contact, and the probe is manually maneuvered over the entire surface of the liver. This needs to be done in a systematic fashion in both cross-sectional and sagittal orientations. During scanning, intrahepatic vasculature is visualized, including the portal vein and its branches as well as the three hepatic veins and their confluence with the inferior vena cava (1a and 1b). Resectability of known disease is determined, and the type of resection can be planned based on the proximity of tumor to major vascular structures. Finally, the remainder of the liver should be scanned to carefully evaluate for occult metastases or other lesions. In most cases, the operating surgeon with experience with IOUS can manipulate the ultrasonic probe and adequately interpret the results. Ultrasound technicians can be helpful in the operating room to assist with or optimize the equipment, and in some situations, a radiologist can be used to aid in interpreting findings.

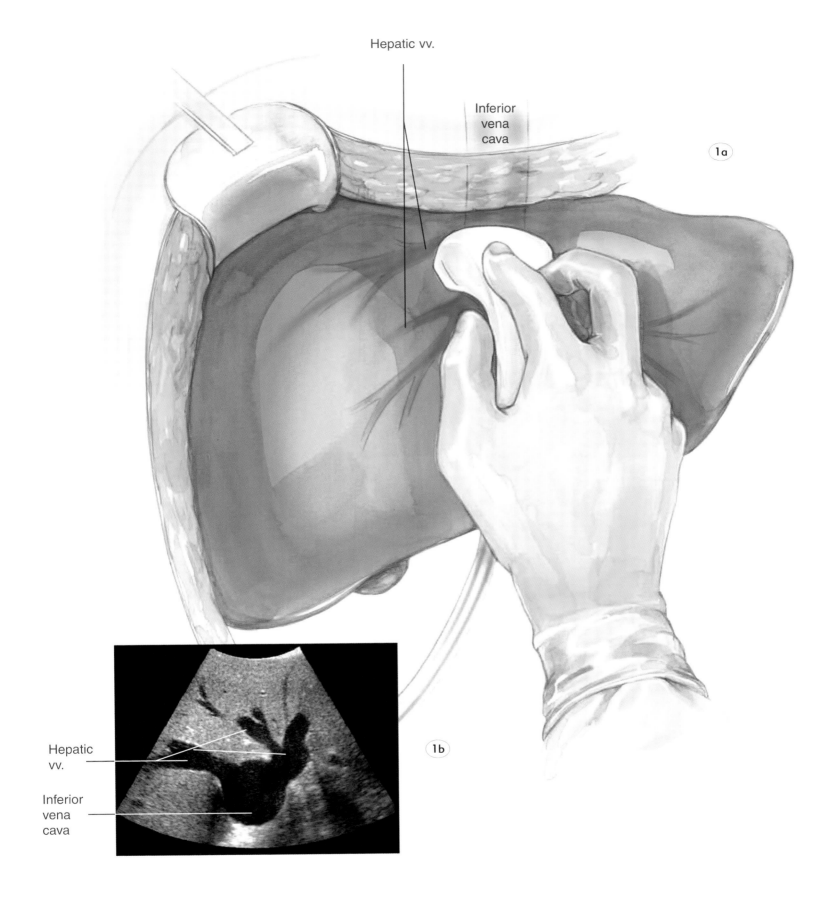

Hepatic vv.

Inferior vena cava

1a

Hepatic vv.

Inferior vena cava

1b

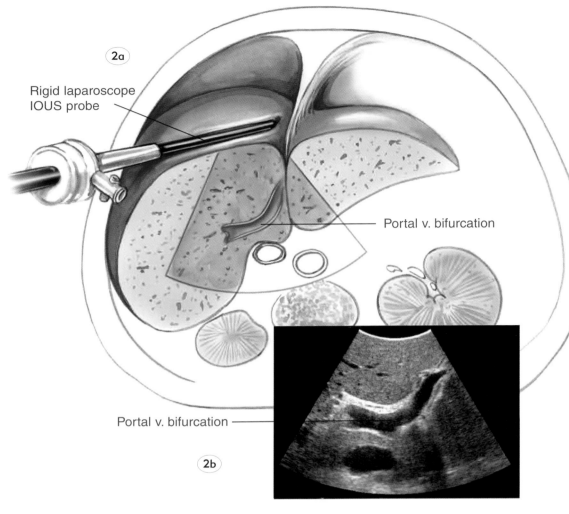

(2a)

Rigid laparoscope
IOUS probe

Portal v. bifurcation

Portal v. bifurcation

(2b)

Laparoscopic IOUS affords the capability of ultrasonographic visualization of the liver using a minimally invasive approach. It can be used for staging and assessment of the liver as well as for guidance of liver lesion biopsy or ablation or for performing laparoscopic liver resection. This technique is done using special ultrasound probes designed for this use. They can be either rigid (2a) or flexible (3) and typically require a 12-mm trocar port. As with open IOUS, the probe is swept over the surface of the liver, visualizing vascular anatomy and seeking otherwise occult lesions (2b).

In cases when the diagnosis of a liver lesion is unknown, IOUS, either open or laparoscopic, can be useful when performing intraoperative needle biopsy. The needle can be inserted directly into a lesion with precision using this technique. Specifically, the IOUS image is oriented in the plane that the biopsy needle will traverse. The needle is visualized in real time during positioning and biopsy. This technique is facilitated by spring-loaded biopsy devices.

Operative tumor ablation using radiofrequency, microwave, or cryotherapy devices is typically done using IOUS (see "Liver Tumor Ablation"). Much like with needle biopsy guidance, the IOUS probe is oriented in the same plane as the target lesion and the anticipated path of the ablation probe. Both probe placement and ablation monitoring uses ultrasound imaging.

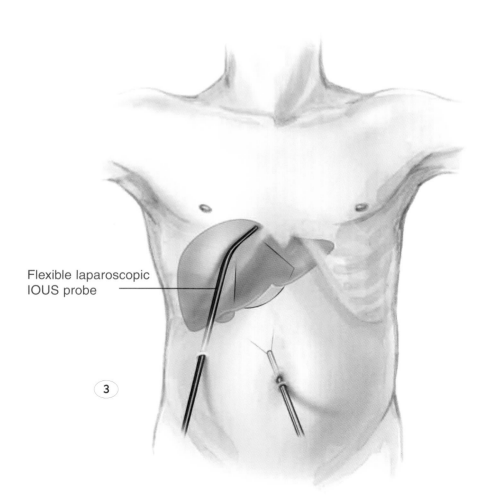

Flexible laparoscopic
IOUS probe

(3)

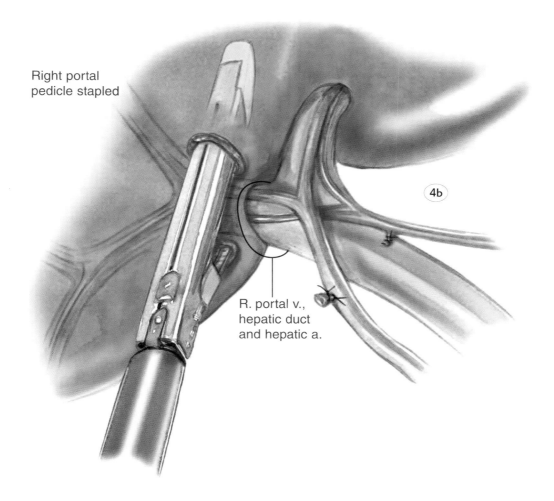

Right portal
pedicle stapled

4b

R. portal v.,
hepatic duct
and hepatic a.

The entire portal pedicle can then be divided within the liver parenchyma using a vascular stapling device (4b). Following ligation or division of the right portal vein, demarcation should be visible between the devascularized right side and the vascularized left hemiliver. At this point, the right hepatic vein is divided using a vascular stapling device, completing the mobilization phase (5).

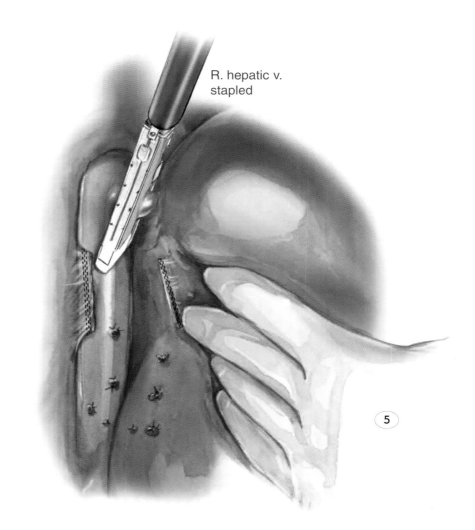

R. hepatic v.
stapled

5

Prior to the parenchymal transection, Glisson's capsule should be scored using electrocautery to map out the line of transection. IOUS can be helpful here in order to confirm adequate margins and to confirm the location of major vascular structures that will be encountered within the liver substance.

Division of the liver can be performed using a variety of methods. Classically, a finger fracture or crush clamp technique was employed in combination with metallic clips or ligatures to control vessels. More commonly, an ultrasonic dissector or water jet device is used to disintegrate and aspirate parenchyma, exposing vascular structures (6). These must then be controlled either with clips, bipolar or monopolar cautery, or using an electrosurgical sealing device. An alternative technique that is gaining popularity is the use of devices that coagulate the parenchyma prior to transection. This technique can utilize saline-enhanced cautery dissector devices or needle-based radiofrequency or microwave ablation devices which precoagulate a plane within the liver before division. Regardless of the device or technique used, the principles are the same—precise division of the liver parenchyma combined with mechanically and/or thermally established hemostasis. Larger pedi-

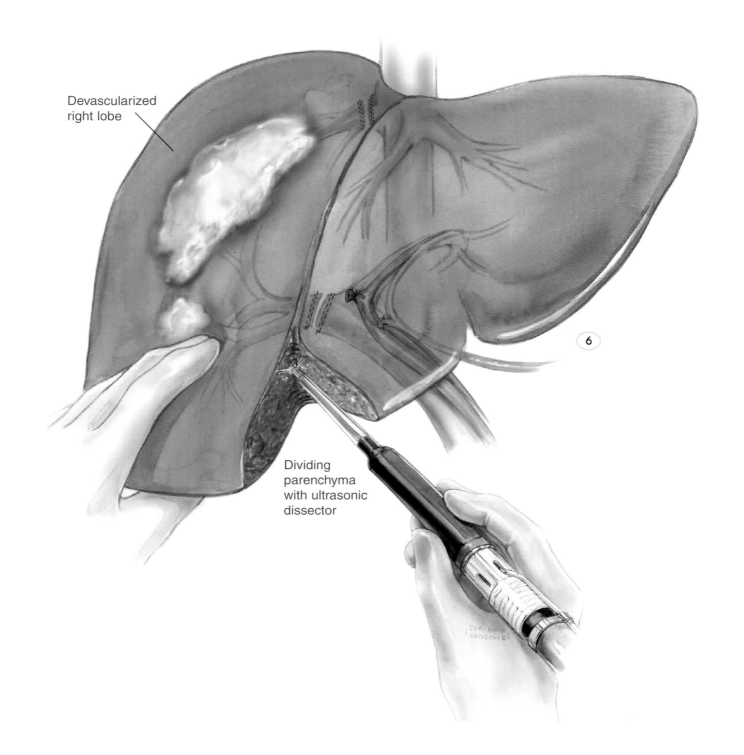

Devascularized
right lobe

Dividing
parenchyma
with ultrasonic
dissector

6

cles and vessels within the liver substance are controlled and divided using clamp ligation or stapling devices. We favor the use of a non-reticulating vascular stapler applied with the small jaw gently introduced within the liver substance (7).

During the parenchymal transection, total inflow occlusion (Pringle maneuver) can be used to temporarily block blood flow to the left liver. To achieve this, a loop tourniquet or non-crushing vascular clamp can be used. While not essential in all liver resections, selected use of total inflow occlusion combined with thermal dissector devices and maintenance of low central venous pressure can significantly lower blood loss during liver resection.

The final steps in performing a right hepatectomy are the management of the liver surface, positioning, final assessment, and closure. More significant bleeding from the resection surface can be controlled using non-absorbable monofilament figure-of-eight sutures applied directly to the bleeding points. Rarely, large absorbable transparenchymal liver U sutures are used when bleeding is excessive.

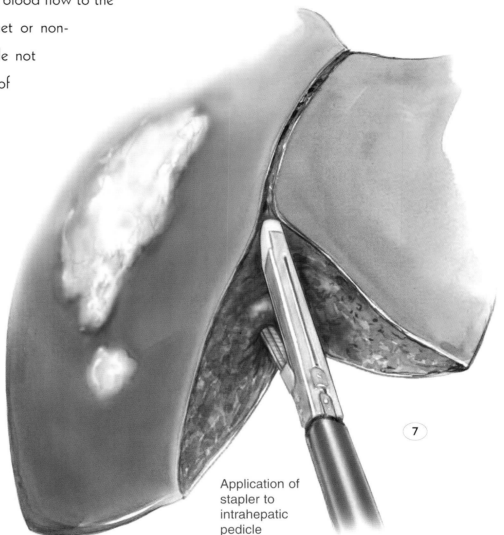

Application of stapler to intrahepatic pedicle

Minor oozing of the surface is controlled using an argon beam coagulating device or other thermal cautery devices (8). Prior to this step, careful inspection and identification of bile leaks are important because the coagulation char can mask small leaks. One useful method to detect small bile leaks on the raw surface is with gentle injection of first saline and then dilute methylene blue dye into the common bile duct via the cystic duct stump. Leaks can then be easily visualized and oversewn. Following surface cauterization, fibrin sealant can be applied to the resection surface in order to further aid in hemostasis and perhaps further reduce the risk of postoperative bile leak. Evidence suggests that the use of perihepatic drains for liver resection, including right hepatectomy, is not necessary. The use of drains can be considered in selected cases where biliary reconstruction is done or there are other concerns of increased risk of bile leak.

In most cases, the liver remnant should be resuspended in a more anatomic position by reattaching the liver at the falciform ligament. This is particularly important when a more extended right hepatectomy is performed, when the left triangular ligament is divided, or when the liver remnant is small. In addition, we advocate repeat visualization of the liver with IOUS. This allows confirmation of patent hepatic arterial, portal, and hepatic venous flow in the remnant.

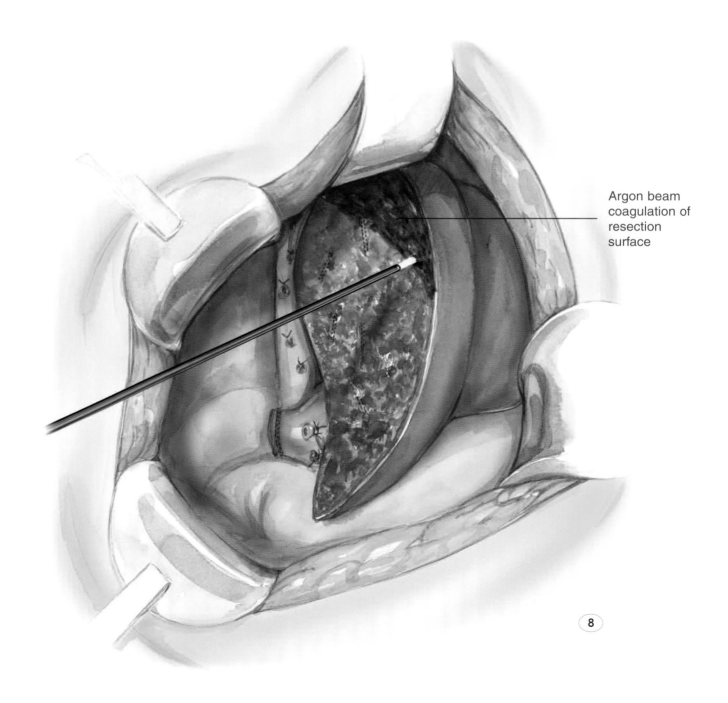

Argon beam coagulation of resection surface

8

Extended Right Hepatectomy (Right Trisectorectomy)

Operative Indications:

An extended right hepatectomy is performed when tumors require right hepatectomy along with a portion of the left liver (1). With this procedure, both the right and middle hepatic veins are divided, leaving only the left hepatic vein to drain the liver remnant. When the entire left medial sector is resected with the right liver, this is called a right trisectorectomy (or sectionectomy). When removing such an extent of liver, it is important to maintain an adequate volume of liver remnant. As with all liver operations, a safe resection requires (1) adequate inflow, (2) sufficient venous outflow, and

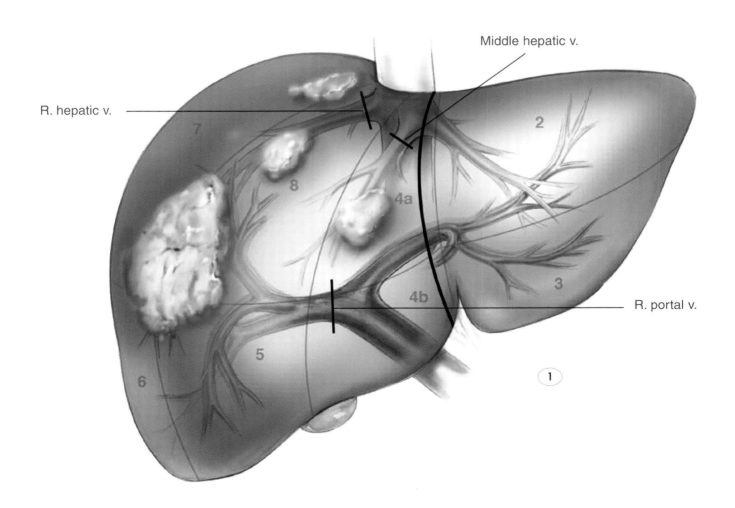

(3) ample liver remnant volume. The necessary liver remnant volume depends on the condition of the liver and should contain at least two contiguous segments. With a healthy liver parenchyma, the ratio of the remnant volume to the total estimated liver volume should be at least 20%. This remnant liver volume should be greater in the presence of cirrhosis or steatosis. In situations in which the anticipated future liver remnant is too small, as measured by preoperative cross-sectional imaging volumetrics, preoperative right portal vein embolization can be done. The goal is to elicit atrophy of the right liver with compensatory hypertrophy of the left liver. This procedure is typically done by the interventional radiologist 5 to 6 weeks prior to surgery, and repeat imaging is done to confirm left liver hypertrophy.

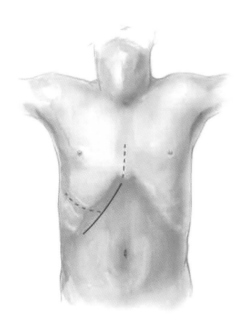

Operative Technique:

Extended right hepatectomy is performed much like that of right hepatectomy. In addition to the right liver (segments 5 to 8), all or part of segment 4 (the left medial sector) is removed in order to achieve tumor clearance. The caudate lobe may or may not be included with this resection.

The operative technique follows the same four basic steps as previously described:

- Exposure and assessment
- Hepatic mobilization and vascular control
- Transection of hepatic parenchyma
- Management of the liver surface, and completion

The exposure of the liver begins with an incision, which allows adequate visualization and manipulation of the liver and surrounding structures. The type of incision is not different than when performing most liver resections, most commonly a right subcostal incision. The assessment phase continues with a careful evaluation of extrahepatic sites within the abdominal cavity. Assessment of the liver is conducted with careful bimanual palpation and visual inspection, followed by intraoperative ultrasonography. As with formal right hepatectomy, particular attention should be paid to assessment of the anatomy of the hepatic veins, the portal pedicles, and proximity of the tumor(s) to these structures.

The operation is then directed at mobilization and vascular control of the right liver. Attachments are divided, including the round, falciform, and right triangular ligaments. Dissection along the posterior right liver and vena cava is conducted sharply, dividing the retrohepatic ligament and isolating the right hepatic vein. The hilar dissection is conducted much like that of a right hepatectomy. The gall bladder is removed and ligation of the right hepatic artery and right portal vein is achieved. The pedicle to the left medial sector is not typically controlled or divided extrahepatically with an extended right hepatectomy but taken as needed intraparenchymally. For this operation, the line of transection is immediately to the right (ipsilateral) of the falciform ligament (1). Care must be taken to stay away from the umbilical fissure in order to maintain the integrity of the pedicle to segments 2 and 3.

As with other hepatectomies, the method of parenchymal transection can vary, including ultrasonic dissection, crush clamp, or preablative transection. Larger pedicles and vessels, including the middle hepatic vein, are divided using a vascular stapler (2). Note that, while the volume of resected liver is greater with this operation, the actual transection surface area following extended right hepatectomy is less than that of a standard right hepatectomy (3) and is often performed in less time. As with other major resections, temporary total inflow occlusion can be used to decrease blood loss during resection.

The final steps are similar to that of a right hepatectomy. It is important with this operation that the liver remnant be resuspended by reattaching the liver at the falciform ligament. If not done, there is a risk of compromising vascular inflow or outflow when the small left remnant falls to the right. Reimaging of the liver with IOUS allows confirmation of hepatic vascular flow in the remnant at the completion of the procedure.

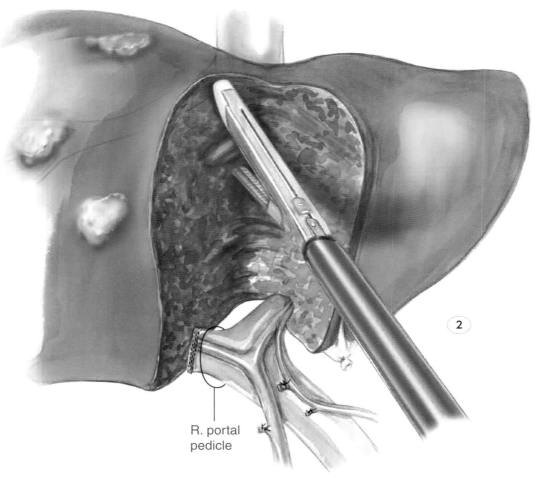

R. portal pedicle

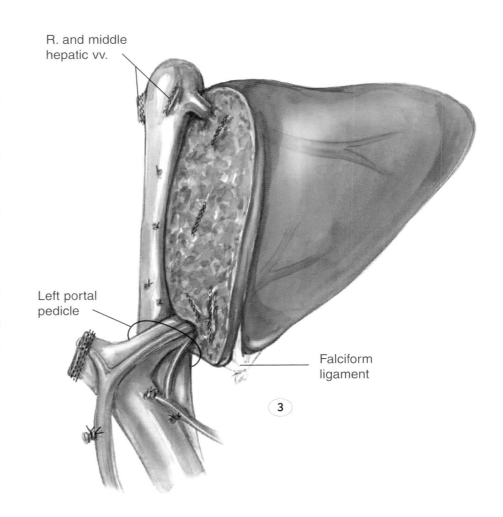

R. and middle hepatic vv.

Left portal pedicle

Falciform ligament

Left Hepatectomy

Operative Indications:

The left liver usually comprises less than 40% of the hepatic volume. Thus, a left hepatectomy is not performed as often as right-sided resections. It is done when complete removal of one or more tumors requires an anatomic resection of segments 2, 3, and 4a and 4b (1). Resection of the caudate lobe can be done with this operation when tumors extend into or involve segment 1. This resection may be indicated for both benign and malignant tumors, including both primary liver cancer and liver metastases.

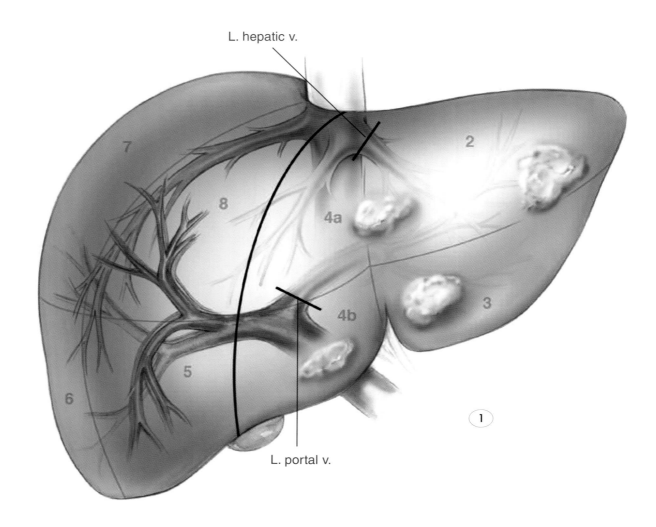

L. hepatic v.

L. portal v.

1

For an extended left hepatectomy, the line of transection is between the anterior and posterior right sectors (1). Care must be taken to not be too close to the right hepatic vein in order to maintain adequate outflow to the liver remnant. For tumors near the hilum, care must be exercised in order not to injure the main right or posterior right pedicle. In some cases, partial preservation of the right anterior sector can be achieved, provided that the right anterior portal pedicle is preserved and adequate tumor margins are achieved. As with other hepatectomies, the method of parenchymal transection can include ultrasonic dissection, crush clamp, or transection with preablation. Vascular staplers should be utilized for larger vessels. The resection surface area of the extended left hepatectomy is the largest, compared to the other major hepatectomies. Temporary total inflow occlusion can be used here, as with other resections, but care must be taken to record the duration of inflow occlusion and consider intermittent release of the clamp every 10 to 15 minutes.

Upon completion of the resection, only the right posterior portal pedicle and right hepatic vein remain (3). Management of the resection surface and closure is similar to that of other major liver resections. With a large surface area, care must be taken to carefully control bleeding and identify any potential bile leaks. Resuspension of the liver is not required, and placement of drains is not necessary.

MINOR RESECTIONS:

Segmental Resection:
Right Posterior Sectorectomy

Operative Indications:

Provided that complete resection of the diseased region can be achieved, anatomic resections of less than a full hemiliver should be considered. This allows for the preservation of a larger liver remnant and increases the probability of a successful repeat hepatectomy in the future if needed. The decision as to whether such a resection can be achieved is largely based on the tumor location relative to the vascular structures, particularly the portal pedicles. A right posterior sectorectomy (6-7 bisegmentectomy, 1) is indicated when a tumor or tumors are in proximity to the right posterior portal pedicle but

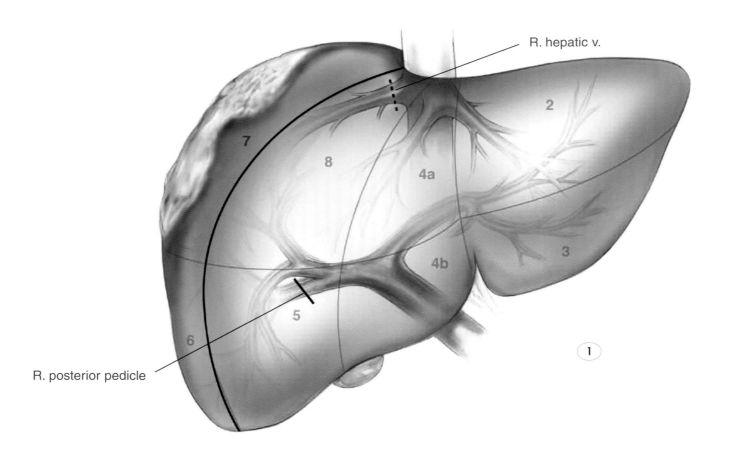

R. hepatic v.

R. posterior pedicle

resection can spare the main and anterior right branches. Similarly, a right anterior sectorectomy can be performed for tumors sparing the posterior pedicle. Careful review of the preoperative cross-sectional imaging and IOUS is important when determining when these operations are indicated.

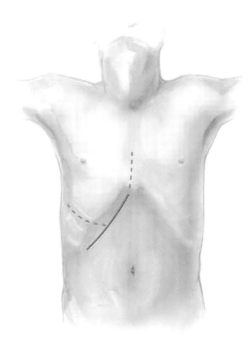

Operative Technique:

The technique of right posterior sectorectomy follows most of the same basic principles employed with all liver resections. The incision and exposure is the same as that of a right hepatectomy. The right hemiliver is fully mobilized, including division of the round ligament, falciform ligament, and the right triangular ligament. Dissection along the posterior right liver and vena cava is conducted sharply, and accessory veins are ligated and divided exposing the retrohepatic ligament just below the right hepatic vein origin. As with the right hepatectomy, the right hepatic vein should be looped and controlled. In many cases, the right hepatic vein will need to be divided with this operation in order to gain adequate tumor clearance.

The hilar dissection begins with a cholecystectomy. The hilar structures, including the hepatic artery and portal vein, are identified. For this resection, however, the dissection is extended into the right hilum, identifying the portal pedicle to the posterior sector. Intraoperative ultrasonography can be helpful in identifying the vascular anatomy, including the length of the main right portal vein and the location of the sectoral branches. The posterior pedicle can be visualized by retracting the right portal vein to the left and dissecting the lateral aspect of the portal vein. Care must be taken to avoid disruption of small branches to the caudate lobe. This can be facilitated, if needed, by looping and applying gentle traction on the main right portal vein.

The technique of ligation or stapling of the posterior portal pedicle en mass is preferred, as these structures come together within Glisson's sheath as they enter the liver parenchyma (2). We have found the proper positioning of the vascular stapler can be confirmed using IOUS before application, avoiding inadvertent injury to the anterior pedicle. Following division of the posterior portal branch, demarcation of the devascularized posterior sector can be readily seen. It is at this point that the right hepatic vein can be divided, if necessary. In such cases, segments 5 and 8 of the liver remnant will usually have adequate venous drainage via the middle hepatic veins.

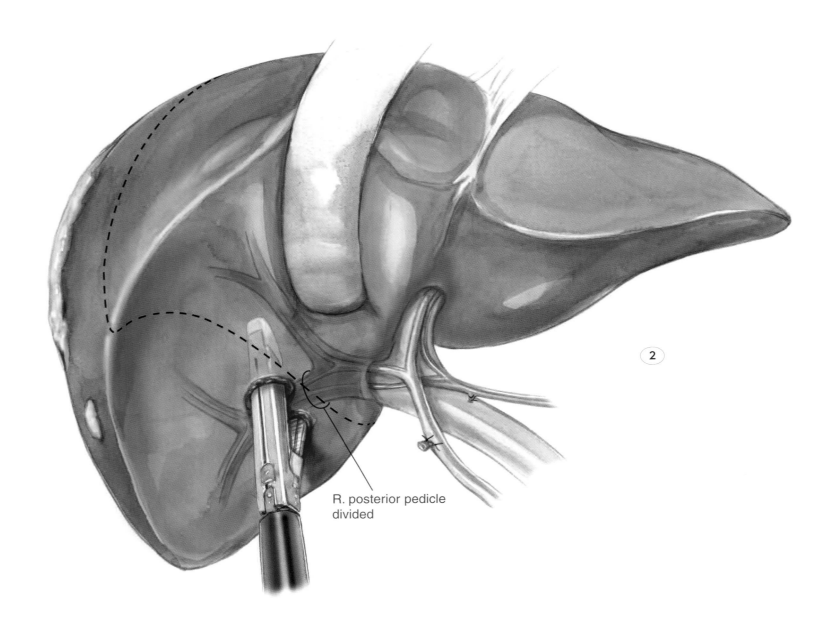

R. posterior pedicle
divided

2

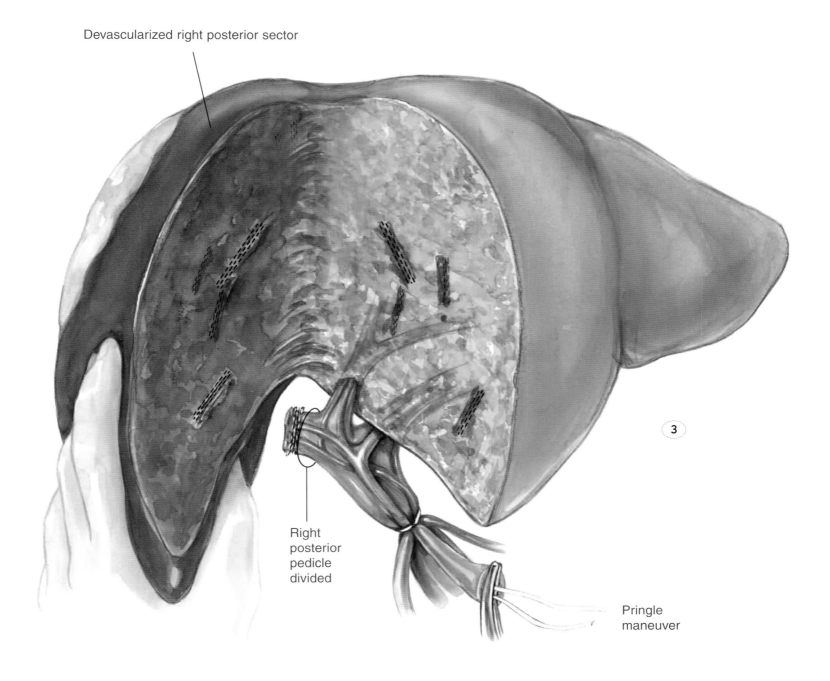

Devascularized right posterior sector

Right
posterior
pedicle
divided

③

Pringle
maneuver

As with other types of resection, the liver substance can be divided using a variety of methods. The crush clamp technique, the ultrasonic dissector, or preablation devices are all options. Temporary total inflow occlusion (Pringle maneuver) can be used for this type of resection as well. To perform this, an umbilical tape and Rommel-type tourniquet can be used (3). Bleeding from the resection surface can be controlled using figure-of-eight sutures applied directly to the bleeding points, and minor bleeding of the surface can be controlled using argon beam coagulation.

Left Lateral Sectorectomy

Operative Indications:

The left lateral sectorectomy (segments 2 and 3) is the most common bisegmentectomy performed (1). It is employed for lesions confined to this portion of the liver where there is no tumor encroachment on the falciform ligament or involvement of the left pedicle at the umbilical fissure. Both benign and malignant tumors in this location may be amenable to this type of resection.

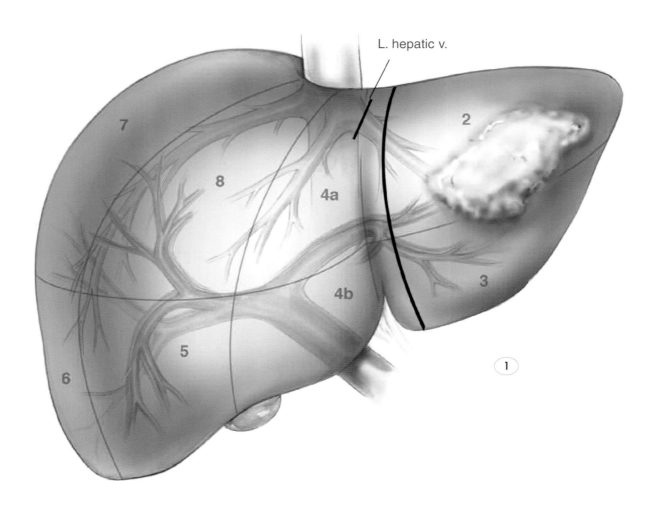

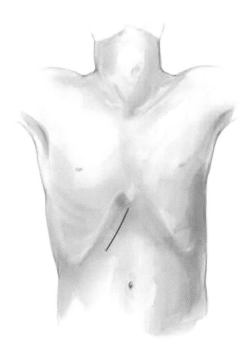

Operative Technique:

The technique of left lateral sectorectomy follows most of the same basic principles employed with all liver resections. The mobilization is relatively easier than other anatomic resections because this is a thinner and more mobile part of the liver. While the incision used for this operation can be any one of the standard incisions, a more limited subcostal or midline incision is often sufficient. Moreover, resection of the left lateral segments can be performed using laparoscopic techniques, with or without hand assistance.

The left liver is mobilized by first dividing the round and falciform ligaments. It is sometimes useful to maintain a long tie on the round ligament in order to maintain traction at the umbilical fissure during the transection. The left triangular ligament is divided (2) and the left lateral sector mobilized with caution so as to not cause injury to the spleen. In most cases, the gastrohepatic ligament is divided in order to facilitate identification of the left hepatic vein. An accessory or replaced left hepatic artery is usually ligated and divided when found. As the left hepatic vein enters segment 2 superiorly, this vessel should be controlled extrahepatically when possible, although it is often more

L. triangular ligament

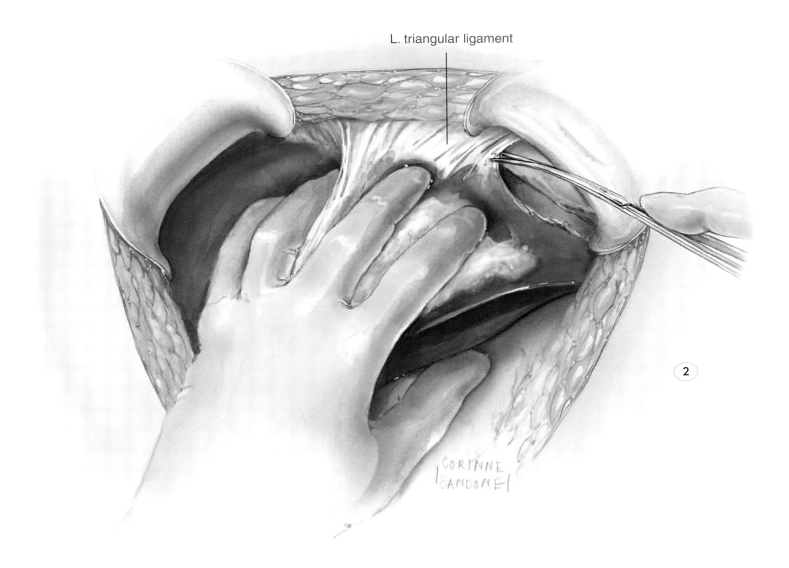

CORINNE
SANDONE

2

difficult to fully control it due to its proximity to the middle vein. In many cases where the tumor is not close to the left hepatic vein, extrahepatic isolation is not required and it can be divided with a vascular stapler within the parenchyma. Sharp dissection along the fissure between the lateral sector and caudate lobe helps to complete the mobilization.

A hilar dissection is not required when performing a left lateral sectorectomy. Traction on the round ligament can facilitate dissection to the left of the umbilical fissure in order to identify the portal pedicles to segments 3 and 2. These are divided intraparenchymally using a vascular stapler or clamps and suture ligatures. The liver capsule is scored approximately 1 cm to the left side of the falciform ligament and along the umbilical fissure (3). The parenchymal dissection is performed beginning from the inferior edge and moving superiorly using any one of the parenchymal transection techniques (4). Linear staplers can be used for the larger vascular branches, including the left hepatic vein.

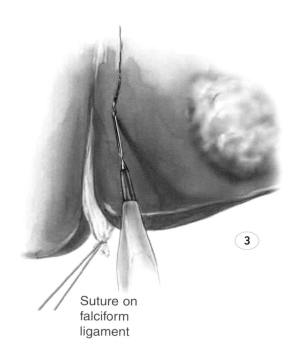

Suture on
falciform
ligament

3

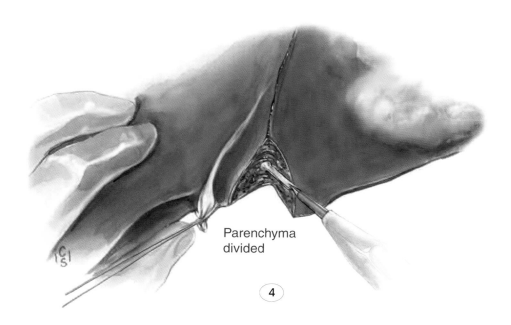

Parenchyma
divided

4

The transection surface is managed with a combination of sutures and thermal coagulation. This surface area is relatively small compared to most other resections (5). Drains are not required.

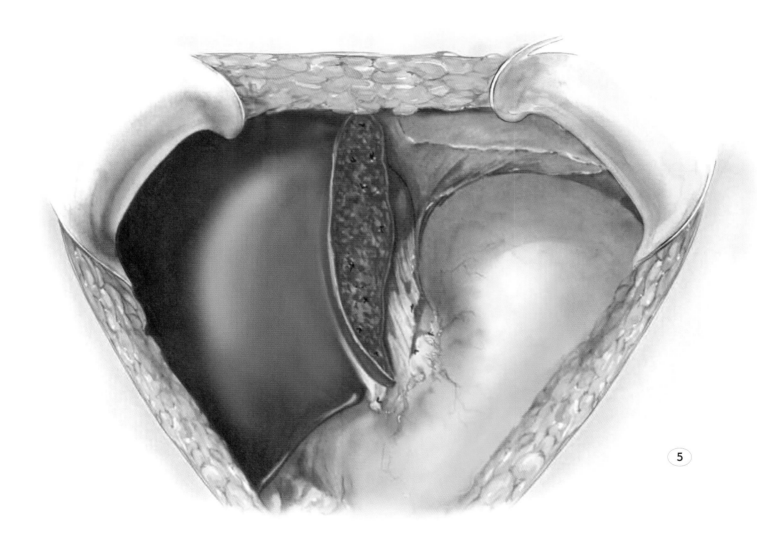

5

Nonanatomic Resection of Liver

Operative Indications:

In addition to anatomic resections of the liver (eg, major resections, bisegmentectomies), resections that do not rely on segmental landmarks and often include less than a complete segment can be performed. Sometimes called wedge resections, these are typically done for small lesions or tumors that are relatively near the liver surface (1). It is not uncommon to perform multiple nonanatomic resections for patients with bilateral tumors, or in some cases combined with anatomic or major resections on the contralateral side. Patients with primary liver cancer, hepatic metastases, or benign tumors all may be candidates for these minor resections.

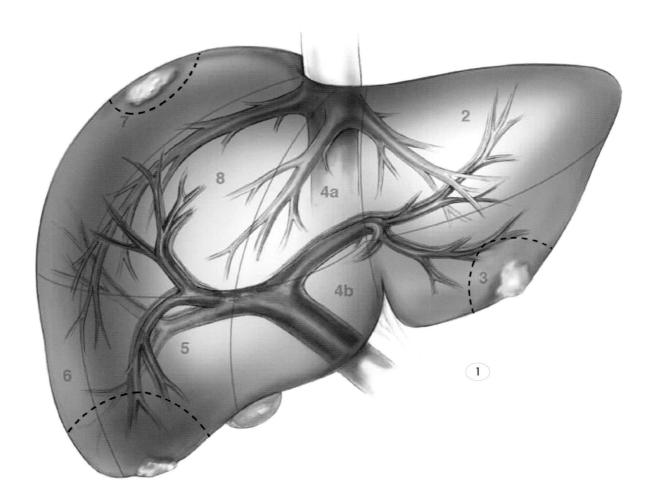

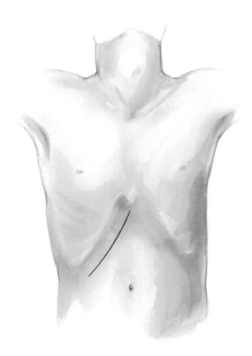

Operative Technique:

When planning a nonanatomic resection, the surgeon still needs to follow the same basic principles employed with all liver resections. The exposure of the liver begins with an incision that allows adequate visualization and manipulation of the liver and surrounding structures. The most common incision is the right subcostal. The extent of visualization and mobilization of the liver depends on the location of the planned resection. Regardless of the location, however, it is still important to fully assess the extent of disease outside of and within the liver before determining the type of resection needed. In some cases, a more limited incision may be used to begin, in order to determine if resectability is feasible. Then, the incision can be enlarged to that which is necessary for resection.

The assessment phase is done much like that of any hepatectomy. Intraoperative ultrasonography is done to determine if additional occult tumors are present and if a nonanatomic resection is feasible and safe. Proximity of a tumor to a major vascular pedicle, which, if taken, would compromise additional liver, is a contraindication to such a resection. Mobilization of the liver and detachment of any suspensory ligaments depends on the location of the planned resection. Ample mobilization is recommended, in most cases, in order to optimize visualization and gain control as needed during the resection. Selective isolation of vascular structures, however, is typically not required for these resections.

A variety of techniques can be employed when performing a nonanatomic resection. As with other more major resections, crushing techniques, dissectors, or precoagulation devices can be used. For smaller resections, standard electrocautery can be used for transecting the liver (2). When near the inferior liver edge, some surgeons make use of large liver sutures placed prior to transection. When using this method, large absorbable transparenchymal liver U sutures are placed in an overlapping fashion approximately 1 cm from the margin of resection (3). Electrocautery is used to perform the parenchymal transection (4) and argon beam coagulation is applied to the surface to achieve complete hemostasis (5).

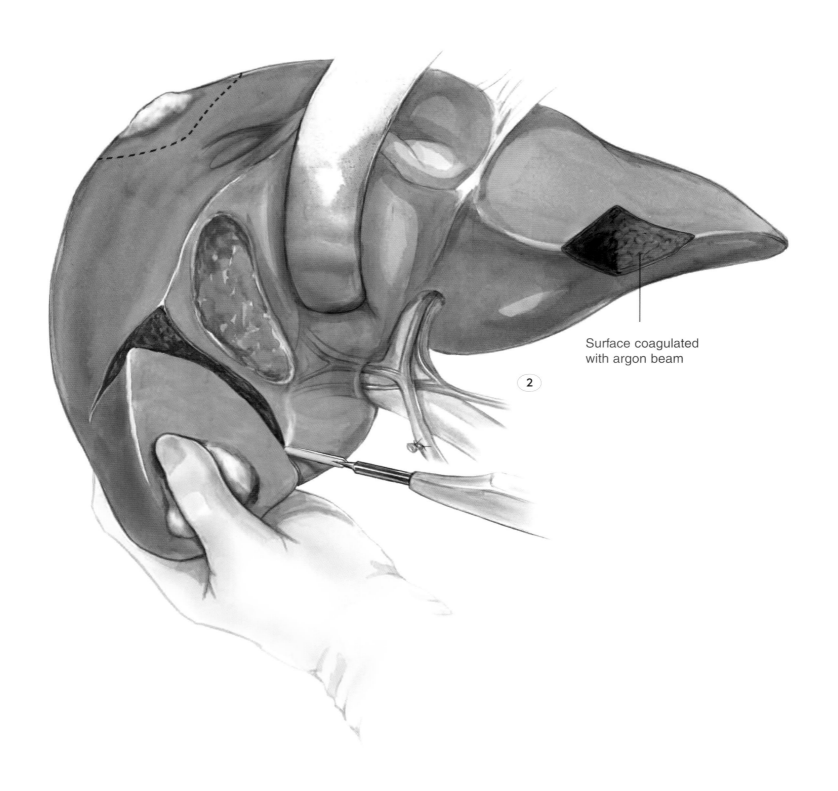

Surface coagulated
with argon beam

2

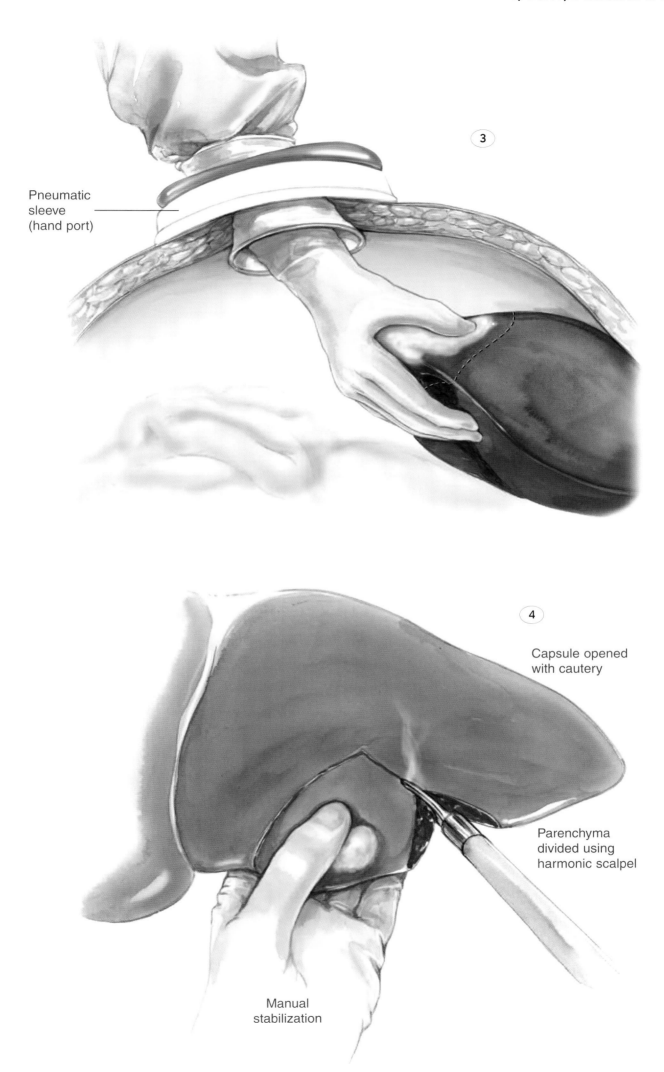

3

Pneumatic
sleeve
(hand port)

4

Capsule opened
with cautery

Parenchyma
divided using
harmonic scalpel

Manual
stabilization

Resection of a Simple Cyst of Liver: Laparoscopic and Open

Operative Indications:

The indications for the treatment of simple cysts are based on symptoms or, in some cases, an equivocal diagnosis. When nonspecific upper abdominal symptoms are present, care must be taken in order to be sure the symptoms are due to the cyst, particularly when the cyst is small and not adjacent to the liver surface. Cyst aspiration, while often performed, results in early recurrences in most cases. Instillation of ethanol or other sclerotic agents can reduce the recurrence rate but can be associated with complications. In some cases, cyst aspiration can be used diagnostically. Patients whose symptoms temporarily resolve with aspiration will likely do well following definitive surgical therapy.

Symptomatic simple hepatic cysts are optimally managed with surgical therapy. Rather than complete resection, partial excision or cyst unroofing is the procedure of choice. In cases where other diagnoses are suspected, complete surgical resection should be considered. The laparoscopic approach should be the operation of choice and can be offered in the majority of cases. Patients with multiple previous upper abdominal operations and dense adhesions, recurrent symptomatic cysts, or polycystic liver disease should be considered for an open procedure, as should those in which the diagnosis is unclear or when complete resection is planned. In addition, cysts located in the superior and posterior right liver or in deeper locations are more difficult to access laparoscopically and may require open surgery.

Operative Technique:

Laparoscopic hepatic cystectomy is done with principles and techniques much like that done for open procedures. Laparoscopic positioning and trocar placement depends on the location and size of the cyst. Typically, two to three subcostal trocars (5 to 12 mm) are used (1). After performing a diagnostic laparoscopy, the cyst is examined to assess the nature, external component and extent. Laparoscopic intraoperative ultrasonography may be useful in assessing the extent and nature of the cyst. Any evidence of septations or papillary projections on ultrasonography should arouse the suspicion of a cystic neoplasm, requiring possible conversion to an open procedure. Intraoperative ultrasonography may also be useful in identifying the hepatic vascular anatomy and the proximity of the cyst to these structures.

Following assurance of the diagnosis by appearance, cyst aspiration can be performed. This can be done by needle aspiration or by entering the cyst with the electrocautery or scissors and then aspirating the fluid contents. The cyst is then opened and examined. It is imperative to operatively confirm the diagnosis of a simple congenital cyst by histologic analysis and identification of a cuboidal epithelial lining. This is accomplished by excising a generous portion of the cyst wall and immediately sending it for frozen section evaluation (2).

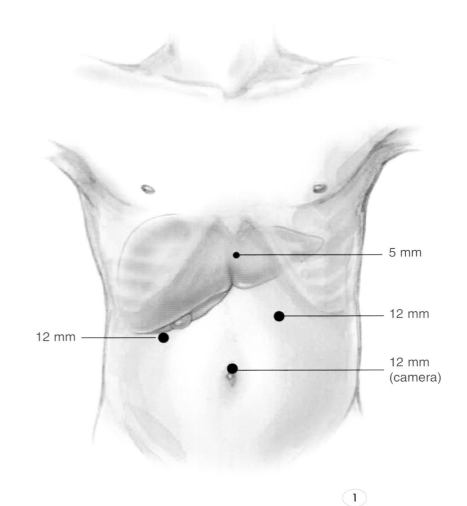

5 mm

12 mm

12 mm

12 mm
(camera)

1

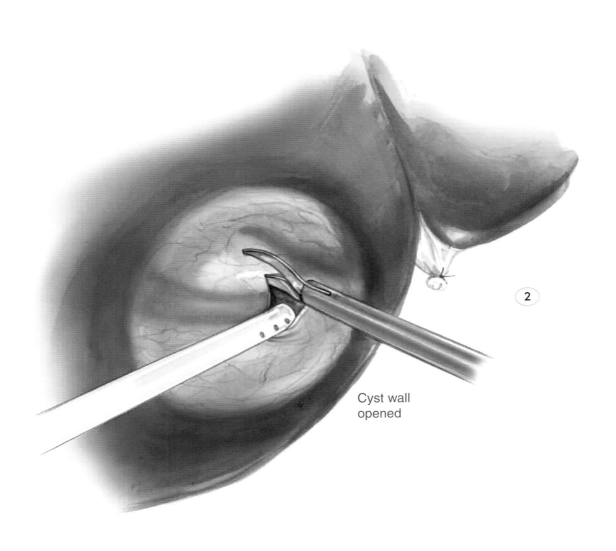

Cyst wall
opened

2

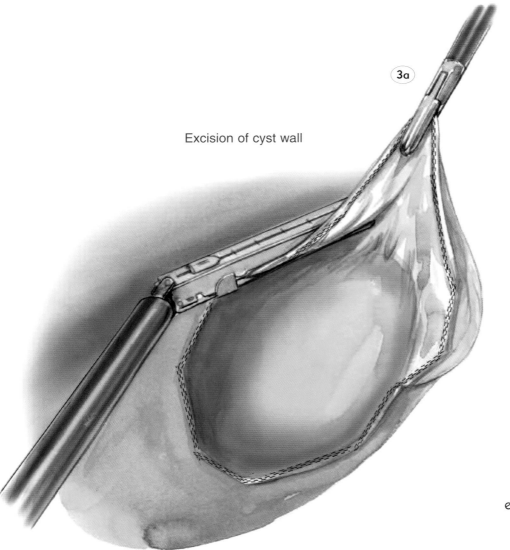

Excision of cyst wall

Once the diagnosis is confirmed, the external portion of the cyst wall should be excised as completely and as close as possible to the cyst–wall-liver interface. This can be performed with the help of endoshears, hook scissors, or harmonic scalpel. Care must be taken, however, to avoid bleeding or bile leakage from the cyst wall edge. Classically, this was achieved by using a running locking suture along the edge of the resected cyst wall, which is difficult when done laparoscopically. More recently, laparoscopic staplers (3a) and bipolar sealing devices (3b) have greatly facilitated excision of the cyst wall. The entire extraparenchy-

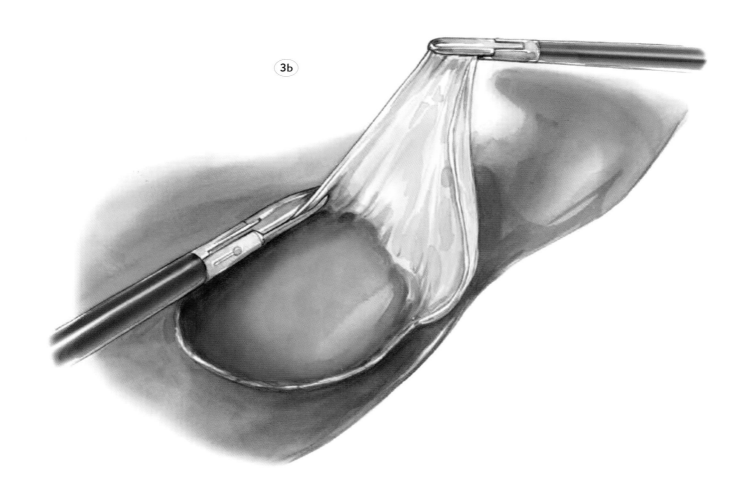

mal component of the cyst needs to be excised completely to minimize the chances of recurrence. Typically, this involves a resection of at least 50% of the cyst wall. Following excision, careful assessment of the remaining cyst wall is important in order to identify any bleeding or bile leaks. Argon beam coagulation, while useful in some cases for hemostasis and ablation of the residual cyst lining, should be used judiciously during laparoscopy in order to avoid injury or gas embolism.

Placement of the omentum within the residual cyst cavity can be useful in order to reduce the risk of recurrence. It may be particularly useful when less than 50% of the surface area could be excised or when there is a significant residual cavity. When performed, the omentum is dissected free from the transverse colon and placed within the residual cavity without tension. It can be fixed in place using clips or sutures. In many cases, a cholecystectomy should be performed in patients with gallstones to avoid returning to the same operative field in the future. In addition, the gall bladder should be removed when it facilitates the cyst resection or if the symptoms could possibly be attributed to it rather than the cyst.

Open surgical fenestration of simple hepatic cysts is done much like that of the laparoscopic operation. For this operation, typically a right subcostal incision is used. Inspection, intraoperative ultrasonography, cyst incision (4), aspiration, and pathologic evaluation of the cyst wall are performed.

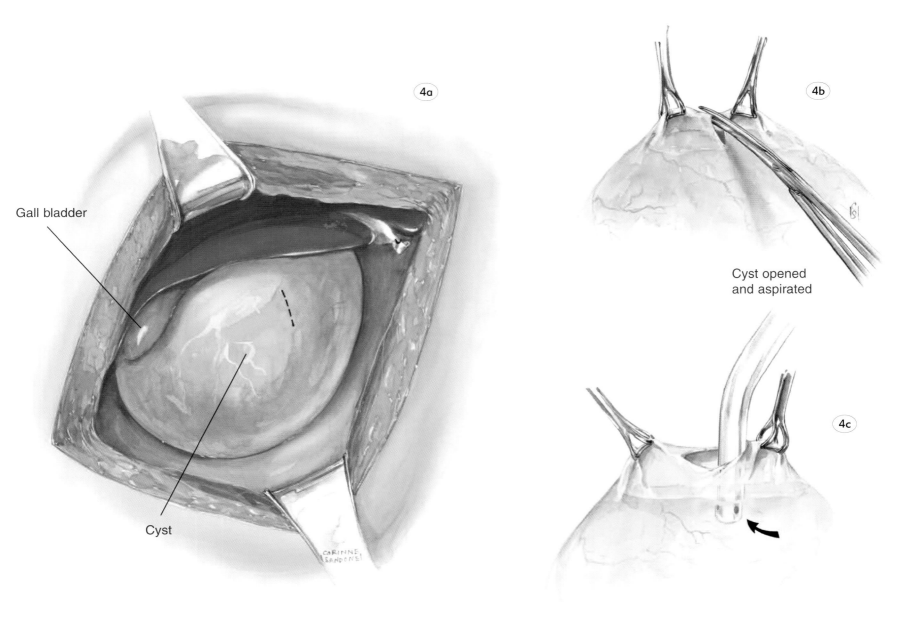

4a

Gall bladder

Cyst

4b

Cyst opened
and aspirated

4c

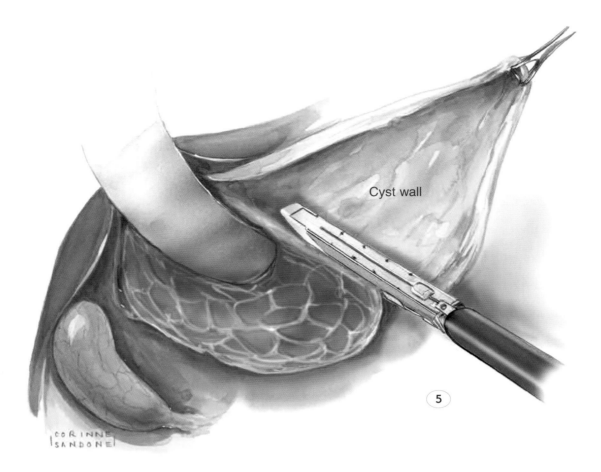

Cyst wall

Resection of as much of the cyst wall as is safely possible is achieved using staplers (5) or a bipolar sealing cautery device. In some cases, sharp excision (6) and use of a running locking suture can be applied to the resection edge (7). Argon beam coagulation can be used on the cut edge and inner residual surface, although care must be undertaken in order to avoid injury to immediately underlying vascular and biliary structures.

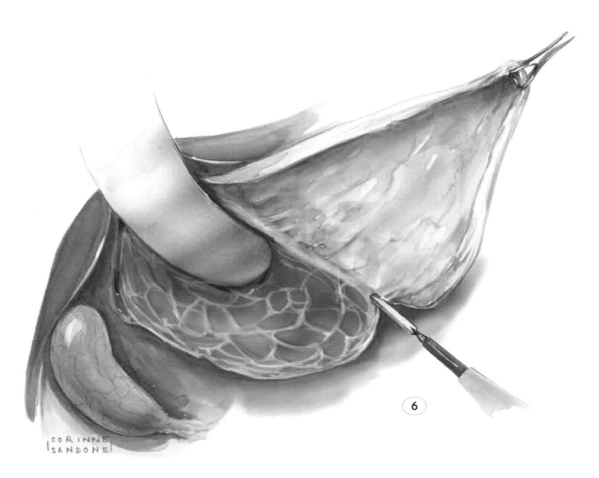

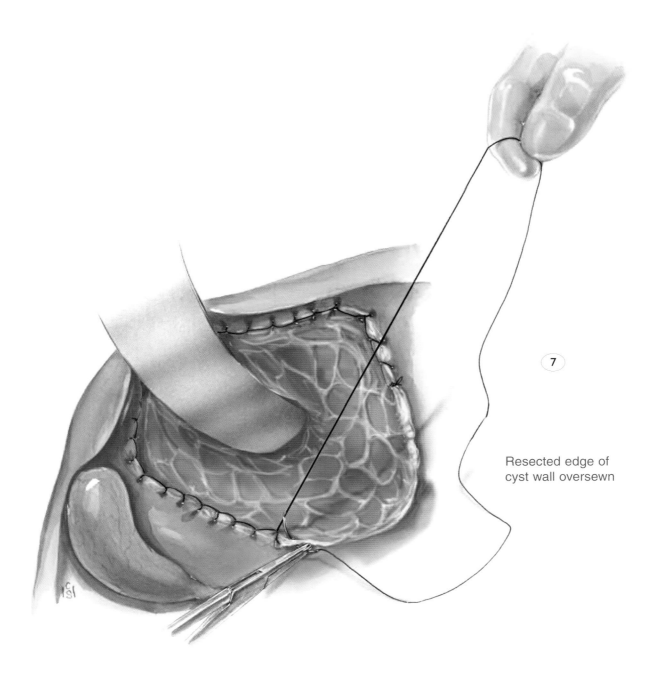

7

Resected edge of
cyst wall oversewn

Management Of Hydatid Cyst

Operative Indications

Cystic echinococcosis, while uncommon in the United States, is endemic in certain parts of the world such as the Middle East and Africa. The infection is often indolent, and the liver and lungs are the most frequently involved organs. Current classification based on ultrasonography reflects the functional state of the parasite. Active cysts demonstrate multiple septations, hydatid sand, and daughter cysts (1); whereas inactive cysts typically reveal heterogeneous hypo- or hyperechogenic degenerative contents and cyst wall calcifications. The diagnosis is suspected based on clinical signs and symp-

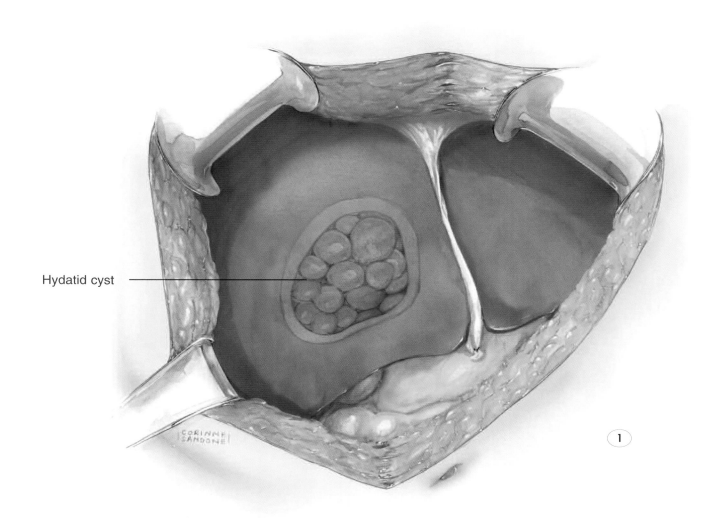

Hydatid cyst

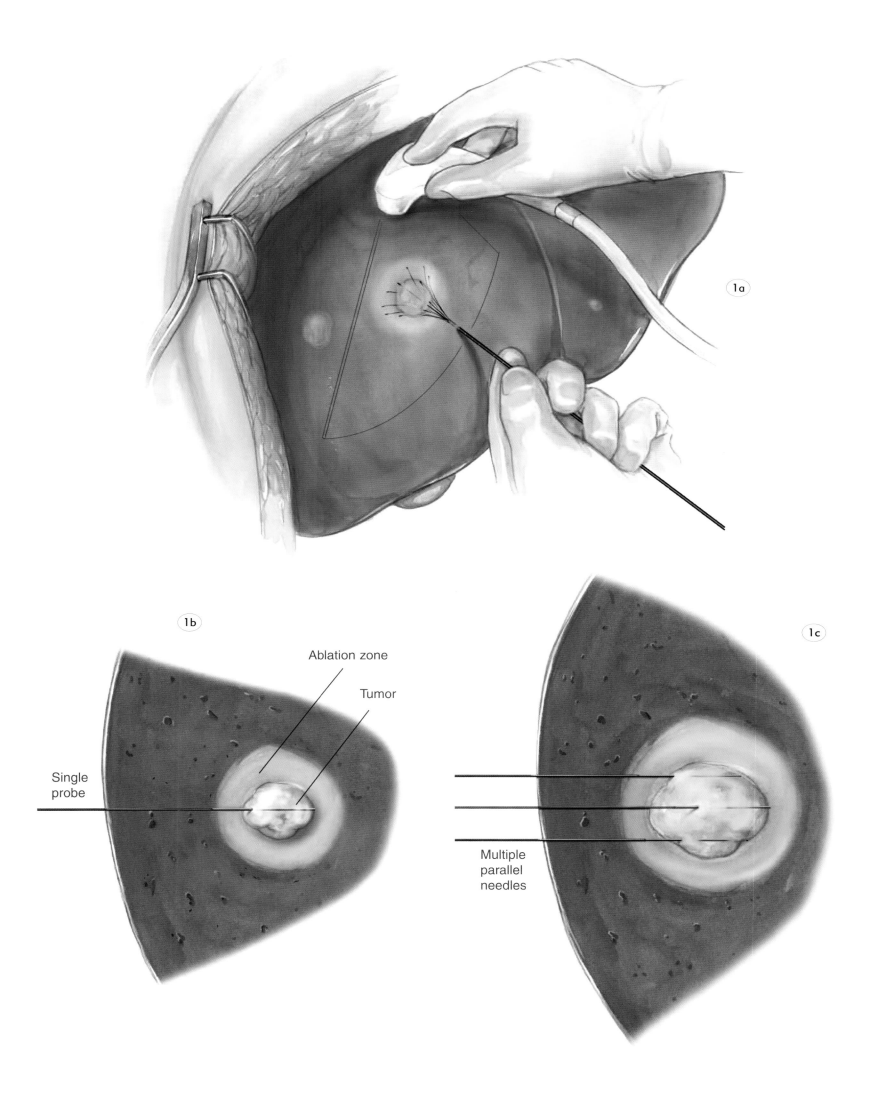

Ablation zone

Tumor

Single
probe

Multiple
parallel
needles

Laparoscopic Radiofrequency Ablation

Laparoscopic RFA offers the advantage of a minimally invasive procedure with the ability to visualize the abdominal cavity and perform the therapy using IOUS. With this approach, patients are treated under general anesthesia, typically in the supine position. In most cases, the procedure can be done with two or three ports (2). The laparoscope is placed in the periumbilical site and the laparoscopic IOUS probe is inserted through a 12-mm port located on the right side. A working port can be added through a 5-mm trocar if needed. The liver is typically partially mobilized, and viscera within 2 cm of the intended ablation zone are moved away. Laparoscopic cholecystectomy can be performed when a target lesion is in proximity to the gall bladder. The RFA electrode is placed into the abdominal cavity immediately below and in parallel to the IOUS probe, either percutaneously or through a 5-mm trocar (2). The needle is placed within the tumor under IOUS guidance, and ablation is performed and monitored as with the open technique (3).

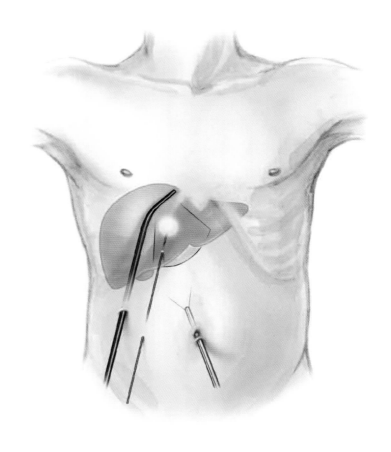

(2)

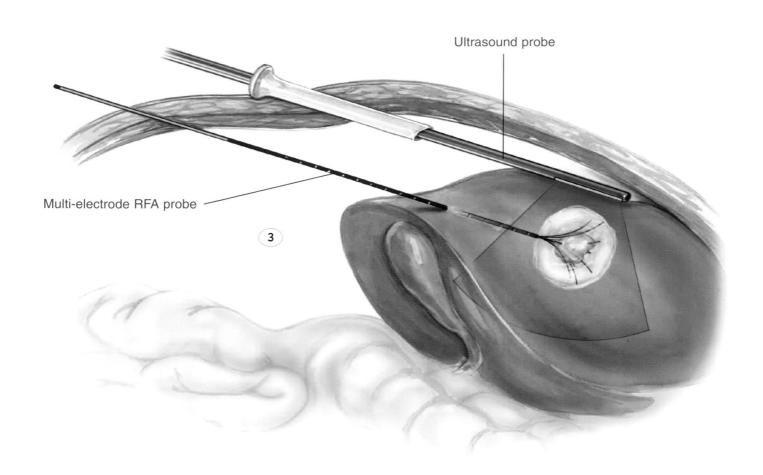

Ultrasound probe

Multi-electrode RFA probe

(3)

Hepatic Artery Infusion Pump

Operative Indications

In selected situations, a hepatic arterial infusion (HAI) pump may be implanted to deliver continuous-infusion regional chemotherapy. Some data indicate that adjuvant regional chemotherapy (with fluorodeoxyuridine) plus systemic chemotherapy following liver resection for hepatic colorectal metastases can reduce the rate of intrahepatic recurrences and possibly improve overall survival. In addition, some have advocated the use of HAI chemotherapy alone or in combination with systemic chemotherapy for patients with unresectable liver-only metastases. Therefore, it is useful for the hepatic surgeon to be facile at implantation of these devices, with or without combined liver resection or ablation.

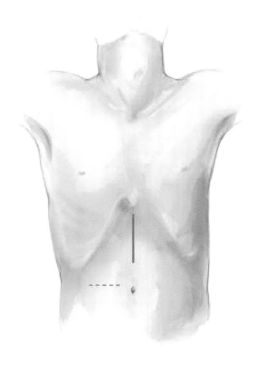

Operative Technique

Prior to proceeding to surgical implantation of such a device, it is important to gain knowledge of the arterial circulation to the liver. In the past, preoperative hepatic arteriography was done in all patients. More recently, high resolution computed tomography or magnetic resonance imaging with arterial visualization (CTA or MRA) has replaced the need for standard arteriography.

In most cases, this procedure can be accomplished through an upper midline incision. When combined with liver resection, the choice of incision will depend on the necessary exposure for the resection. As with other operations for malignancy, the abdomen should be carefully examined to be certain there is no evidence of tumor outside the liver. This is particularly important when implanting such a device for metastatic colorectal cancer as there is little indication for HAI in patients with evidence of extrahepatic disease.

Arterial anatomy can be quite variable, including replaced or accessory vessels from the left gastric artery or superior mesenteric artery. In most cases, the classic hepatic arterial anatomy is present, with a common hepatic artery arising from the celiac axis, which gives off a right gastric artery and the gastroduodenal artery (GDA) prior to bifurcating into the right and left hepatic arteries (1). First, a cholecystectomy is performed. It is imperative to remove the gall bladder in all cases where HAI chemotherapy is being considered.

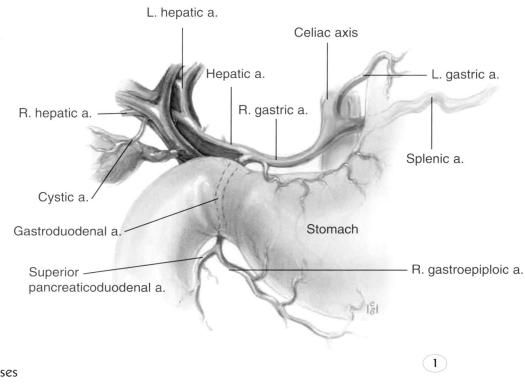

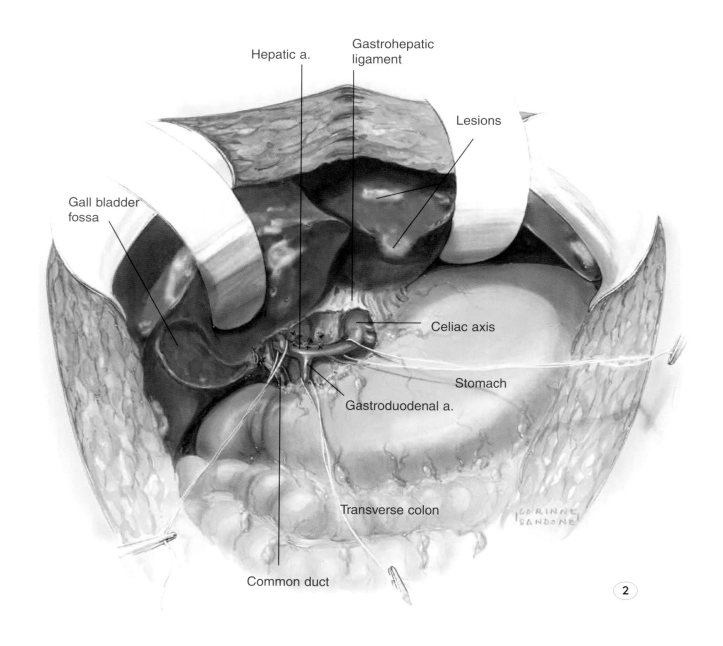

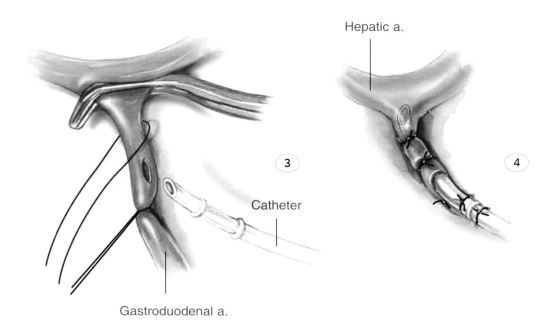

Hepatic a.

3

4

Catheter

Gastroduodenal a.

If not, severe chemotherapy-induced cholecystitis will occur. Next, the common hepatic artery, the GDA, and the proper hepatic artery are all dissected and encircled with vessel loops (2). It is important to divide all supraduodenal and other arterial branches arising from the hepatic artery that do not supply the liver, in order to avoid any chance of the chemotherapeutic agents entering vessels perfusing structures other than the liver. If this is not successfully performed, significant gastritis and duodenitis will result from exposure to the chemotherapeutic agents.

Once the arterial anatomy has been identified, dissected, and made ready for catheter insertion, the subcutaneous pocket is created. To accomplish this, a small transverse incision is made at approximately the level of the umbilicus only long enough to accommodate the device, creating a pocket inferiorly at the level above the fascia. Once the pocket has been created, the fully primed and warmed infusion pump is inserted, bringing the catheter through the fascia within the peritoneal cavity (5). Care must be exercised to avoid redundant catheter within the pocket in order to prevent injury to the catheter during subsequent pump accessions. The device is then anchored to the rectus fascia with non-absorbable, high-strength suture (eg, 0-polypropylene).

The pump catheter is first trimmed in order to position the flanges near the tip. The catheter is then introduced retrograde into the GDA. To accomplish this, the GDA is fully mobilized and then ligated distally close to the duodenum and at least 2 cm from the origin. Maintaining this suture for counter-traction can be useful during catheter insertion. The hepatic artery at the junction of the GDA is then occluded with a small atraumatic curved vascular clamp (3). A small arteriotomy is then made in the GDA approximately 1 cm from the origin, and the catheter is inserted and triply ligated in place (4). Care must be taken to place the catheter tip at the artery origin without obstructing the hepatic arterial flow. In addition, overtightening of ligatures should be avoided in order to prevent catheter occlusion.

Two of the ligatures should be placed immediately in front of and behind the first catheter flange in order to prevent migration. Upon completion, the catheter should lie tension-free within the abdominal cavity and without kinks (5).

Replaced or accessory right or left hepatic arteries can be ligated, in most cases, provided it is not the dominant blood supply to the liver. If present, it cannot remain patent, as non-infused circulation to the liver will limit the efficacy of the regional chemotherapy. Following inserting and securing the catheter, the bolus port of the pump is then injected with heparinized saline via a Huber needle to document unobstructed flow. Care should be taken to avoid backflow of blood into the catheter and pump as this may limit the long-term flow of the device. Fluorescein dye is then injected into the bolus port, and the liver and upper abdomen are observed under an ultraviolet (Woods) lamp. This step is used to rule out evidence of extrahepatic perfusion and document good bilobar distribution.

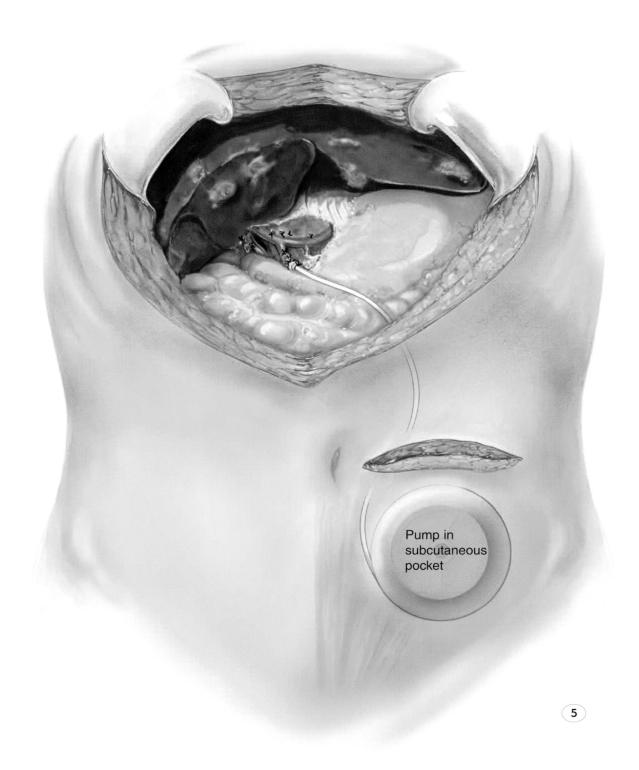

Pump in subcutaneous pocket

5

Surgical Drainage of Liver Abscess

Operative Indications

The diagnosis of a liver abscess in any patient with fever is readily made by ultrasonography or cross-sectional imaging, despite the fact that there may be very little in the way of physical findings. They are most commonly associated with biliary tract pathology. Colonic diverticular disease and other intra-abdominal septic processes may also produce liver abscesses and, not infrequently, they can be of unknown etiology. In most cases, liver abscesses are successfully managed using a percutaneous approach. In some cases, however, liver abscesses are multilocular, recurrent, or fail attempted percutaneous management. In such cases, they may require laparotomy and open drainage.

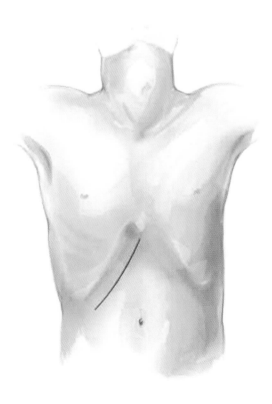

Operative Technique

Patients are generally explored through a right subcostal incision. If the pathology is in the left lobe of the liver, the incision can be extended across the midline. Exposure can be maximized by the use of a self-retaining retractor. The liver is exposed and any adhesions divided using the electrocautery.

Intraoperative ultrasonography can be useful in cases of deep-seated abscess in order to identify the location, extent, and site with the closest proximity to the liver surface (1).

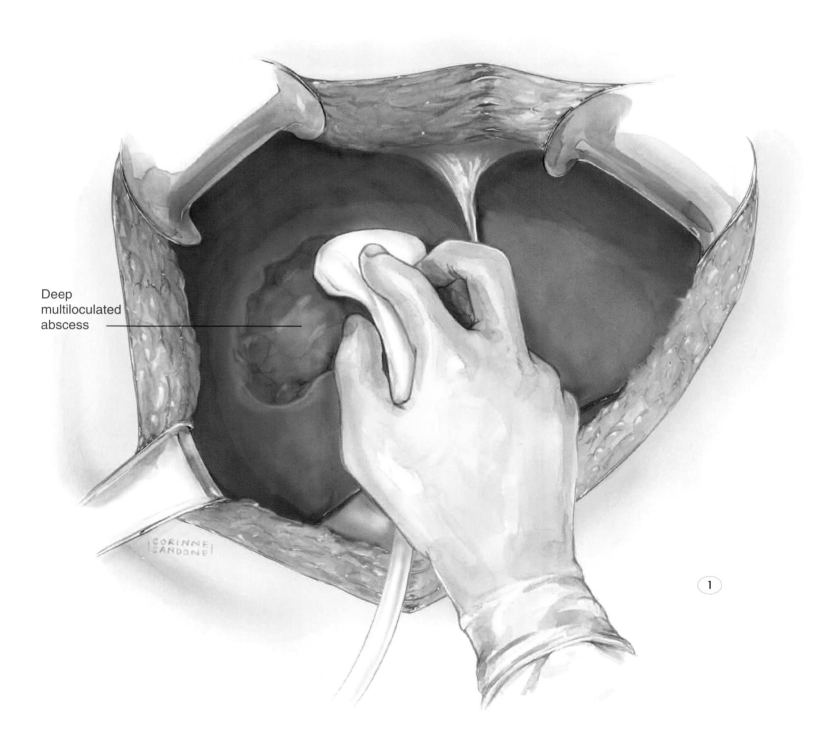

Deep
multiloculated
abscess

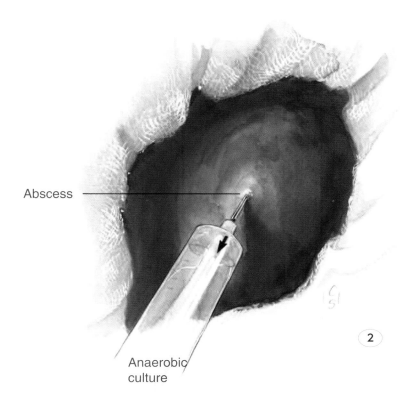

Abscess

Anaerobic culture

2

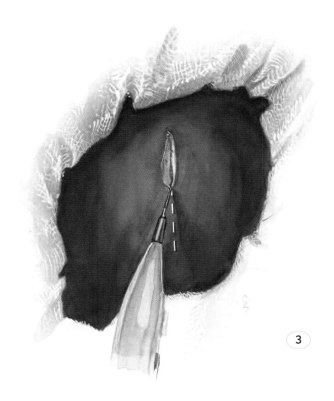

3

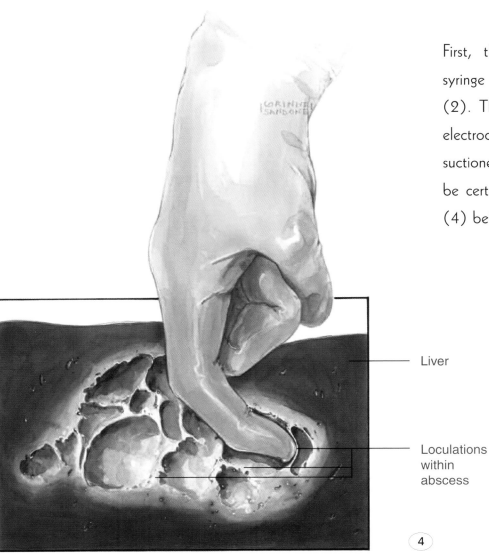

First, the abscess should be aspirated using a syringe and sent for aerobic and anaerobic culture (2). The abscess cavity is then opened with the electrocautery (3) and the contents completely suctioned out. The cavity is explored manually to be certain that there are no undrained loculations (4) before irrigating the cavity.

Liver

Loculations within abscess

4

If the remnant abscess cavity is large or deep, placement of an omental pedicle (5) should be considered to minimize the risk of recurrence. Drains should be placed within the cavity and in the perihepatic space.

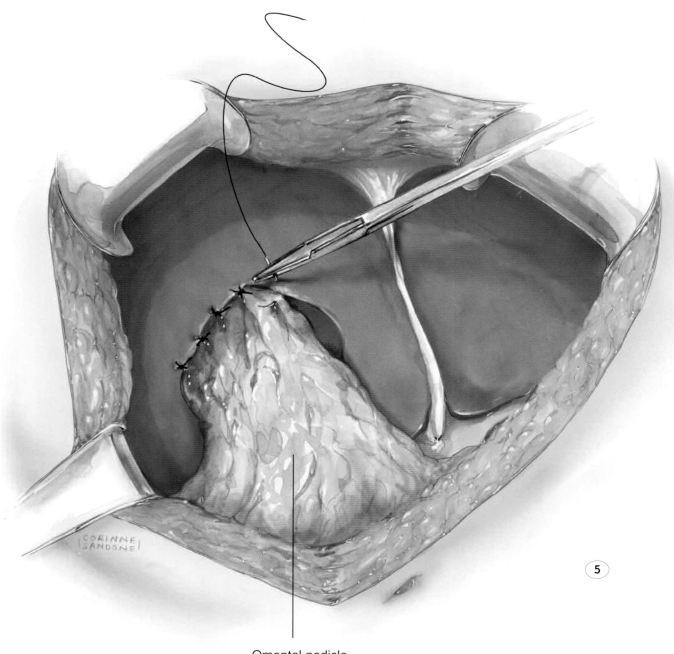

Omental pedicle

5

SHUNTS

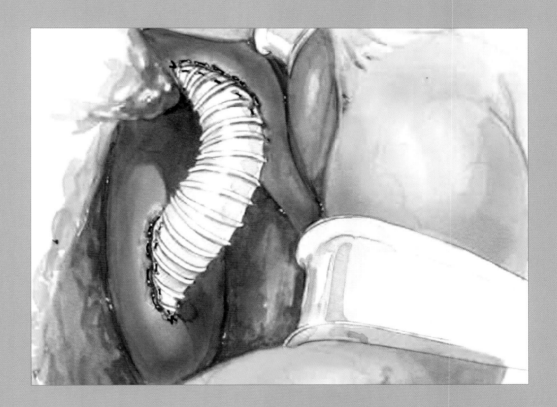

Interposition Mesocaval Shunt

The management of patients with portal hypertension has changed substantially over the past decade. Most patients with liver disease, portal hypertension, and bleeding esophageal varices are managed with sclerotherapy or variceal banding. Others with advanced liver disease are managed by hepatic transplantation. Many of these patients are managed initially during their acute bleeding phase with the insertion of a transjugular intrahepatic portasystemic shunt (TIPS) if they cannot be controlled with sclerotherapy. The introduction and increased usage of the TIPS procedure has virtually eliminated the need for emergency portasystemic shunting. This procedure is generally used today in patients who are transplant candidates, but whose bleeding cannot readily be controlled with sclerotherapy as a bridge to liver transplantation. There still remains, however, a very small group of patients with portal hypertension and bleeding varices that cannot be controlled adequately with sclerotherapy, but who still have enough hepatic reserve and synthetic capacity that they are not yet candidates for hepatic transplantation. These patients are candidates for a mesenteric systemic venous shunt.

The mesocaval shunt is a total shunt utilized to decompress the portal venous system in the face of portal hypertension and bleeding varices. It has been used extensively in patients with portal hypertension secondary to cirrhosis. When initially proposed, it was suggested that this shunt allowed continued prograde flow through the portal system into the liver, while at the same time achieving an adequate decrease in portal pressure. This contention has been debated extensively, and is still not resolved to everyone's satisfaction. Although, in some patients, prograde flow to the liver may continue, in most instances, the shunt is total, and all portal flow passes into the systemic venous system, bypassing the liver. Retrograde flow in the portal vein from the liver also occurs. The interposition mesocaval shunt is the easiest, quickest, and safest of all the mesenteric systemic decompression operative procedures. For this reason, many surgeons have adopted it as their shunt of choice in those instances where mesenteric-systemic decompression is chosen as the means of management. It used to be performed in the emergent or semi-emergent situation, but in most instances now, if sclerotherapy is not effective, a TIPS procedure is resorted to. Because it is a total shunt, many feel the risk of encephalopathy post-shunt is high. Many series, however, have shown a low incidence of encephalopathy, and thus, some continue to support use of this shunt in the elective situation when a portasystemic decompression procedure is required. This is particularly true when intractable ascites is present. Construction of a functional side-to-side total shunt, such as the mesocaval interposition shunt, is an effective treatment for ascites, whereas a selective shunt is not.

In our estimation the mesocaval interposition shunt is the procedure of choice for the unusual form of portal hypertension that is secondary to hepatic vein thrombosis: Budd-Chiari syndrome. In Budd-Chiari syndrome, there is no route of egress for portal venous and hepatic arterial inflow. The liver becomes markedly congested, central lobular necrosis occurs because of the marked congestion, and patients present with massive ascites. Successful management requires conversion of the portal vein into an outflow track. Although some utilize the side-to-side portacaval shunt, which will be demonstrated subsequently, the markedly congested liver and the often hypertrophied caudate lobe frequently make the side-to-side portacaval shunt difficult, and in some instances impossible. For that reason the mesocaval shunt, which is performed well below the liver and well away from the hypertrophied caudate lobe, has been adopted by many as the shunt of preference for patients with Budd-Chiari syndrome, provided there is no inferior venous cava compression or obstruction.

In many patients with portal hypertension who are considered candidates for a mesenteric-systemic shunt, hepatic vein catheterization is carried out. Measuring the wedged hepatic vein pressure confirms the diagnosis of portal hypertension in patients with parenchymal liver disease. Demonstrating occluded hepatic veins confirms the diagnosis of Budd-Chiari syndrome in patients with hepatic vein thrombosis. Mesenteric angiography used to be performed routinely so that, on the venous phase of angiography, patency of the superior mesenteric and portal veins could be confirmed. But now, with magnetic resonance imaging (MRI) or a three-dimensional computed tomography (CT) scan, mesenteric vessels can be clearly delineated, and angiography is no longer necessary. In patients with Budd-Chiari syndrome, however, inferior vena cavography and pressure measurements still need to be carried out to be certain that compression of the vena cava by a hypertrophied caudate lobe, or even thrombosis of the inferior vena cava, is not present precluding a mesocaval shunt.

Operative Technique:

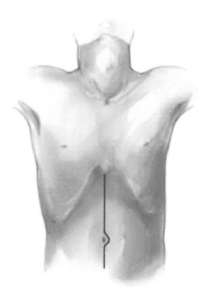

A mesocaval shunt can be performed through either a bilateral subcostal or midline incision. We prefer the midline incision. Once the peritoneal cavity is entered, and any ascites suctioned free, the abdomen is thoroughly explored. If a liver biopsy has not been performed, one is performed at the beginning of the operative procedure. If the mesocaval shunt is being performed for portal hypertension, secondary to cirrhosis, the liver should be carefully examined for evidence of a hepatoma. Suspicious areas should be biopsied.

The transverse colon and omentum are reflected cephalad (1). A transverse incision is made in the peritoneum at the root of the transverse mesocolon (2) to initiate dissection of the superior mesenteric vein. There are no landmarks to lead one to the superior mesenteric vein. It generally is a midline structure, but the transverse mesocolon has to be opened widely and the dissection deepened in an effort to identify the vein. The superior mesenteric artery is generally to the left of the superior mesenteric vein and posterior in location. The anatomic relationship of the superior mesenteric vein and the superior mesenteric artery, however, is inconstant and palpating for the superior mesenteric artery rarely helps in identifying the superior mesenteric vein. As the dissection in the root of the transverse mesocolon is deepened, however, the superior mesenteric vein is always readily identified.

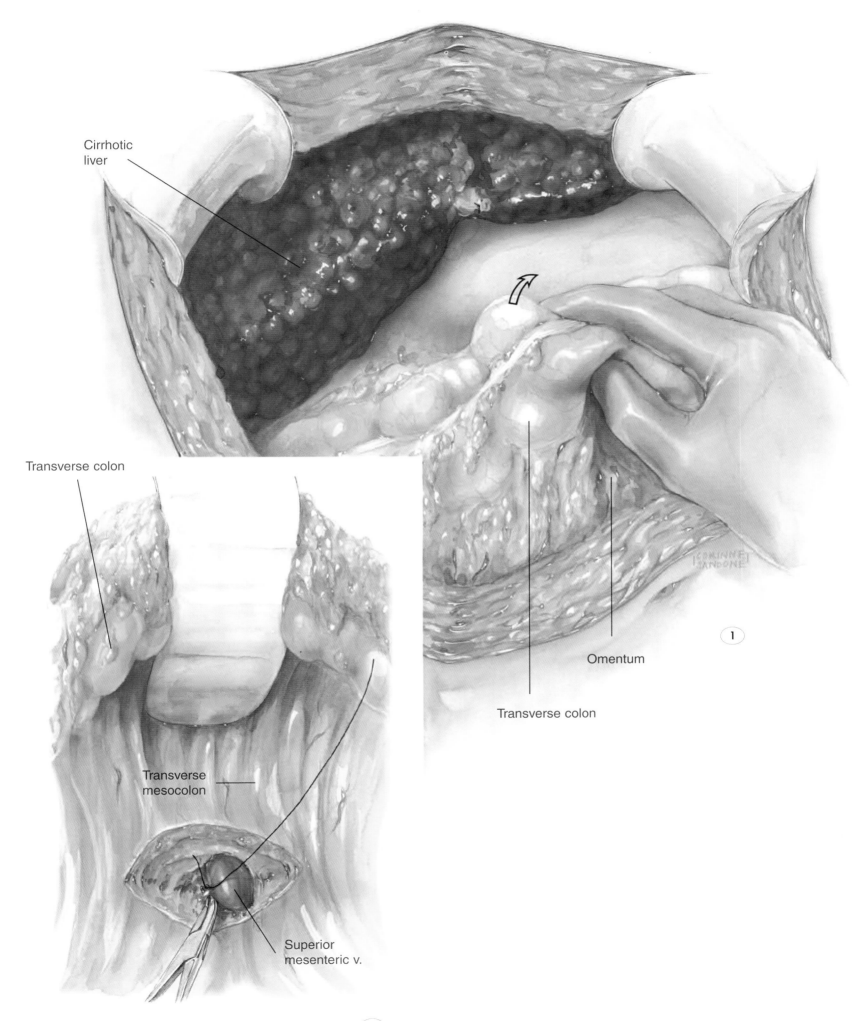

Cirrhotic
liver

Transverse colon

Omentum

Transverse colon

Transverse
mesocolon

Superior
mesenteric v.

1

2

In the dissection of the superior mesenteric vein, one often encoun-
ters large lymph nodes and hypertrophied lymphatic channels.
The larger lymphatic channels should be ligated prior to division. Lymph flow through these large lymphatic channels is
brisk and, unless controlled, will keep the operative field surrounding the superior mesenteric vein flooded with lymph and
will contribute significantly postoperatively to ascites formation.
Once the anterior surface of the superior mesenteric vein is identified, it is completely mobilized and cleaned for a length of at least
6 cm. Small branches are ligated and divided and large branches are controlled with a vessel loop (3). The vein should be completely mobilized circumferentially cephalad up to the point where is passes posterior to the neck of the pancreas. Distally,
the vein should be mobilized until it starts its major branching, generally at the inferior border of the third
portion of the duodenum. In a significant percentage of patients, the inferior mesenteric vein joins the left lateral
aspect of the superior mesenteric vein and does not enter the splenic vein directly. Although it can be safely ligated and
divided, the inferior mesenteric vein can also easily be preserved. It should be mobilized and then doubly looped with a vessel loop for control prior to opening the superior mesenteric vein.

It is always possible to clean a 6 or 7 cm length of large diameter superior mesenteric vein, beginning at the inferior
border of the pancreas and extending caudally, prior to major branching. As one dissects the superior mesenteric vein cephalad, there are often sizable branches from the uncinate process and head of the pancreas that enter the vein posteriorly and
into its right lateral border. These should be carefully ligated and divided. Often, there is also a major mesenteric branch
that directly enters posteriorly and slightly to the right. This is a constant branch with a very wide diameter that is difficult
to ligate and divide because of its posterior location. This is the first jejunal branch joining the superior mesenteric vein. It
is nearly always present and should be controlled by double looping with a vessel loop (3).

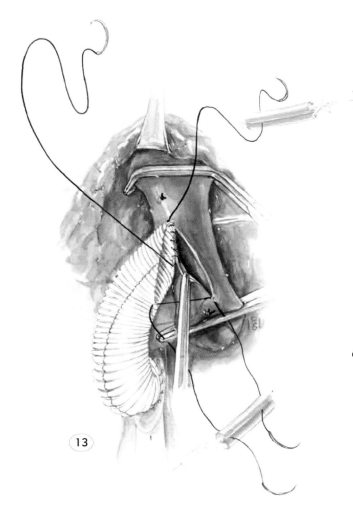

The prosthesis is anastomosed to the superior mesenteric vein with 5-0 synthetic non-absorbable suture material. Sutures are placed at each end of the anastomosis, passing from outside in on the superior mesenteric vein and from inside out on the prosthesis. The right lateral suture line is run first; it is run from within the prosthesis and vein. The superior suture is tied and then passed from outside the prosthesis to within before being run. This suture line should incorporate very small bites of superior mesenteric vein and prosthesis, in order not to invert a significant suture line that will subsequently interfere with flow (13). The suture line is run down to the inferior limit of the venotomy. It is sometimes possible, depending upon the orientation of the superior mesenteric vein and the prosthesis, to insert this suture line from outside the prosthesis and superior mesenteric vein. This eliminates the inevitable inversion of the right lateral suture line into the anastomosis. Generally, however, this is not possible, and the suture line has to be placed from within the superior mesenteric vein and prosthesis.

The inferior stay suture is then secured, and the suture that has been run down from above is passed from within to without the prosthesis and then secured to the inferior suture. The left lateral anastomotic line is then run from above down, and down upwards to meet at the midportion of the suture line (14).

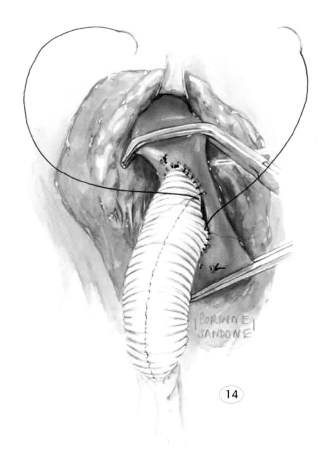

A large bore needle is passed into the most anterior portion of the prosthesis, and the clamps removed slowly from the superior mesenteric vein
(15). The clamp on the inferior vena cava is left in place. This allows
the prosthesis to fill with blood, with the needle acting as a vent for
the release of air.

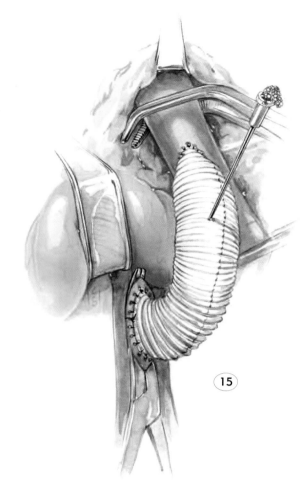

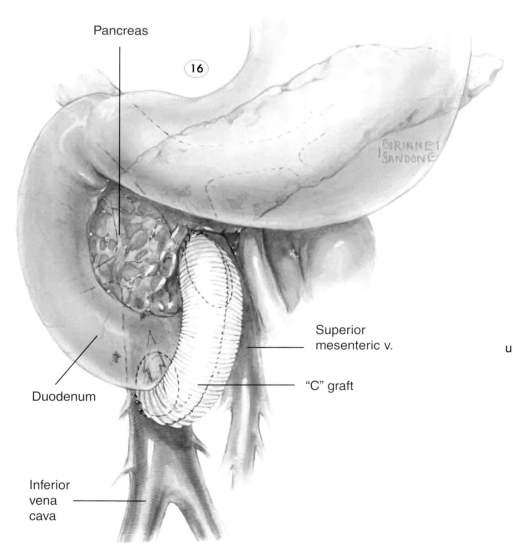

Pancreas

Duodenum

Superior
mesenteric v.

"C" graft

Inferior
vena
cava

Once the prosthesis has completely
filled with blood, the clamp is removed
from the inferior vena cava, and flow
through the prosthesis established. The
course of the prosthesis assumes a "C" configuration (16).

The anastomosis between the prosthesis and inferior vena cava is actually partially underneath the third portion of the duodenum (17). The prosthesis has to pass inferiorly as well as anteriorly to pass below the third portion of the duodenum. It then passes on top of the third portion of the duodenum, on top of the uncinate process of the pancreas, to be anastomosed obliquely to the anterior surface of the superior mesenteric vein. This "C"

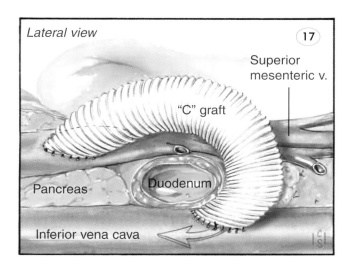

configuration allows the prosthesis to be anastomosed to the anterior aspect of the superior mesenteric vein, well above where the superior mesenteric vein branching occurs. Thus, one is always assured of superior mesenteric vein with a large diameter. Furthermore, since the anastomosis is oblique, it tends to be very large. In addition, since the anastomosis is to the anterior aspect of the superior mesenteric vein, it is technically easy to perform. This is in contrast to the old mesocaval "H" shunt, which runs directly anteriorly from the inferior vena cava, below the lower border of the third portion of the duodenum, and joins the posterior aspect of the superior mesenteric vein. The "H" shunt anastomosis is harder to perform and is often performed to a segment of the superior mesenteric vein that is already branched.

Mesenteric venous pressure can be measured post-shunt, by inserting a 19-gauge needle, connected to a manometer, into the prosthesis. Pressures can be measured with the prosthesis toward the vena cava clamped and unclamped.

Distal Splenorenal Shunt

Operative Indications:

The distal splenorenal shunt is a selective shunt, in contrast to the mesocaval and portacaval shunts, which are total shunts. The distal splenorenal shunt is constructed so that mesenteric blood continues to flow antegrade into the liver, while gastroesophageal varices are decompressed retrograde through the vasa brevia and left gastroepiploic vessels into the spleen, and out the splenic vein into the systemic venous system. This shunt was introduced in an attempt to eliminate the portasystemic encephalopathy that some patients develop after a total shunt. With the acceptance of sclerotherapy and variceal banding as the first line of management for gastroesophageal variceal bleeding secondary to portal hypertension, the need for elective portasystemic decompression has decreased. The introduction and increased usage of the transjugular intrahepatic portasystemic shunt (TIPS) procedure has also further decreased the need for operative portasystemic decompression procedures. Even though the TIPS procedure has been used principally for the short-term control of bleeding varices and as a bridge to liver transplantation, in some instances, patency has been such that it has proven to be a longer term solution.

Nevertheless, there are situations in which an elective portasystemic shunt is indicated. Many surgeons have accepted the selective distal splenorenal shunt as the procedure of choice in the elective situation. Patients with intractable ascites are not candidates for the distal splenorenal shunt. Since sinusoidal pressure is not decreased by the distal splenorenal shunt, massive ascites is not treated effectively by this procedure. Technically, the distal splenorenal shunt is a difficult operative procedure and should not be attempted in the emergency setting. But patients with liver disease, portal hypertension, and a history of bleeding esophageal varices, but still with good liver reserve and who are considered candidates for an elective shunt, are good candidates for the distal splenorenal shunt. Many patients with severe liver disease and no liver reserve, who in the past were considered candidates for the distal splenorenal shunt, are now considered candidates for liver transplantation.

Although the anterior suture line can also be placed in a continuous fashion, we usually place a series of interrupted 5-0 synthetic non-absorbable sutures to avoid purse stringing (7). Before the final suture is secured in the anterior row of the anastomosis, the DeBakey bulldog clamp is removed from the splenic vein, with the Cooley clamps still in place on the renal vein, to fill the anastomosis with blood and to evacuate air. The Cooley clamps are then removed from the renal vein.

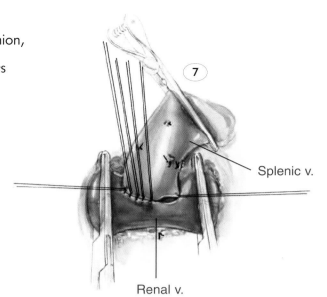

Splenic v.

Renal v.

A modification of the distal splenorenal shunt can be performed whereby the body and tail of the pancreas are completely mobilized off the splenic vein all the way to the splenic hilum. This modification was introduced in an attempt to prevent the development of vascular collaterals between the mesenteric venous system providing prograde flow to the liver and venous channels leading to the spleen that are decompressed through the distal splenorenal shunt. The development of such collaterals through the pancreas can obviate the selectiveness of this shunt and result in mesenteric blood entering the systemic venous system and bypassing the liver. In performing this modification, the mobilization and cleaning of the splenic vein circumferentially proceeds towards the splenic hilum until the body and tail of the pancreas are actually completely free all the way to the hilum (8). This prolongs the procedure, but is felt by some to be necessary to ensure long-term success of the distal splenorenal shunt.

Entire length of splenic v.

Spleen

Pancreas

Renal v.

Ligated inferior mesenteric v.

When one successfully constructs a selective distal splenorenal shunt, portal hypertension persists in the mesenteric system, and prograde flow continues through the portal vein and into the liver. In contrast, the pressure in the gastroesophageal varices has been lowered by decompression through the vasa brevia and left gastroepiploic vessels into the spleen, out the splenic vein, and into the left renal vein. These two portal beds are further disconnected by ligating the right gastroepiploic, the coronary, and the right and left gastric veins (9). If the coronary vein has not been ligated at its junction with the portal vein, it should be interrupted at the superior border of the pancreas. The umbilical vein is also ligated at the point where the abdominal incision crosses the ligamentum teres.

Portacaval Shunt

Operative Indications:

Today, most patients with liver disease, portal hypertension, and bleeding esophageal varices are managed nonoperatively with sclerotherapy or variceal banding. Others, with advanced liver disease and no hepatic reserve, are managed by liver transplantation. In addition, the introduction of TIPS has eliminated the need for emergent surgical intervention in those patients whose bleeding esophageal varices cannot be controlled by sclerotherapy or banding. Even though long-term patency of the TIPS procedure remains a problem, many patients are being managed utilizing TIPS for intermediate or even long-term control of the portal hypertension. There remains, however, a small group of patients with portal hypertension and bleeding varices that cannot be controlled long-term with sclerotherapy or banding, but who have enough hepatic reserve and synthetic function that they are not yet candidates for liver transplantation. These patients are candidates for a mesenteric systemic venous shunt. In addition, the rare form of portal hypertension, Budd-Chiari syndrome, is still considered an indication in some instances for mesenteric systemic venous shunting.

Which shunt to use when mesenteric systemic venous shunting is indicated remains controversial, despite decades of data collection and debate. The first shunts to be used successfully were the end-to-side and side-to-side portacaval anastomoses. Although used infrequently today, these shunts still have their advocates. The end-to-side portacaval shunt can be performed with moderate speed and only moderate blood loss. This shunt is contraindicated in patients with intractable ascites, since sinusoidal pressure is not reduced with this procedure. However in an occasional patient with no ascites, and who angiographically has been demonstrated as having retrograde flow out the portal vein, this shunt has some theoretical advantage. The incidence of encephalopathy following an end-to-side portacaval shunt is significant, but its incidence compared to the side-to-side portacaval shunt is probably less. Even though all prograde flow to the liver through the portal venous system is obviously interrupted following an end-to-side shunt, retrograde flow out the portal vein does not occur. Many feel that end-to-side portacaval shunting carries with it a lower incidence of encephalopathy than the side-to-side shunt, and it has a clear theoretical advantage in the patient who preoperatively already has retrograde flow.

The side-to-side portacaval shunt can be used in the presence of intractable ascites. Mesenteric pressure is not only reduced, but the portal vein is converted into an outflow tract, and sinusoidal pressure is lowered, thus effectively eliminating ascites formation. Technically, it is perhaps a more difficult shunt to perform, and partial resection of the caudate lobe is often necessary to approximate the portal vein and inferior vena cava. Some surgeons also feel that the side-to-side portacaval shunt is the shunt of choice for Budd-Chiari syndrome, that unusual form of portal hypertension that presents with hepatic vein thrombosis. When it is used, however, since the caudate lobe is often hypertrophied in Budd-Chiari syndrome, the shunt may be technically difficult, and actually require a partial caudate lobe resection to carry it out.

The newest of the portacaval shunts is the interposition H graft. This involves interposing a prosthesis between the portal vein and inferior vena cava. If these prostheses are of sufficiently small diameter, advocates of this procedure claim that the shunt is selective and that prograde flow through the portal vein into the liver continues. Drops in portal pressure are more modest when small-diameter interposition H grafts are used, but in most instances the drop is sufficient to eliminate subsequent esophageal bleeding. In some instances, early thrombosis of these H grafts occurs, but usually percutaneous transhepatic, or trans—inferior-vena-cava procedures in the catheter laboratory can effectively de-clot them, and long-term patency is excellent.

It is important to note that the presence of any type of portacaval shunt will significantly increase the technical difficulty of hepatic transplantation. This is not true of the mesocaval shunt, which is well away from the porta hepatis, and can be easily ligated at the time of liver transplantation. Whichever type of portacaval shunt is anticipated, patients should undergo catherization of the hepatic veins preoperatively, so that estimation of portal pressure can be obtained by a wedged hepatic venous pressure. In the past, mesenteric angiography was also performed, but with MR angiography, and three-dimensional CT scans, the mesenteric venous system can easily be imaged noninvasively.

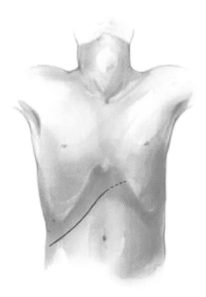

Operative Technique:

End-to-Side:

These portacaval shunt procedures are best performed through a long right subcostal incision, often extended over to the left costal margin. The patient should be rotated 15 degrees to the left. Upon entering the abdomen, any ascitic fluid is suctioned free and the abdomen is carefully examined for evidence of other pathology. If the liver has not been biopsied preoperatively, a biopsy is performed. The diseased liver is carefully examined for any evidence of suspicious nodules that could indicate a hepatoma. Opening the hepatoduodenal ligament laterally exposes the portal vein.

The biliary tree, which resides anterior and slightly lateral to the portal vein, is gently retracted medially (1). The gall bladder is often thickened and somewhat tense because of the lymphatic hypertension. One should not confuse this with acute cholecystitis, because removing the gall bladder unnecessarily will add to the morbidity of the procedure. The hepatoduodenal ligament should be opened widely from the duodenum to the hepatic hilum. The portal vein should be mobilized and cleaned circumferentially from the duodenum to the portal vein bifurcation. Amazingly few branches will require division. There is often a small branch from the right branch of the portal vein into the posterior segment of the right lobe of the liver that should be divided to avoid injury. In addition, the coronary vein may be encountered if the dissection proceeds far enough under the first portion of the duodenum and head of the pancreas. This vein should be preserved.

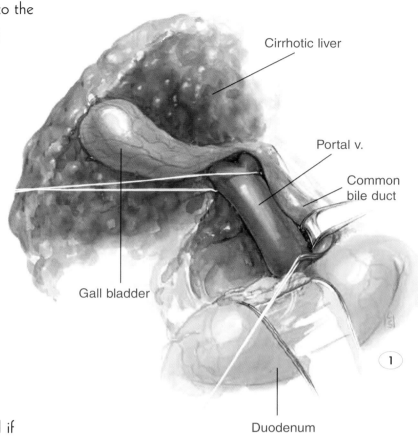

Once an adequate length of portal vein has been mobilized, the inferior vena cava is exposed. The duodenum is kocherized. The overlying serosal and areola tissue should be clamped and ligated before division (2). The retroperitoneum is rich with enlarged lymphatic and venous channels. The electrocautery is usually not adequate to control bleeding and the escape of lymph.

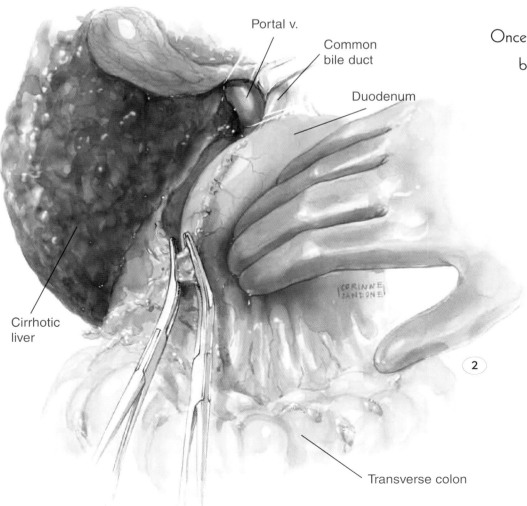

The duodenum is extensively mobilized to expose the inferior vena cava from the level of the renal veins up to the point where is passes posterior to the caudate lobe (3). It is not necessary to completely mobilize the inferior vena cava circumferentially or to surround it with a vessel loop. The inferior vena cava will be partially occluded with a Satinsky clamp along its anterior and lateral surfaces, and circumferential mobilization is not necessary. Following circumferential mobilization of the portal vein and cleaning of the anterior and lateral surfaces of inferior vena cava, one is prepared to perform the end-to-side portacaval shunt.

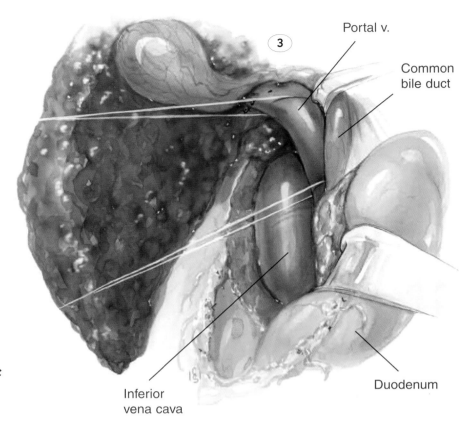

Obtain as much length as possible on the portal vein. This is accomplished best if the right and left branches of the portal vein are identified, cleaned, and ligated with 2-0 silk. The portal vein can then be occluded with a straight Cooley clamp at the point where it arises from behind the pancreas. The portal vein is divided just prior to its bifurcation into the right and left branches (4). It is helpful for subsequent orientation to mark the inferior and superior borders of the portal vein with fine traction sutures. The portal vein is trimmed to the appropriate length. This is an important step as one does not want either redundancy or a portal vein that is too short and results in tension. Often a slight bevel is required on the end of the portal vein, but this varies and is determined by the anatomic relationships between the portal vein and inferior vena cava. The inferior vena cava is partially occluded with a Satinsky clamp. An ellipse is removed from the anterior wall of the inferior vena cava. It is important not to make this venotomy too long; otherwise, the portal vein will be stretched into a slit-like orifice.

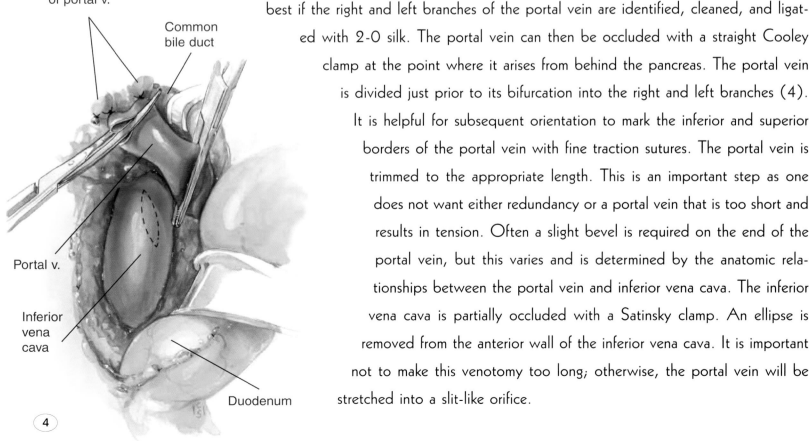

The anastomosis is performed with continuous 5-0 synthetic nonabsorbable suture material. Stay sutures are placed from outside the portal vein to within, and from inside the inferior cava to without, on both the superior and inferior ends of the anastomosis. The superior suture is secured and then passed outside in on the inferior vena cava. The lateral suture line is run from within the anastomosis (5). It is then passed back outside at the inferior limit of the suture line and secured to the inferiorly placed stay suture. The right lateral anastomosis is performed by suturing from above downward, and then from below upward, meeting midway (6). Before these two sutures are secured, the Cooley clamp on the portal vein is slowly opened to allow the anastomosis to fill with blood and air to be extruded. The completed shunt is a total portasystemic shunt (7), completely diverting all mesenteric flow into the inferior vena cava. Obviously, however, no retrograde flow of liver blood occurs via the portal vein.

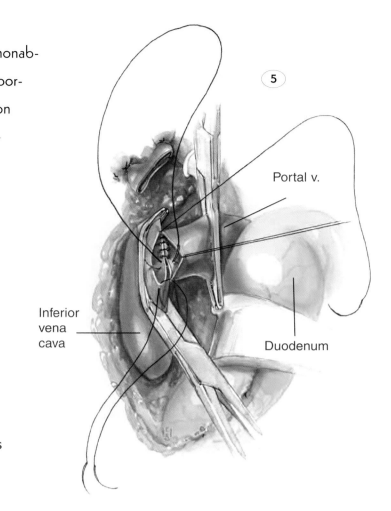

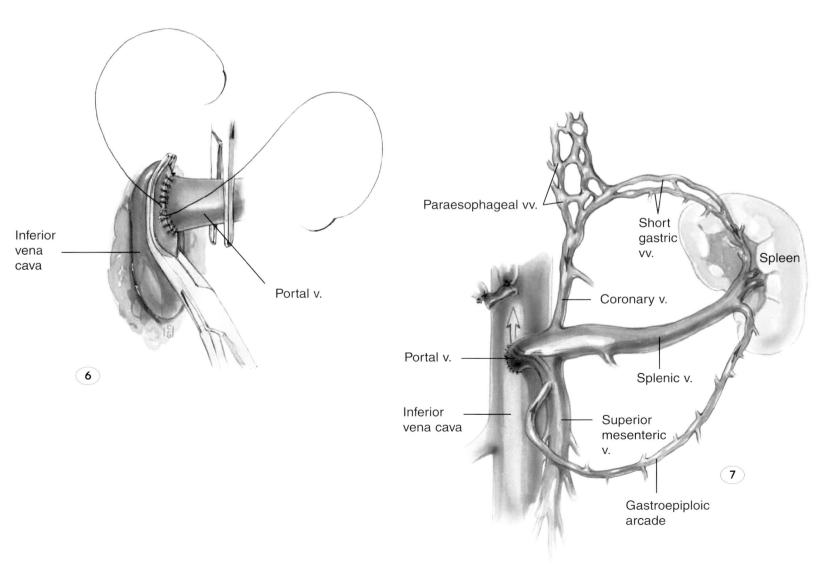

Side-to-Side

Some surgeons prefer a side-to-side portacaval shunt over an end-to-side shunt. This may be driven by personal preference or by massive intractable ascites that would not be helped by an end-to-side portacaval shunt. Long-term patency rates are probably highest for this shunt. In addition, when Budd-Chiari syndrome is present, the side-to-side portacaval shunt can effectively convert the portal vein into an outflow tract, thus decompressing the massively congested liver. When performing a side-to-side portacaval shunt for Budd-Chiari syndrome, it may be necessary to perform a partial resection of the hypertrophied caudate lobe.

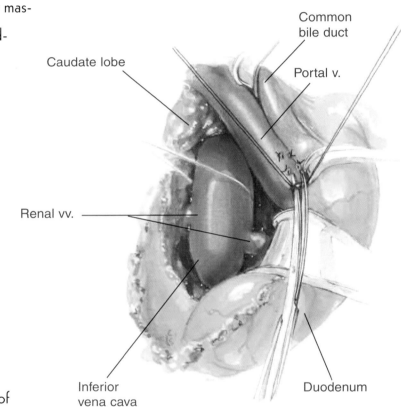

The initial steps in performing a side-to-side portacaval shunt are identical to those in performing an end-to-side portacaval shunt. The portal vein, however, should be mobilized for a greater length under the first portion of the duodenum and under the head of the pancreas to allow more mobility (8). This usually involves ligating and dividing several branches that pass from the portal vein into the caudate lobe of the liver, and into the head and uncinate process of the pancreas (8). In addition, more mobilization of the inferior vena cava is required, and this often means circumferential mobilization with the passage of vessel loops. The caudate lobe is usually interposed between the most cephalad portion of the portal vein and the inferior vena cava.

THE PANCREAS

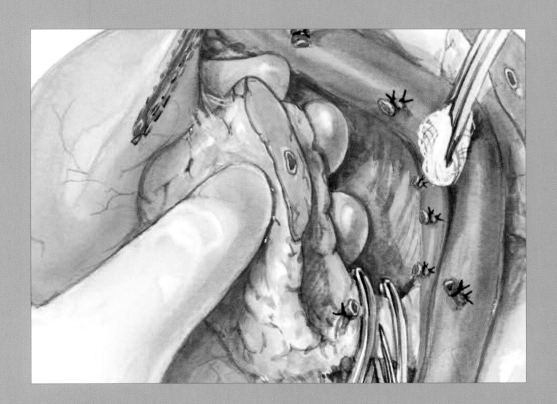

Longitudinal Pancreaticojejunostomy: Puestow Procedure

Operative Indications:

Patients with chronic pancreatitis, abdominal pain, and a dilated pancreatic duct are candidates for a longitudinal pancreaticojejunostomy, or the Puestow procedure. In addition, patients with recurrent attacks of acute pancreatitis and a dilated pancreatic duct can also be considered for the Puestow procedure. It is not absolutely clear whether these patients respond with a decrease or elimination of their recurrent attacks, but it is clear that patients with chronic pancreatitis and chronic abdominal pain do respond. Of the patients with chronic pain, 75 to 85% achieve significant relief. Patients with markedly dilated pancreatic ducts, and with calcification in their pancreas, appear more apt to benefit from this operation than patients without calcification or smaller ducts. Patients with pancreatic duct dilatation of 5 or 6 mm in diameter (or greater) are considered candidates for this operation. Unfortunately, less than 50% of patients with chronic pancreatitis have a dilated pancreatic duct. Patients without a dilated pancreatic duct with abdominal pain from chronic pancreatitis, or from recurrent acute attacks, are candidates for an ablative procedure if surgery is required.

Operative Technique:

The "chain of lakes" pattern of pancreatic duct dilatation, when present, lends itself well to the Puestow procedure. In fact, a dilated duct with multiple intervening strictures, the so-called "chain of lakes," is an unusual pattern. Most patients with chronic pancreatitis and a dilated duct have dilatation virtually throughout the entire duct (1).

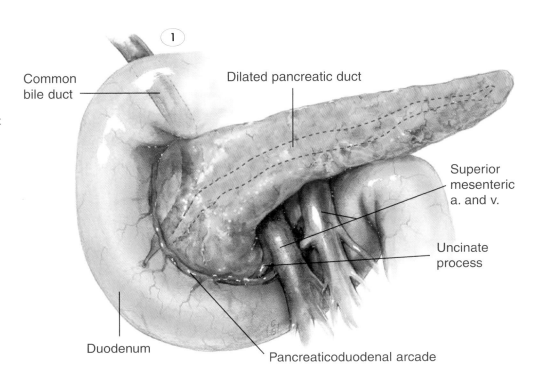

① Common bile duct — Dilated pancreatic duct — Superior mesenteric a. and v. — Uncinate process — Pancreaticoduodenal arcade — Duodenum

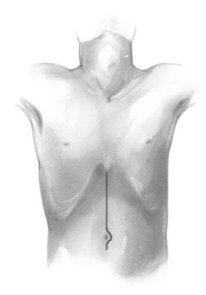

The operative procedure can be done either through a midline or bilateral subcostal incision. Once the abdomen is entered, the pancreas is exposed by removing the greater omentum from the transverse colon (2). This means of entering the lesser sac is preferred over that in which the omentum is just divided in its midportion. The entire pancreas is exposed and palpated through the lesser sac. The duodenum is then kocherized, and the head and uncinate process carefully palpated. Once the tail, body, neck, head, and uncinate process of the pancreas have been exposed, the dilated pancreatic duct frequently can be identified by finger palpation along the anterior surface of the gland. Its position is confirmed by aspirating with a 20-gauge needle and a 10-ml syringe (3). At times, it may be surprisingly difficult to identify a dilated pancreatic duct, which has been demonstrated preoperatively by computed tomography (CT) scan or endoscopic retrograde cholangiopancreatography. Intraoperative ultrasound will be of help in these situations.

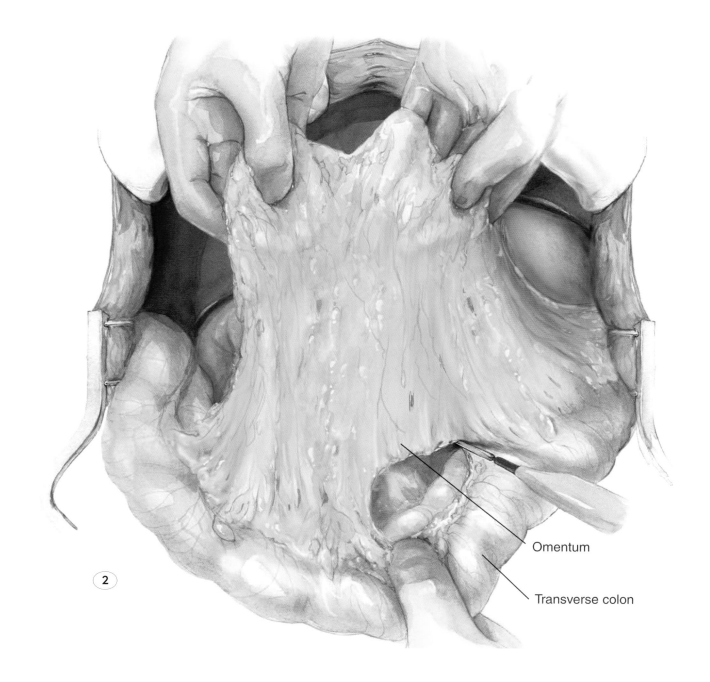

Omentum

Transverse colon

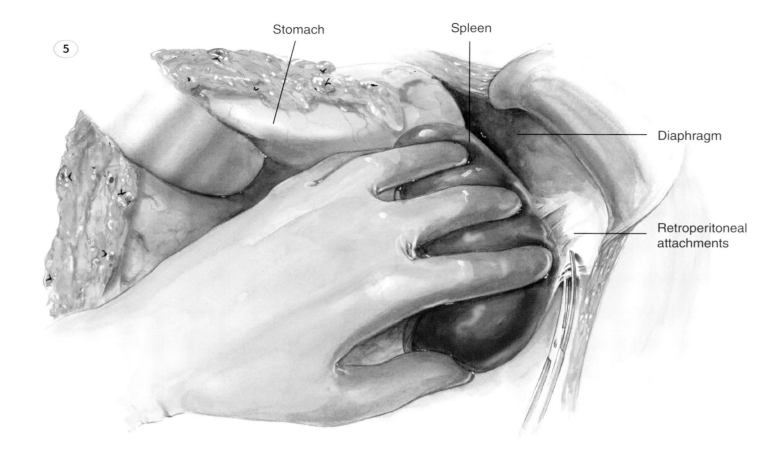

5

Stomach

Spleen

Diaphragm

Retroperitoneal
attachments

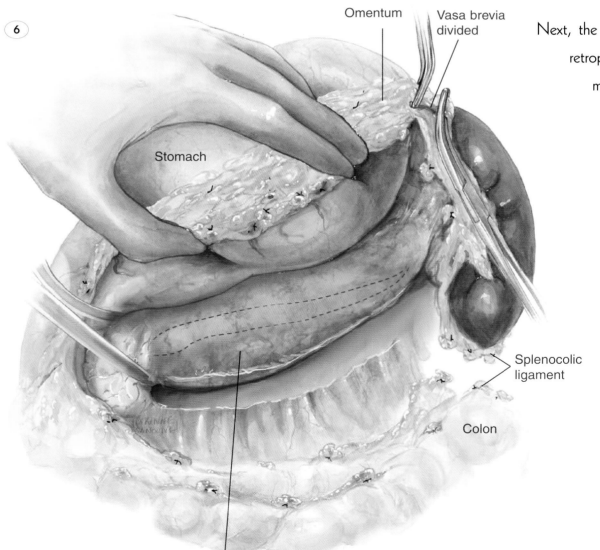

6

Omentum

Vasa brevia
divided

Stomach

Splenocolic
ligament

Colon

Pancreas

Next, the spleen is mobilized out of the retroperitoneum (5). The attachments between the lower pole of the spleen and the omentum and the splenic flexure of the colon are doubly clamped, divided, and ligated with 2-0 silk. The omentum is then further divided between Kelley clamps and ligated with 2-0 silk anterior to the splenic hilum. The vasa brevia are divided between Reinhoff clamps, and ligated with 3-0 silk (6).

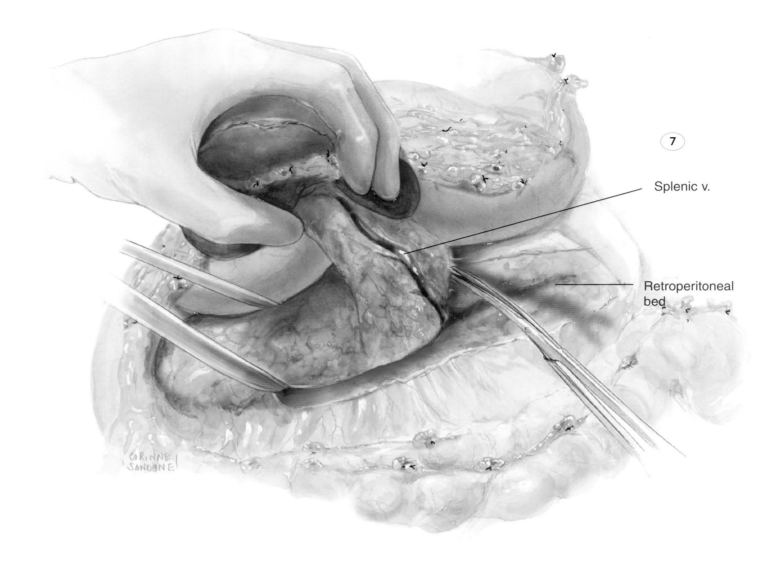

⑦

Splenic v.

Retroperitoneal bed

L. gastric a.

Celiac axis

Hepatic a.

Splenic a.

⑧

The spleen, and the tail and body of the pancreas are mobilized out of the retroperitoneum (7). Care should be taken to avoid injury to the inferior mesenteric vein and its junction with the splenic vein. The inferior mesenteric vein frequently will join the superior mesenteric vein directly and not the splenic vein. If it joins the splenic vein, an attempt should be made to preserve it. If this proves difficult, the inferior mesenteric vein can be clamped, divided, and ligated with impunity.

Once the tail and body of the pancreas have been mobilized out of the retroperitoneum, the splenic artery is identified at its origin from the celiac axis. One has to be certain of carefully identifying the splenic artery. The takeoff of the hepatic artery from the celiac axis is often more prominent and more easily palpated and visualized than is the splenic artery (8).

Splenic a.
divided

9

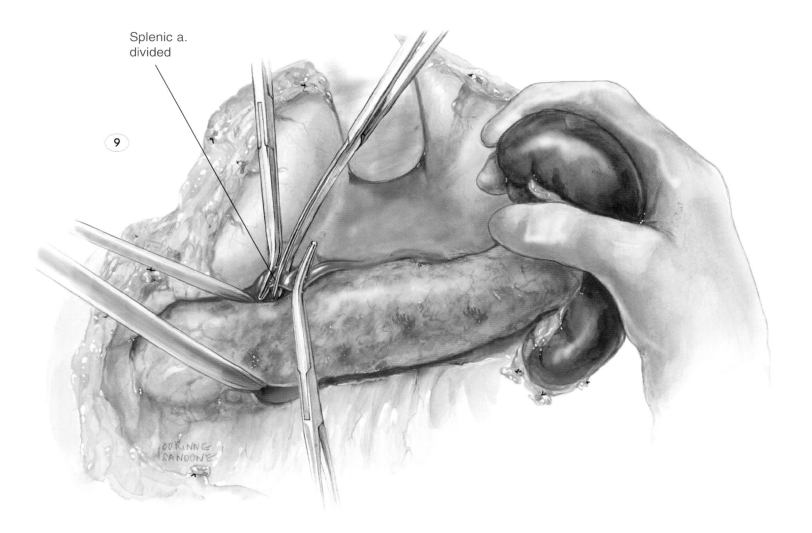

Splenic a.
looped

10

One has to be absolutely certain that one does not mistake the hepatic artery for the splenic artery. The splenic artery is clamped, divided and ligated and then suture ligated (9).

If the splenic vein has thrombosed secondary to the chronic pancreatitis, one may wish to identify the splenic artery early in the operative procedure, prior to mobilizing the spleen out of the retroperitoneum. If one identifies the splenic artery early along the superior border of the body of the pancreas and loops it with a vessel loop (10), if bleeding becomes a problem in mobilizing the spleen and tail of the pancreas subsequently, the splenic artery can be ligated early in the dissection.

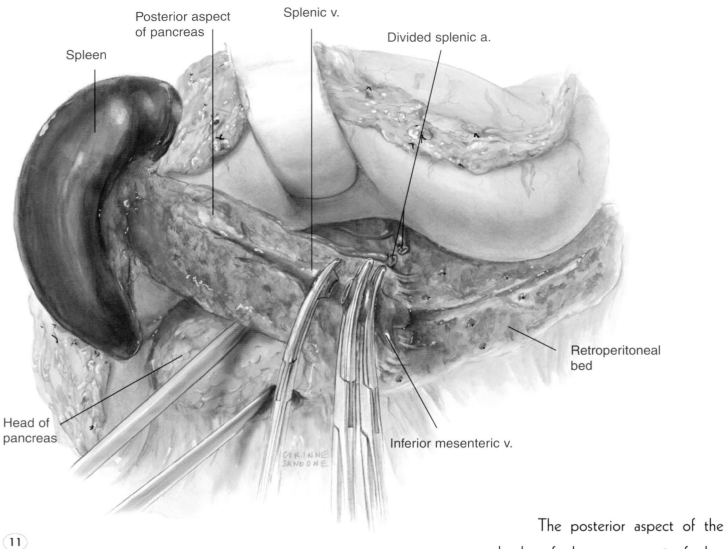

Spleen

Posterior aspect
of pancreas

Splenic v.

Divided splenic a.

Retroperitoneal
bed

Head of
pancreas

Inferior mesenteric v.

11

The posterior aspect of the body of the pancreas is further mobilized out of the retroperitoneum until the point of the inferior mesenteric vein joining the splenic vein is clearly identified. At this point, the splenic vein is mobilized off the posterior aspect of the pancreas, distal to its junction with the inferior mesenteric vein, and is triply clamped, divided, and triply ligated (11). From this point on, the splenic vein should be preserved and carefully dissected away from the posterior aspect of the pancreas (12). Much of this can be done bluntly, but there are small veins between the pancreas and the splenic vein that need to be identified, ligated, and divided. Again, if this part of the dissection proves difficult, it is acceptable to clamp, divide, and ligate the inferior mesenteric vein and leave the splenic vein on the back of the pancreas until one reaches the superior mesenteric vein.

Once the body and neck of the pancreas have been completely mobilized, the junction of the splenic vein and superior mesenteric vein is clearly identified. If the splenic vein has not previously been ligated, it is done at this point. Prior to dividing the neck of the pancreas, a row of 3-0 synthetic absorbable horizontal mattress sutures is placed across the proximal neck (13).

If the pancreatic duct is only minimally dilated, the anastomosis can be performed with a single layer of interrupted 3-0 silk sutures with the knots left on the outside (6).

This modification of the Puestow procedure is of particular value when there is a large inflamed of the head of the pancreas. In these instances, the head and uncinate process of the pancreas may not be adequately decompressed with just a Puestow procedure, and adding the Frey modification of a local head resection is an excellent idea. Two closed suction Silastic drains are left to the site of the lateral pancreaticojejunostomy and are brought out through stab wounds in the left upper quadrant. The Roux-en-Y loop is tacked to the rent in the transverse mesocolon with interrupted 3-0 silks. The defect in the small bowel mesentery is closed with a continuous 4-0 silk.

Alternate: Duct less than 1 cm in diameter

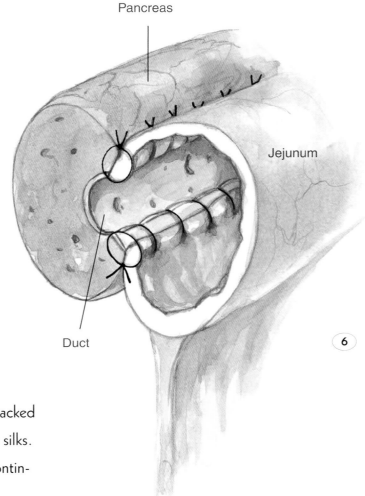

Pancreas

Jejunum

Duct

6

Duodenal Preserving Pancreatectomy for Chronic Pancreatitis (The Beger Procedure)

Operative Indications:

In patients with chronic pancreatitis, and abdominal pain, with a small fibrotic gland with a dilated pancreatic duct, the Puestow procedure is an excellent operation. One should be certain during the performance of the lateral pancreaticojejunostomy that a Bakes dilator can be passed through the open pancreatic duct down through the ampulla into the duodenum. If there is an enlarged head of the pancreas, a substantial inflammatory mass, and/or one cannot pass a Bakes dilator easily through the proximal pancreatic duct, through the ampulla and into the duodenum, then a local head resection and lateral pancreaticojejunostomy (the Frey procedure) is an excellent operation. Many patients, however, have a very large inflammatory mass in the head of the pancreas but no dilated pancreatic duct. These patients can be treated with the duodenal-preserving pancreatectomy, or the Beger procedure. This operation has gained significant popularity in Europe and, in many areas, is the most frequently performed operation for chronic pancreatitis. It has been slow to catch on in the United States, and is not nearly as frequently performed as the Puestow procedure, the Frey procedure, and the pylorus-preserving pancreaticoduodenectomy. It is an operation that requires a good deal of experience to perform.

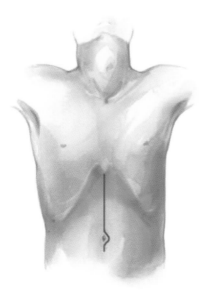

Operative Technique:

The abdomen is entered either through a bilateral subcostal or an upper midline incision. The abdomen is first explored for other pathology. The omentum is then removed from the transverse colon, and the neck, body and tail of the gland examined. We prefer to perform an extensive kocherization, although the originator of the operative procedure does not kocherize the duodenum. This operation is ideally suited for patients with a very large inflammatory mass in the head of the pancreas. The first step in the procedure is to be certain one is not dealing with an adenocarcinoma of the head of the pancreas. One should

Once the papilla is opened, the ductal and duodenum mucosa are approximated with interrupted 5-0 synthetic absorbable sutures (3, 4). When the papillotomy is completed, the largest lacrimal duct probe and/or the smallest Bakes dilator should be accommodated. Following the papillotomy, pancreatic juice, which initially spurts out of the accessory papilla with a stream, flows out easily and rapidly, unimpeded. The duodenotomy is closed with an inner continuous layer of synthetic absorbable 3-0 suture material placed in a Connell fashion. The outer layer is placed using interrupted 3-0 silk sutures. The duodenotomy may be drained with a closed suction Silastic drain.

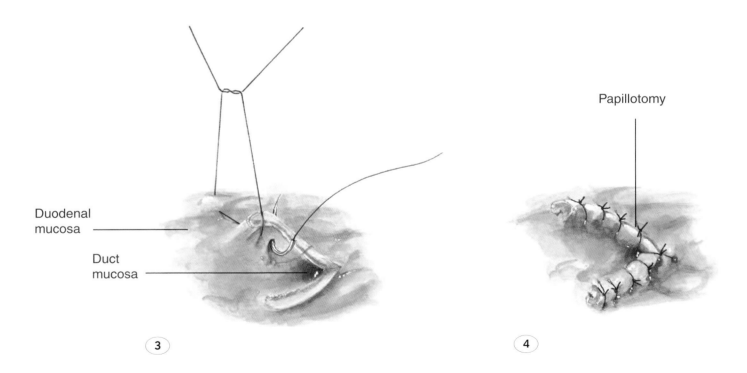

Duodenal
mucosa

Duct
mucosa

Papillotomy

3

4

Drainage of Pancreatic Pseudocyst into a Roux-en-Y Jejunal Loop

Operative Indications:

A pancreatic pseudocyst results from disruption of the main pancreatic duct. This is often associated with an episode of acute pancreatitis, but a pseudocyst can also develop in the setting of chronic inflammation. Even less common, a pancreatic pseudocyst can develop following trauma or distal to a pancreatic neoplasm. Many pancreatic pseudocysts resolve spontaneously. The duct disruption will cicatrix and close and the pancreatic secretions in the cyst will be rapidly reabsorbed. If the cyst does not resolve, operative drainage may be required. Pseudocysts 5 or 6 cm in diameter or less are generally asymptomatic and do not result in life-threatening complications. Pseudocysts over 6 cm in diameter, however, can potentially cause life-threatening complications.

Pseudocysts can cause pain, duodenal obstruction, and biliary obstruction; they can erode into adjacent structures, most commonly the colon or duodenum; they can become secondarily infected; they can be associated with life-threatening hemorrhage, often from a false aneurysm bleeding into the cyst. For these reasons, most pseudocysts over 6 cm in diameter that do not spontaneously resolve after a period of observation and/or remain symptomatic, should be considered for drainage. The drainage procedure of choice, if the cyst can be drained dependently, is through the transverse mesocolon into a Roux-en-Y jejunal loop. One can also drain pseudocysts percutaneously, or internally using endoscopic techniques. However, complications are significant and recurrences common. We therefore continue to favor open internal drainage.

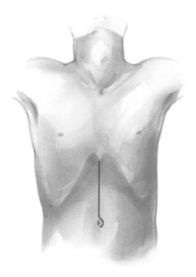

Operative Technique:

Either a bilateral subcostal or midline incision can be used. The abdomen is examined to rule out other pathology.

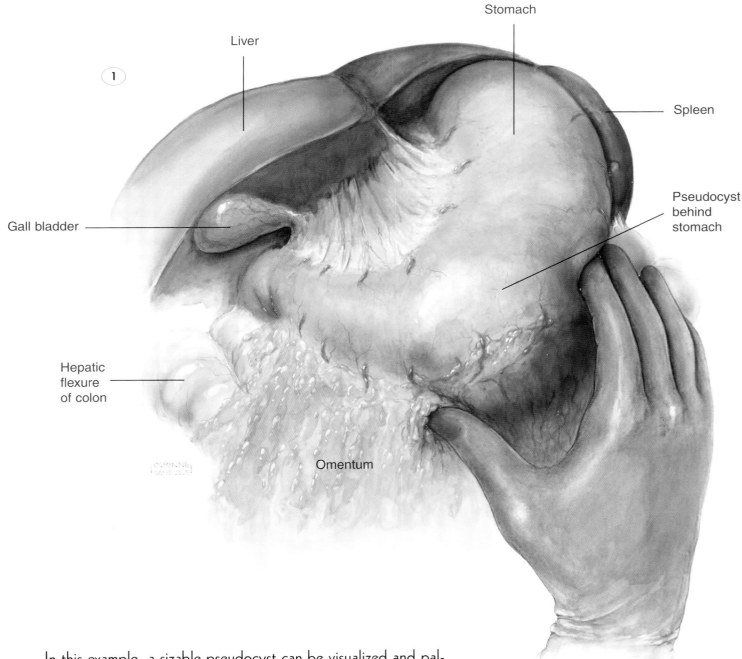

In this example, a sizable pseudocyst can be visualized and palpated posterior to the stomach (1). Since the cyst is directly
behind the stomach with the posterior wall of the stomach comprising the anterior wall of the cyst, it could easily be drained by a cystogastrostomy. To avoid the constant alkaline bathing of the antrum
that results following a cystogastrostomy, and owing to the small
incidence of bleeding, we favor a cystojejunostomy into a Roux-en-
Y jejunal loop as the treatment of choice whenever possible.

After retracting the transverse mesocolon in a cephalad direction, the pseudocyst can be seen and felt to be presenting through the transverse mesocolon. This allows ideal access for dependent drainage into a Roux-en-Y jejunal loop. At
this point, generally the cyst is aspirated to confirm its presence in the area palpated (2). In addition, at some point the
cyst wall should be biopsied to be certain that one is not dealing with a cystic neoplasm. If there is any discrepancy
between the size of the mass that is palpated and the size of
the cyst identified on CT scan, a cystogram can be performed by injecting contrast media into the cyst and taking an operative x-ray. This operative x-ray should produce an image that corresponds to the size of the
palpable mass. If it does not, one has to be concerned that there may be a second pseudocyst
or a loculated pseudocyst that would not be
drained entirely through the access route
identified with the needle aspiration.

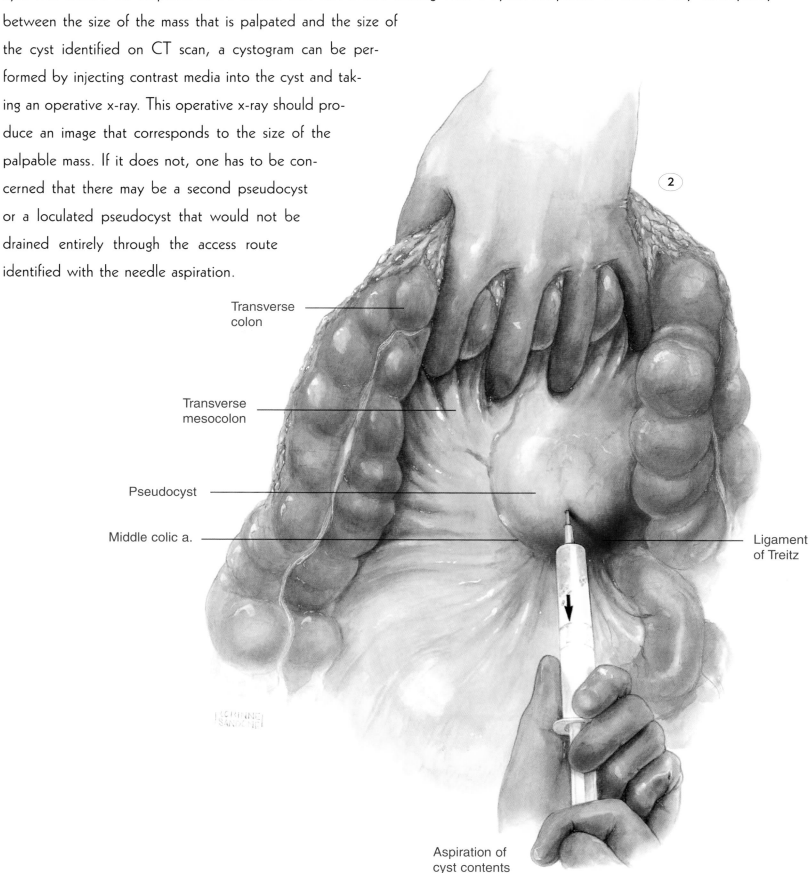

Transverse colon

Transverse mesocolon

Pseudocyst

Middle colic a.

Ligament of Treitz

Aspiration of cyst contents

Drainage of Pancreatic Pseudocyst into the Stomach

Operative Indications:

The operative indications for drainage of a pseudocyst into the stomach are the same as listed for drainage of a pancreatic pseudocyst into a Roux-en-Y jejunal loop. Drainage of a pseudocyst into a Roux-en-Y loop is our preferred approach. In some instances, however, the cyst resides high in the abdomen and does not present through the transverse mesocolon, so dependent drainage with a Roux-en-Y jejunal loop is not possible. In most of these instances, the cyst is adherent to the posterior wall of the stomach; the posterior wall of the stomach makes up the anterior wall of the pancreatic pseudocyst (2). In this circumstance cystogastrostomy is the procedure of choice.

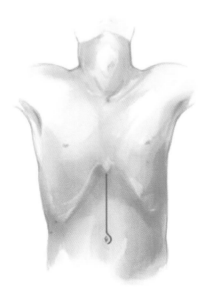

Operative Technique:

Either a bilateral subcostal or midline incision is appropriate. Once the abdomen is entered, the pseudocyst can be easily palpated and visualized displacing the stomach.

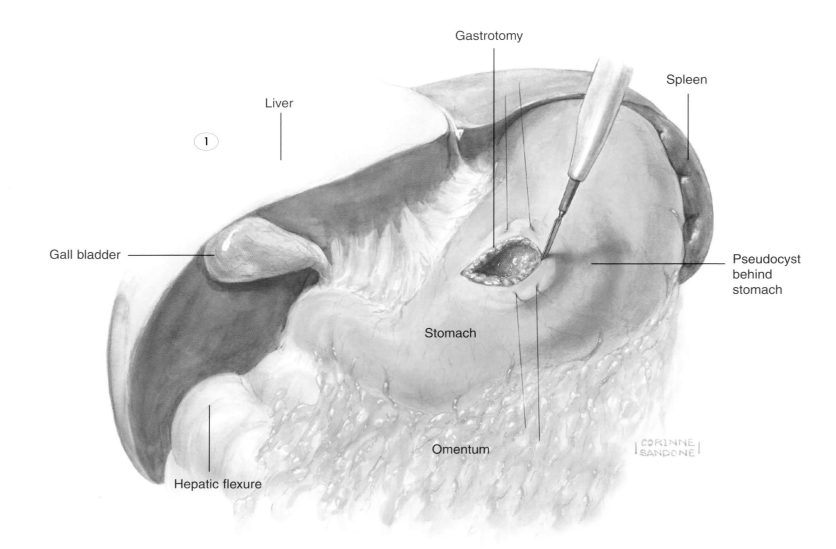

Gastrotomy

Spleen

Liver

1

Gall bladder

Pseudocyst behind stomach

Stomach

Omentum

Hepatic flexure

CORINNE SANDONE

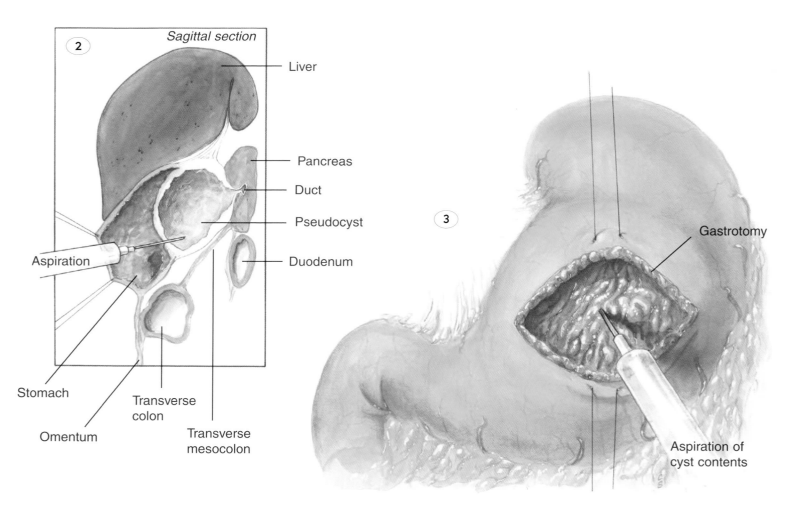

2   *Sagittal section*

Liver

Pancreas

Duct

Pseudocyst

Duodenum

Aspiration

Stomach

Transverse colon

Omentum

Transverse mesocolon

3

Gastrotomy

Aspiration of cyst contents

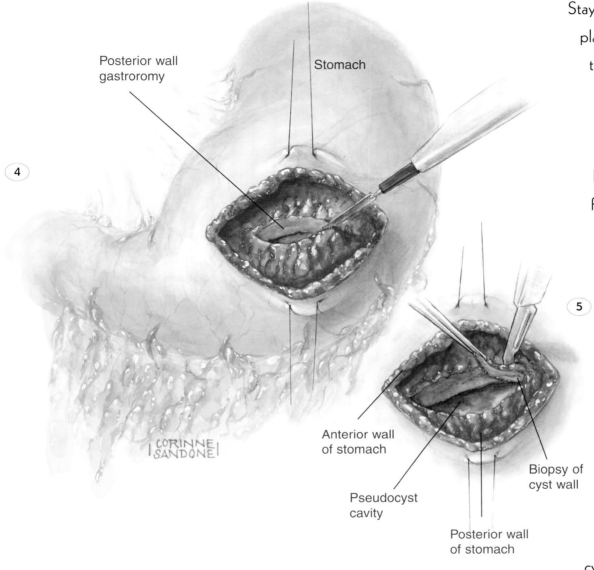

Posterior wall
gastroromy

Stomach

4

CORINNE
SANDONE

5

Anterior wall
of stomach

Pseudocyst
cavity

Biopsy of
cyst wall

Posterior wall
of stomach

Stay sutures of 3-0 silk are placed in the anterior wall of the stomach and a gastrotomy is performed with the electrocautery directly over the pseudocyst (1). The location of the cyst is confirmed by aspirating through the posterior wall of the stomach into the cyst with a 20-gauge needle and a 10-ml syringe (2, 3).

Not all of the cyst contents should be aspirated, as this will make subsequent entry into the cyst more difficult.

If there is a discrepancy between the size of the palpable mass and the size or number of pseudocysts as identified preoperatively by CT scan, a cystogram can be performed by injecting contrast media into the cyst and performing an operative radiograph. The cross-section demonstrates the anatomic relationships between the pancreas, the disrupted pancreatic duct, the pseudocyst, and the stomach (2). Note that the posterior wall of the stomach comprises a portion of the anterior wall of the pseudocyst. This diagram also nicely demonstrates that the pseudocyst does not present through the root of the transverse mesocolon. After the position of the pseudocyst has been confirmed by needle aspiration, the cyst is entered by incising through the posterior wall of the stomach using the electrocautery (4). A portion of the cyst wall is sent for frozen section to be certain that one is not dealing with a cystic neoplasm (5). If the incision into the cyst does not appear to gape widely open, an ellipse of stomach and cyst wall can be excised.

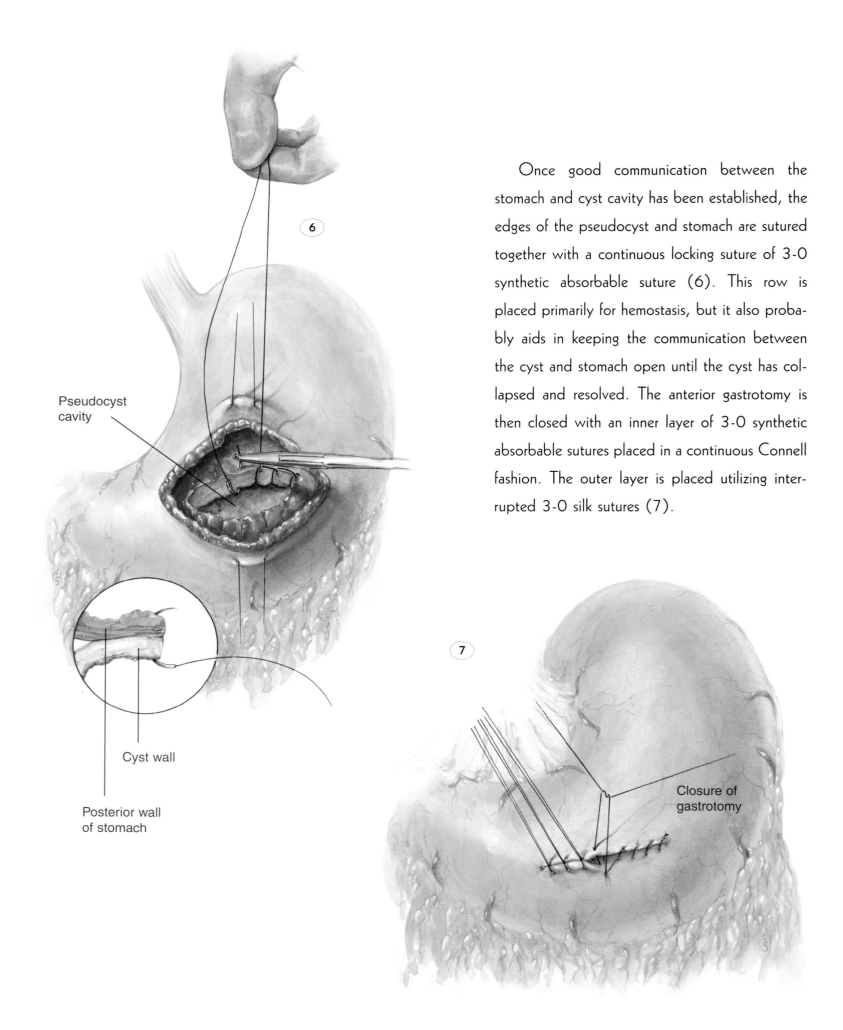

Pseudocyst
cavity

Cyst wall

Posterior wall
of stomach

Once good communication between the stomach and cyst cavity has been established, the edges of the pseudocyst and stomach are sutured together with a continuous locking suture of 3-0 synthetic absorbable suture (6). This row is placed primarily for hemostasis, but it also probably aids in keeping the communication between the cyst and stomach open until the cyst has collapsed and resolved. The anterior gastrotomy is then closed with an inner layer of 3-0 synthetic absorbable sutures placed in a continuous Connell fashion. The outer layer is placed utilizing interrupted 3-0 silk sutures (7).

Closure of
gastrotomy

Drainage of Pancreatic Pseudocyst into the Duodenum

Operative Indications:

The vast majority of pseudocysts can be drained into a Roux-en-Y jejunal loop or into the stomach. Rarely, however, a pseudocyst is located in the head of the pancreas so that the only option for drainage is into the adjacent duodenum. The same indications for cyst drainage that were outlined for cystojejunostomy and cystogastrostomy pertain to drainage of a pseudocyst into the duodenum.

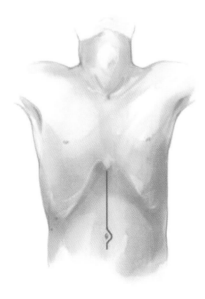

Operative Technique:

The abdomen is entered through either a right subcostal or upper midline incision. The pseudocyst which resides in the duodenal C loop in the head of the pancreas is exposed (1), and the omentum is cleaned from the anterior wall of the cyst. The duodenum is kocherized. A posterior row of interrupted 3-0 silk sutures is placed between the cyst and the medial aspect of the duodenum. After the cyst location has been identified by needle aspiration as depicted for cystojejunostomy and cystogastrostomy, an opening into the pseudocyst is made with the electrocautery. A portion of the cyst wall is sent for frozen section to be certain one is not dealing with a cystic neoplasm.

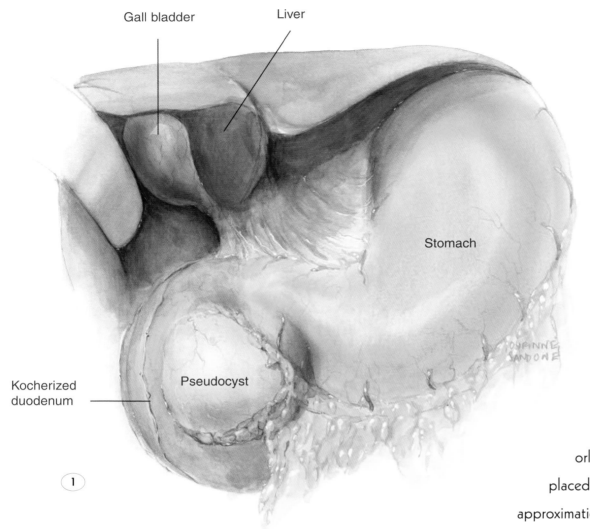

Gall bladder

Liver

Stomach

Kocherized duodenum

Pseudocyst

1

A parallel opening into the duodenum is made, also with the electrocautery (2). A posterior inner continuous locking layer of 3-0 synthetic absorbable suture is placed (3) and then brought anteriorly in a Connell fashion. This row is placed for hemostasis, as well as for good approximation of the cyst wall and duodenum.

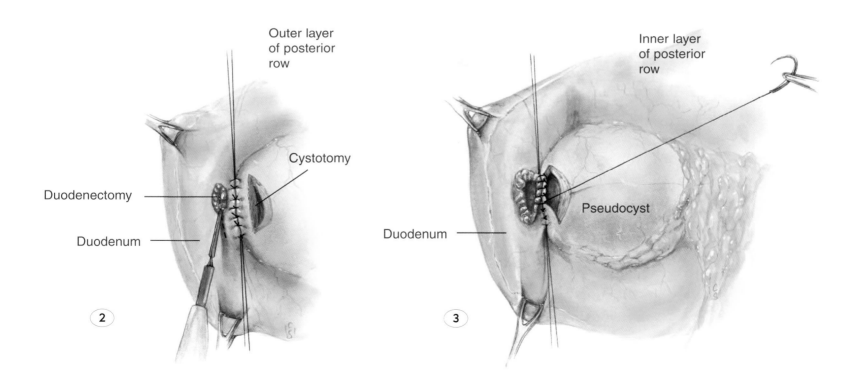

Outer layer of posterior row

Cystotomy

Duodenectomy

Duodenum

2

Inner layer of posterior row

Duodenum

Pseudocyst

3

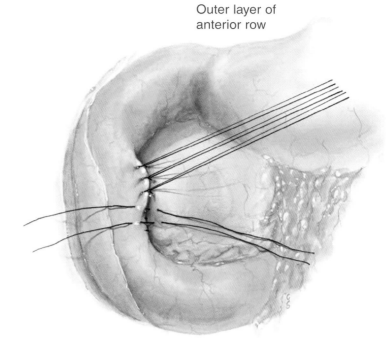

Outer layer of
anterior row

4

The outer layer of the anterior row is placed,
again utilizing 3-O silk sutures (4). The anastomosis is drained with a closed suction drain. The
inset demonstrates the anatomic relationship
between the head of the pancreas and the pancreatic duct, the pseudocyst, and the duodenum with
the cystoduodenostomy (5).

Another approach for draining a pseudocyst into the
duodenum involves performing a duodenotomy, and then
entering the pseudocyst via the medial aspect of the duodenum.
In our estimation, this results in potential risk to either the bile duct or
pancreatic duct, and the description provided here is a much safer technique.

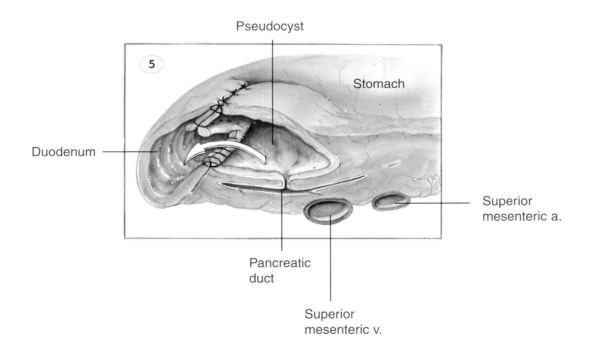

Pseudocyst

5

Stomach

Duodenum

Superior
mesenteric a.

Pancreatic
duct

Superior
mesenteric v.

Pancreaticoduodenectomy (Pylorus-Preserving Whipple Procedure)

Operative Indications:

Pancreaticoduodenectomy, or the Whipple procedure, may be indicated for a variety of benign and malignant diseases. It is most commonly performed for one of the four periampullary adenocarcinomas arising in the head of the pancreas, the ampulla, the distal bile duct, or the duodenum. The procedure is also utilized for less common neoplasms that may arise in the head of the pancreas. These include the cystic neoplasms, both serous and mucinous cystadenomas and mucinous cystadenocarcinomas, intraductal papillary mucinous neoplasms, islet cell tumors (both benign and malignant), and solid and pseudopapillary neoplasms (Hamoudi tumor). Benign ampullary and duodenal adenomas may also occasionally require a pancreaticoduodenectomy for management. There are also a handful of rare tumors, including gastrointestinal stromal tumors and acinar cell tumors, that are treatable by pancreaticoduodenectomy. Some pancreatic surgeons feel that pancreaticoduodenectomy is the procedure of choice for chronic pancreatitis when a dilated duct is not present and a Puestow procedure, therefore, cannot be performed. It is a particularly attractive operation for chronic pancreatitis when the disease is most severe in the head and uncinate process, with less extensive involvement of the body and tail of the gland. Rarely, pancreaticoduodenectomy may be indicated for extensive pancreatic and duodenal trauma, when it is felt that duodenal repair and pancreatic drainage would be inadequate surgical management. In most instances, however, a pancreaticoduodenectomy is performed for a malignant neoplasm arising in the periampullary region. The pylorus-preserving modification of the classic Whipple procedure has become our standard, and it is utilized in over 80% of the pancreaticoduodenectomies done for neoplasms.

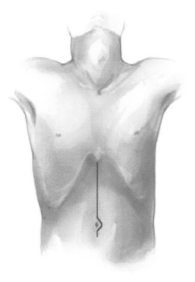

Operative Technique:

The operative procedure can be performed through either a bilateral subcostal or an upper abdominal midline incision. Once the abdomen is entered, a thorough exploration must be

Alternative: Roux-en-Y hepaticojejunostomy

An alternative way of performing the double bypass is to create a Roux-en-Y jejunal loop distal to the gastrojejunostomy (5). Alimentary tract continuity is reestablished with an end-to-side jejunojejunostomy performed with an inner continuous layer of 3-0 absorbable synthetic suture material and an outer interrupted layer of 3-0 silk. The Roux-en-Y loop should be approximately 60 cm in length. Again, a cholecystectomy is performed, and the common hepatic duct divided. The distal end of the biliary tree is oversewn. An end-to-side hepaticojejunostomy is performed with a single layer of interrupted 4-0 absorbable synthetic suture material. The Roux-en-Y jejunal loop is sutured to the rent in the transverse mesocolon with interrupted 4-0 silk sutures.

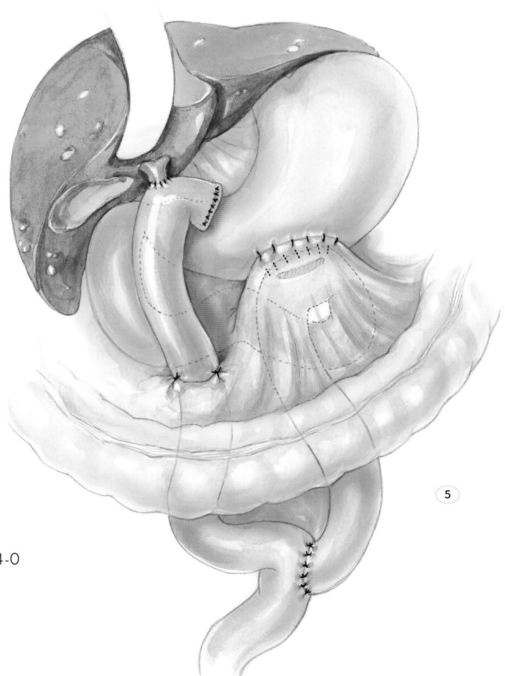

5

Distal Pancreatectomy for Tumor

Operative Indications:

The majority of adenocarcinomas of the pancreas arise in the head, neck and uncinate process. Approximately 25%, however, arise in the body and tail of the gland. The resectability rate of lesions in the body and tail is somewhat less than in the head because patients do not develop obstructive jaundice to signal the presence of a tumor. Generally, weight loss and pain occur and result in imaging studies that diagnose the lesion. In addition to adenocarcinomas, serous and mucinous neoplasms arise in the body and tail of the pancreas, as do intraductal papillary mucinous neoplasms. Neuroendocrine, or islet cell tumors, both benign and malignant, as well as Hamoudi tumors, occur in the body and the tail of the gland.

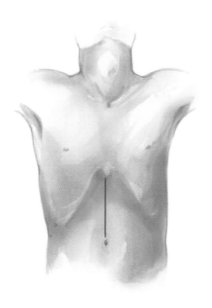

Operative Technique:

An upper midline incision is used. Once the abdomen is entered, evidence of tumor dissemination is looked for. If there are no liver metastases, or serosal implants, the tumor is exposed by removing the omentum from the transverse colon. When the tumor is exposed in the lesser sac, it can be grasped to see if it is mobile. These tumors often extend up toward the neck of the pancreas. Therefore, the superior mesenteric and portal veins should be exposed to be certain that the tumor does not involve these structures.

The inferior border of the neck of the pancreas is mobilized, and the superior mesenteric vein identified. The superior mesenteric vein is carefully dissected bluntly off the posterior aspect of the neck of the pancreas. The portal vein is identified by opening up the areolar plane along the superior border of the neck of the pancreas. Once it is identified, the dissection of the portal vein is connected to the superior mesenteric vein dissection, and the neck of the gland is looped with a small Penrose drain (1). Next, one has to be certain that the tumor does not involve the celiac axis and the hepatic artery (2). A short segment of splenic artery at its takeoff from the celiac axis needs to be free to be ligated and divided. Once it is demonstrated that these structures are not involved by tumor, the operation proceeds.

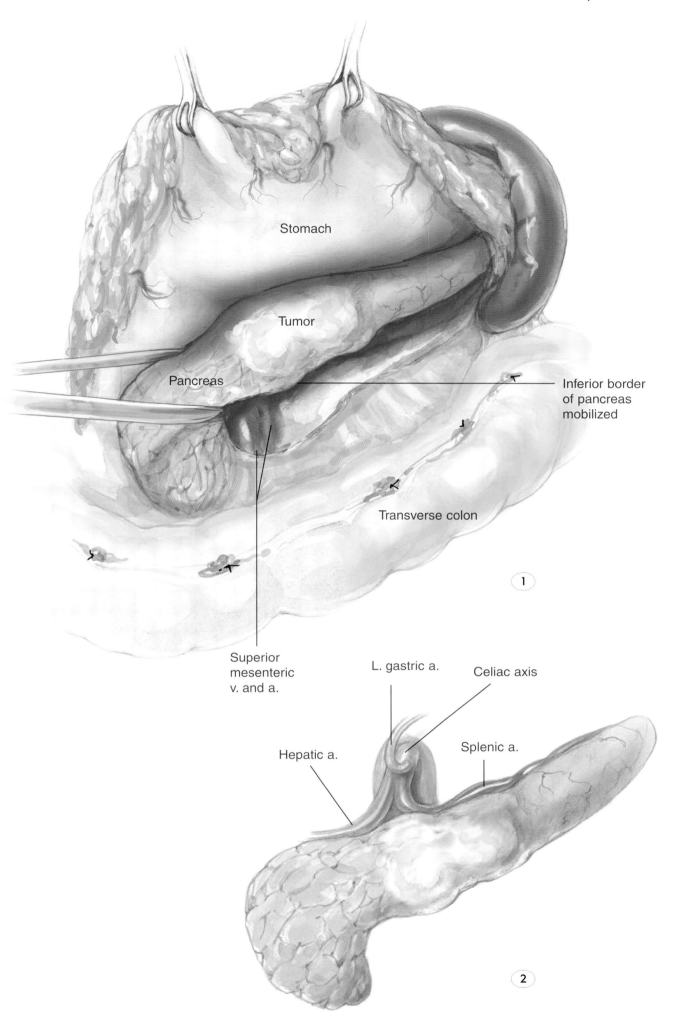

Stomach

Tumor

Pancreas

Inferior border
of pancreas
mobilized

Transverse colon

①

Superior
mesenteric
v. and a.

L. gastric a.

Celiac axis

Hepatic a.

Splenic a.

②

The removal of the omentum from the transverse colon proceeds up along the splenic flexure of the colon, and the splenic flexure of the colon is mobilized and retracted inferiorly. At this point, the omentum is divided anterior to the hilum of the spleen between Kelly clamps, and ligated with 2-0 silks. The vasa brevia are then divided between Reinhoff clamps, and ligated with 2-0 silks (3).

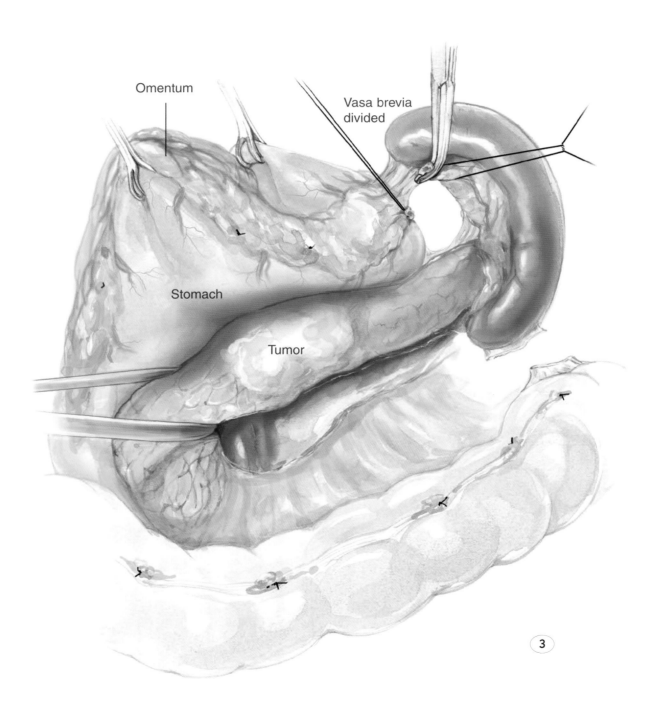

3

Next, the spleen is mobilized out of retroperitoneum by dividing the serosal attachments between the lateral and posterior aspects of the spleen, and the retroperitoneum. This generally proceeds relatively bloodlessly. During the dissection and mobilization of the tail of the gland, one has to be certain that the left adrenal gland, which is adjacent to the tail of the pancreas, is not injured (4). Bleeding from the left adrenal gland can be troublesome to control.

If the splenic vein is involved with tumor and is thrombosed, and splenomegaly is present, or if the tumor is particularly large, before mobilization of the spleen and tail of the pancreas, one might want to identify the splenic artery after its takeoff from the celiac axis and ligate it immediately (5). One needs to be absolutely certain not to confuse the hepatic artery with the splenic artery. The splenic artery can be difficult to identify, as it often passes posterior to the pancreas immediately after arising from the celiac axis, and the only prominent artery above the superior border of the pancreas is the hepatic artery.

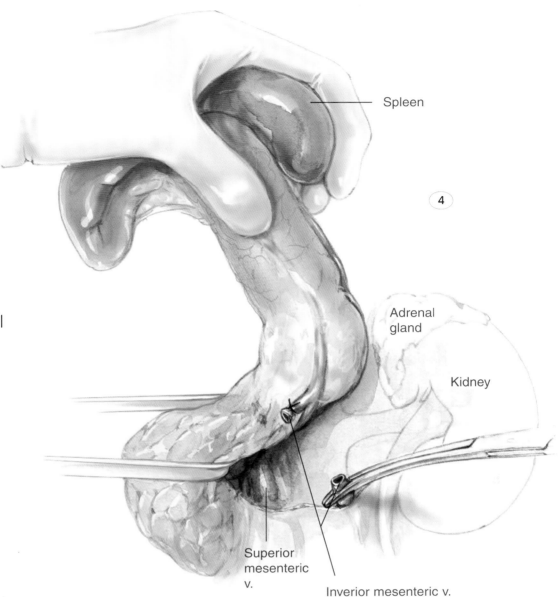

Spleen

4

Adrenal gland

Kidney

Superior mesenteric v.

Inverior mesenteric v.

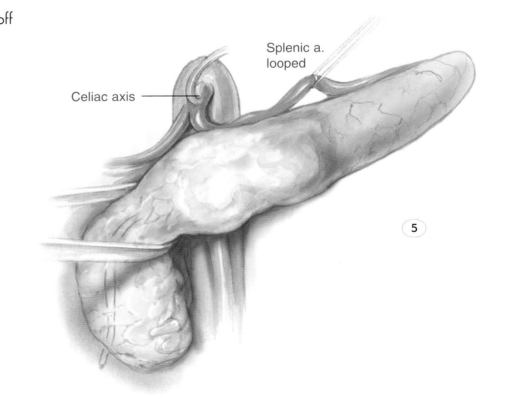

Splenic a. looped

Celiac axis

5

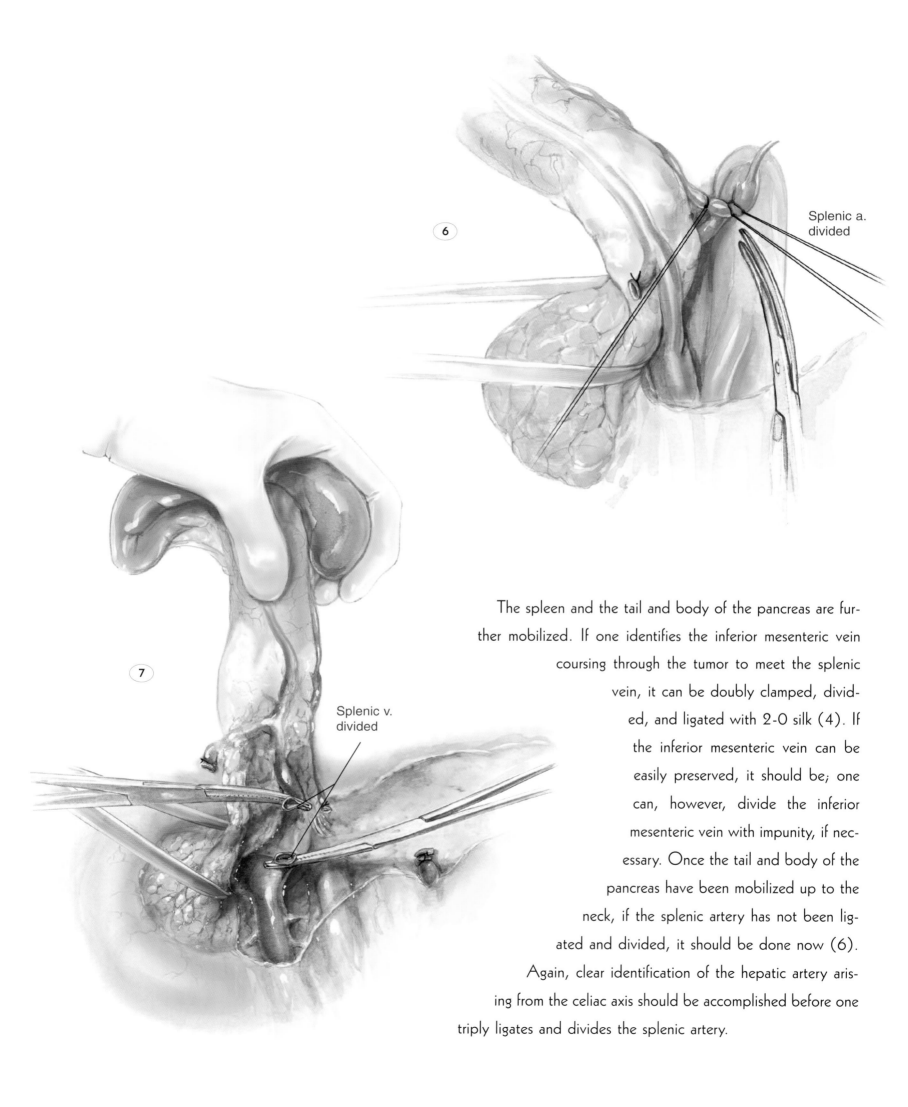

Splenic a. divided

Splenic v. divided

The spleen and the tail and body of the pancreas are further mobilized. If one identifies the inferior mesenteric vein coursing through the tumor to meet the splenic vein, it can be doubly clamped, divided, and ligated with 2-0 silk (4). If the inferior mesenteric vein can be easily preserved, it should be; one can, however, divide the inferior mesenteric vein with impunity, if necessary. Once the tail and body of the pancreas have been mobilized up to the neck, if the splenic artery has not been ligated and divided, it should be done now (6). Again, clear identification of the hepatic artery arising from the celiac axis should be accomplished before one triply ligates and divides the splenic artery.

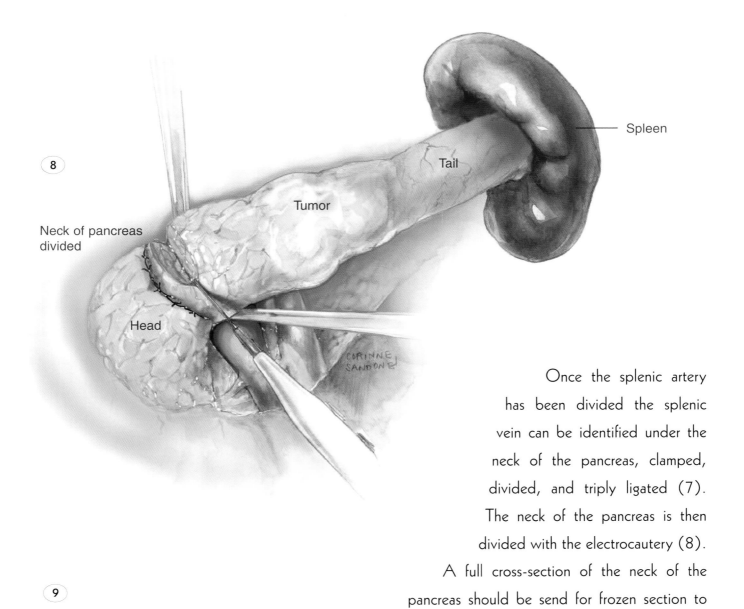

Spleen

8

Tail

Tumor

Neck of pancreas
divided

Head

9

Once the splenic artery
has been divided the splenic
vein can be identified under the
neck of the pancreas, clamped,
divided, and triply ligated (7).
The neck of the pancreas is then
divided with the electrocautery (8).
A full cross-section of the neck of the
pancreas should be send for frozen section to
be certain there is a clear margin (9).

The pancreatic duct should be identified in the proximal remnant. The incidence of pancreatic cutaneous fistulas is
actually higher for distal pancreatectomies than it is following a
Whipple resection. The incidence can be kept to a minimum if the
pancreatic duct is identified and suture ligated.

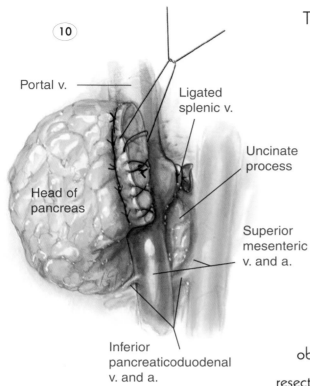

⑩

Portal v.

Ligated splenic v.

Uncinate process

Head of pancreas

Superior mesenteric v. and a.

Inferior pancreaticoduodenal v. and a.

The end of the pancreatic remnant is closed with two layers of interrupted 3-0 synthetic absorbable suture; the first is an overlapping horizontal mattress suture, and the second is a figure-of-eight suture (10). Two closed suction Silastic drains are left to drain the pancreatic remnant. A specific lymphadenectomy is not performed as a rule during distal pancreatectomy. But wide soft-tissue margins are included, particularly in the retroperitoneum, to be sure that the posterior margin of the tumor is negative.

Rarely, even in the face of celiac axis involvement by tumor, the tumor may be resectable via distal pancreatectomy. If good hepatic artery flow is provided by the gastroduodenal artery via its collaterals with the superior mesenteric artery, as demonstrated either preoperatively by angiogram or, at the time of surgery, by clamping the celiac axis and observing a pulse in the hepatic artery distal to the gastroduodenal artery, a resection can be performed that includes a distal pancreatectomy and splenectomy, and resection of the celiac axis and proximal hepatic artery (11).

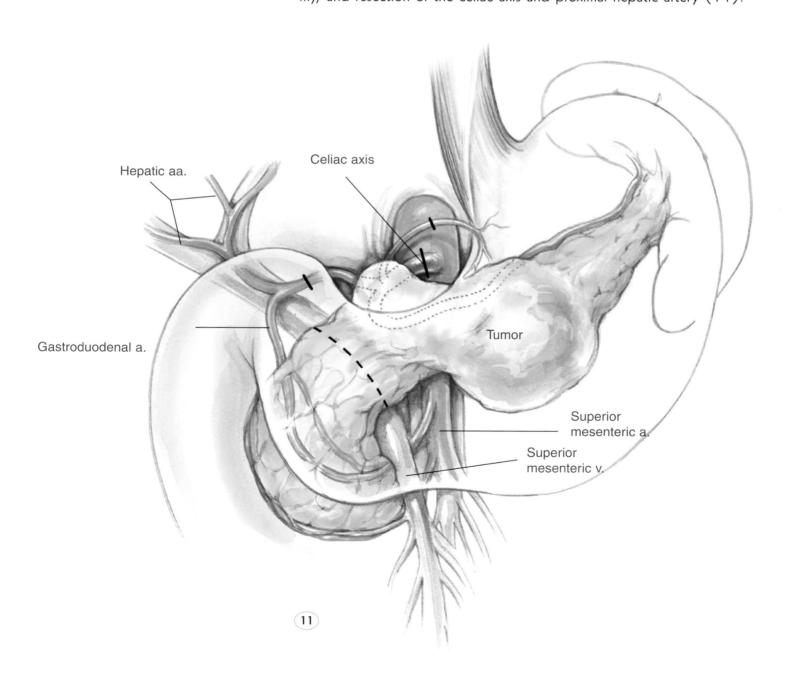

Hepatic aa.

Celiac axis

Gastroduodenal a.

Tumor

Superior mesenteric a.

Superior mesenteric v.

⑪

Central Pancreatectomy with Pancreaticogastrostomy

Operative Indications:

There are instances when small benign, or low-grade malignant, tumors arise in the neck or proximal body of the pancreas, leaving one undecided as to whether to perform a pancreaticoduodenectomy or a distal pancreatectomy. If one performs a pancreaticoduodenectomy, one is doing a very extensive operative procedure for a small lesion that probably does not require it. If one were to do a distal pancreatectomy, 85% of the gland would be removed, again for a small benign or low-grade malignant lesion. In these instances, a central resection seems appropriate. Small benign serous or mucinous cystadenomas, small islet cell tumors that cannot be shelled out, or an occasional intraductal papillary mucinous neoplasm, are examples of tumors in the neck and proximal body that might be amenable to a central pancreatectomy. In addition, instead of constructing a Roux-en-Y loop in which to drain the distal pancreatic remnant, we feel it is preferable—and quicker— to perform a pancreaticogastrostomy. The back wall of the stomach rests on the anterior surface of the body and tail of the pancreas, and this adjacency makes a pancreaticogastrostomy between the distal pancreatic remnant and the back wall of the stomach very feasible.

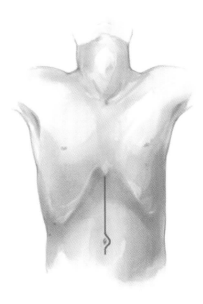

Operative Technique:

The patient can be explored either through a midline incision or a transverse bilateral subcostal incision. Once the abdomen is entered, a thorough exploration is carried out to be certain there is no pathology elsewhere. The lesser sac is entered by removing the omentum from the transverse colon. The pathology is easily identified in the neck and/or proximal body of the pancreas. The rest of the pancreas should be thoroughly explored through the lesser sac, by mobilizing the neck, body and tail of the pancreas along the inferior border. The duodenum should also be kocherized and the head, neck and unci-

nate process palpated from the right side. When one is satisfied that one is dealing with a small benign or low-grade malignant tumor, such as an islet cell tumor, one can proceed with a central pancreatectomy.

The inferior border of the neck and proximal body of the pancreas is mobilized after incising the serosal attachment onto
the inferior border of the pancreas. The superior mesenteric vein is easily identified. The anterior surface is carefully dissected from the posterior aspect of the neck of the pancreas. The superior border of the pancreas along its neck is next mobilized by incising the serosal reflection. The portal vein is identified and dissected from the posterior aspect of the neck of the
pancreas and connected to the superior mesenteric vein dissection. The neck of the pancreas is looped with a small Penrose
drain (1). The central portion of the pancreas is then reflected anteriorly, and the splenic vein identified. The splenic vein
has to be carefully dissected from the undersurface of the neck and proximal body of the pancreas. There are a few small
venous branches that have to be carefully dissected free, doubly ligated, and then divided. The splenic artery is often separate from the neck and proximal body of the pancreas, and
does not have to be dissected. But if it does arise and
join the superior border of the neck and proximal
body, it also needs to be dissected free. There
may be several small arterial branches that have
to be doubly ligated and divided.

Once the central portion of the pancreas has been mobilized, it can be divided
with the electrocautery proximally at the
junction of the neck and head of the pancreas, and distally such that there is at
least a 2 cm margin on either side of
the tumor (1). The specimen
should be sent for frozen section,
and both margins checked.

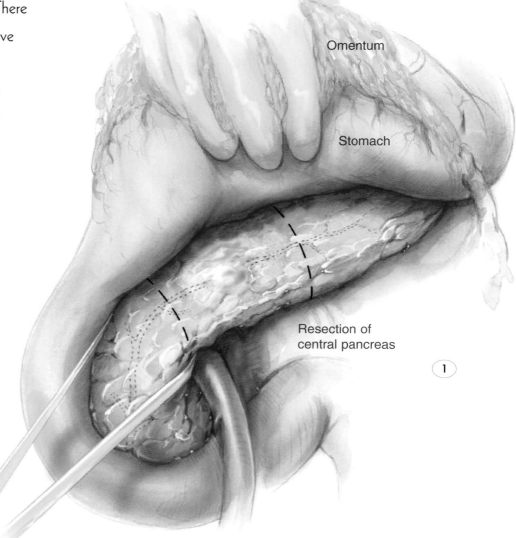

Omentum

Stomach

Resection of
central pancreas

(1)

The proximal pancreatic remnant should be oversewn with two layers of 3-0 synthetic absorbable suture. The first layer is placed in an overlapping horizontal mattress fashion, and the second layer is placed in a figure-of-eight fashion. An attempt should be made to identify the pancreatic duct in the proximal pancreatic remnant, as its ligature with a mattress suture (2) will decrease the likelihood of a pancreatic cutaneous fistula.

An end-to-side pancreaticogastrostomy is performed between the distal pancreatic remnant and the posterior wall of the stomach. It is performed in two layers: an outer interrupted layer of 3-0 silk and an inner continuous layer of 3-0 synthetic absorbable suture material. The pancreatic duct may or may not be dilated. In either case, it is incorporated in the inner continuous layer of 3-0 synthetic absorbable suture. If the duct is of normal caliber, often two (or at the most three) throws can incorporate the duct, both inferiorly and superiorly. If it is dilated, several throws of the inner layer can incorporate the dilated pancreatic duct (3).

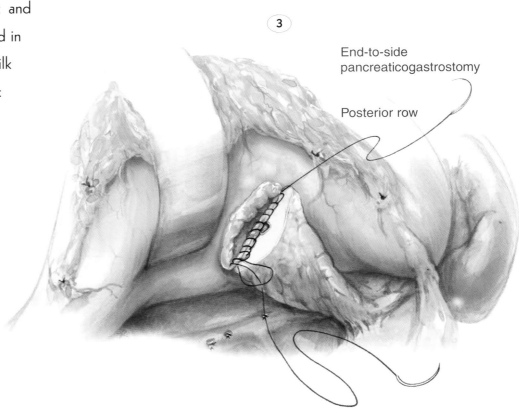

Pancreatic duct closed

End-to-side pancreaticogastrostomy

Posterior row

The outer interrupted layer of the left lateral anastomotic site is placed first. A gastrotomy is then fashioned of the appropriate length. The inner continuous layer of 3-0 absorbable suture is then placed running down the left lateral side of the anastomosis first in a locking fashion (3), and then passing along the right lateral inner layer in an over-and-over suture. The anastomosis is completed when one places the outer interrupted layer of 3-0 silk sutures along the right lateral anastomotic border (4).

These patients are particularly prone to developing pancreatic cutaneous fistulas out through the drains, since often both the proximal and distal pancreatic remnants are normal soft tissue. We generally use three Silastic closed suction drains for a central resection. One drain each is placed on either side of the pancreaticogastrostomy and a third drain at the proximal pancreatic remnant. This central resection maximally preserves pancreatic parenchyma in patients in whom one is not concerned about doing a radical resection or including a large amount of surrounding soft tissue or lymph nodes.

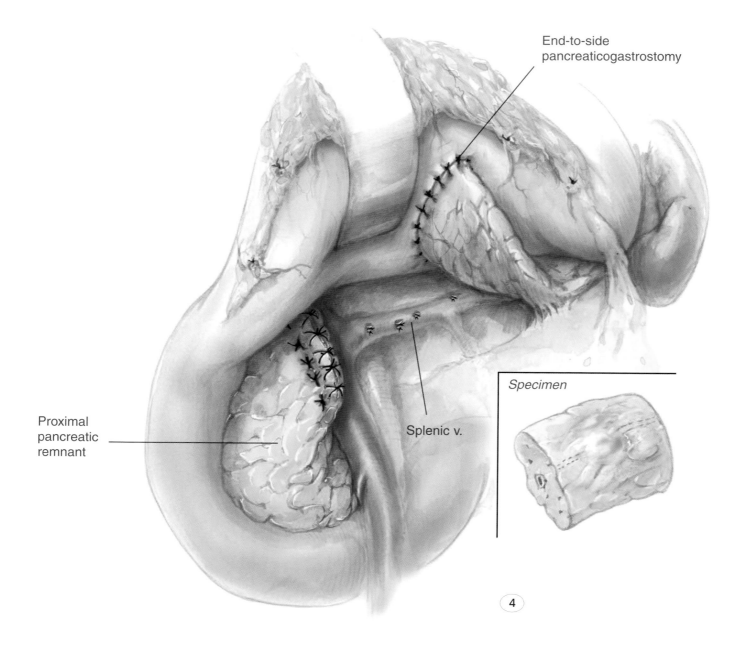

End-to-side
pancreaticogastrostomy

Proximal
pancreatic
remnant

Splenic v.

Specimen

4

Laparotomy for Insulinoma

Operative Indications:

Once the diagnosis of an insulinoma has been confirmed on the basis of serum glucose and insulin levels, there are a variety of options in attempting to localize the tumor. In the past, angiography was used routinely. It is rarely performed today. Three-dimensional, thin-section CT scans often will be able to identify the location of the insulinoma. The use of magnetic resonance imaging has shown promise; however, the most accurate means of tumor identification pre-operatively is with endoscopic ultrasound. Even with these more accurate means of identifying the location of an insulinoma, in some instances the patient will be explored with the diagnosis of insulinoma, but without knowing its exact location.

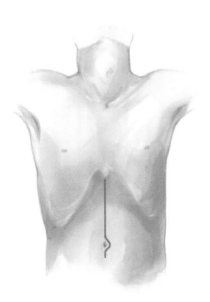

Operative Technique:

Either a bilateral subcostal or midline incision can be used. Once the abdomen has been entered, a thorough exploration is carried out for evidence of other pathology. Because most insulin-secreting neuroendocrine tumors are benign, however, only rarely would one find evidence of metastatic disease.

Kocherized
duodenum

Stomach

Head of
pancreas

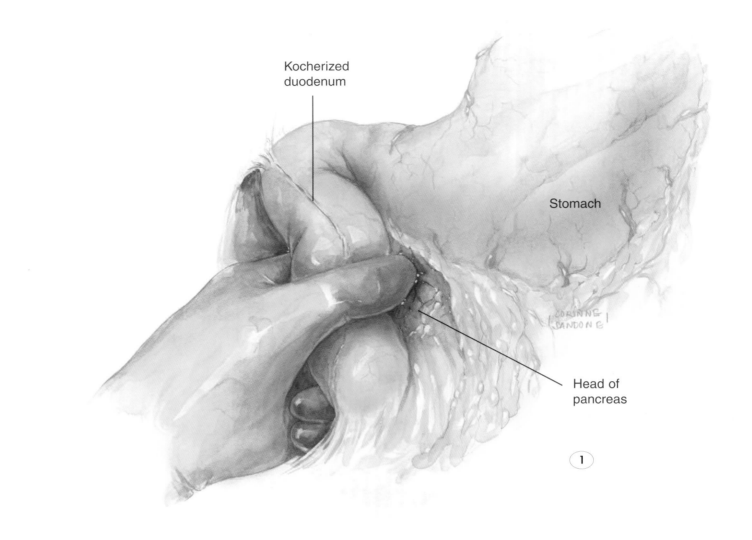

①

Duodenum

②

Body of
pancreas

Head of
pancreas

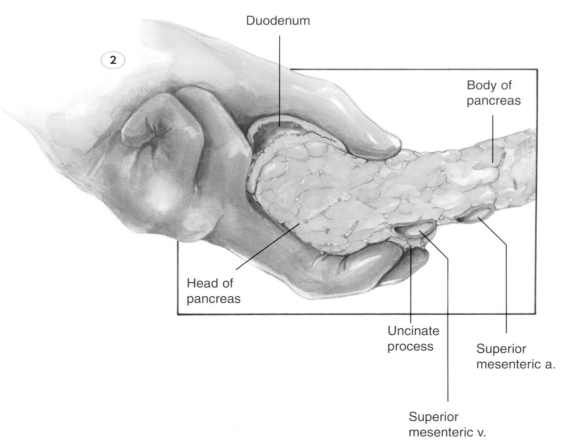

Uncinate
process

Superior
mesenteric a.

Superior
mesenteric v.

The duodenum is extensively kocherized and the head, uncinate process, and neck of the pancreas carefully palpated for evidence of tumor (1, 2). The head is the thickest portion of the pancreas, and a small tumor may be particularly difficult to palpate in this location. The lesser sac is then entered by removing the greater omentum from the transverse colon. The peritoneal reflection along the inferior border of the pancreas is incised, and the neck, body and tail of the

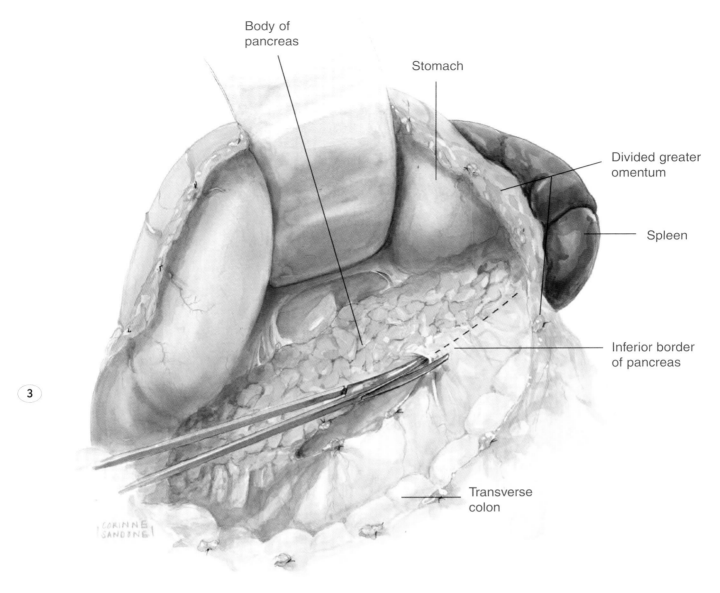

Body of pancreas

Stomach

Divided greater omentum

Spleen

Inferior border of pancreas

Transverse colon

3

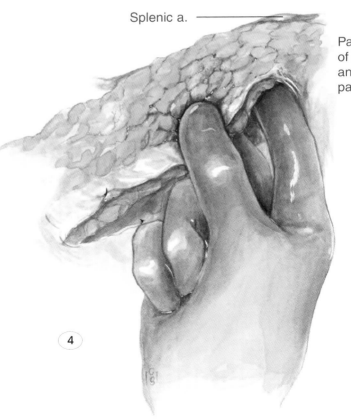

Splenic a.

Palpation of body and tail of pancreas

4

gland are mobilized out of the retroperitoneum (3). This can generally be done rapidly, bluntly, and bloodlessly. It is particularly important when exploring a patient for an insulinoma that one be able to visualize and palpate the entire pancreas. Once the body and tail have been mobilized, one can easily palpate both anteriorly and posteriorly for evidence of a mass (4). If, after careful visualization and palpation of the entire pancreas, the lesion cannot be identified, intraoperative ultrasound should be used. Of all the pre- and intraoperative imaging devices that are available, this is the most accurate. Most insulinomas will be identifiable.

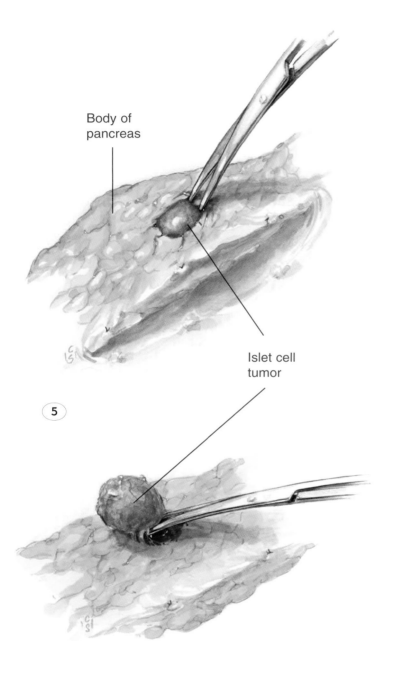

Body of
pancreas

Islet cell
tumor

5

6

When the insulinoma is identified, it often can be shelled out without performing a formal pancreatic resection. Some insulinomas, however, are malignant; and if such a lesion is encountered, a formal pancreatic resection will be necessary. In addition, even with some benign lesions, the adherence of the lesion to surrounding pancreatic tissue and/or its size may make a formal resection necessary. If the lesion is in the head, this might require a pancreaticoduodenectomy. If the lesion is in the body or tail and cannot be shelled out, a distal pancreatectomy will be necessary. If it is in the neck of the gland, or in the proximal body, a central resection might be possible.

Because of the relatively thin nature of the pancreas, and because insulinomas are soft and spherical, usually a part of the neoplasm will be evident underneath the capsule of the pancreas. It will usually appear to have a darkish coloration although, occasionally, lesions are flesh-colored. Such lesions will usually shell out with a combination of blunt and sharp dissection (5). A variety of techniques can be used (6).

Placing small ligaclips on the pancreas side and cauterization toward the insulinoma side will provide for a rapid bloodless mobilization of the lesion (7). Once the lesion is removed (8), one should examine the bed of the tumor carefully to be certain there is no evidence of a major pancreatic duct injury that occurred during the dissection. If not, the remaining portion of the gland should be carefully examined again to be certain that a second lesion is not present. Closed-suction Silastic drains are left in the area of the insulinoma removal, and brought out through stab wounds in the left upper quadrant.

In the past after thorough examination, if an islet cell tumor could not be identified, many surgeons felt that performing a distal 85% pancreatectomy was appropriate. Other surgeons, however, actually felt one should perform a pancreaticoduodenectomy because the head of the gland is the thickest portion of the gland and is more likely to hide an insulinoma and make it undetectable. Today, however, very few surgeons feel that a blind pancreatectomy of any sort should be performed. If an insulinoma cannot be identified after thorough examination and the extensive use of intraoperative ultrasound, the patient should be closed and other means of insulinoma identification subsequently carried out.

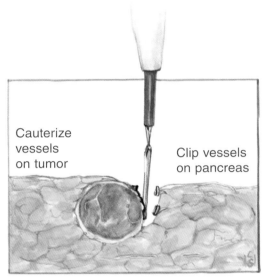

Cauterize vessels on tumor

Clip vessels on pancreas

Shelling out of Islet Cell Tumor

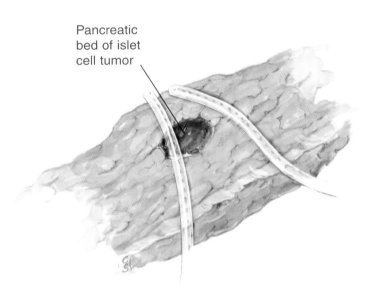

Pancreatic bed of islet cell tumor

8

Débridement and Drainage of Pancreatic Abscess

Operative Indications:

The development of a pancreatic abscess is the major cause of morbidity and mortality following an episode of severe acute pancreatitis. Early diagnosis is essential if pancreatic débridement and drainage are to be performed early enough to prevent life-threatening complications. With three-dimensional CT scanning to identify peripancreatic fluid collections and areas of necrotic pancreas with or without air bubbles, and with the ability of fine-needle aspiration of fluid collections to look for bacteria, the diagnosis of a pancreatic abscess can now be made relatively early in the development. When the diagnosis is made, the patient should be stabilized and taken to the operating room as soon as possible. There are instances in which there are large collections of fluid in association with an infected pancreatic necrosis that can be drained percutaneously. In some instances, percutaneous drainage will allow the patient to be stabilized, and subsequently undergo pancreatic débridement under more favorable conditions. There perhaps are unusual instances in which the pancreatic necrosis and abscess can be managed entirely percutaneously, but these instances are rare, and most patients with infected pancreatic necrosis require surgical intervention.

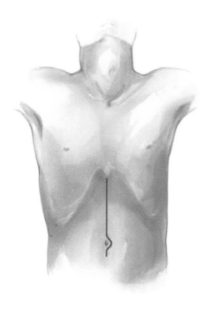

Operative Techniques:

Either a long midline or a bilateral subcostal incision can be used. Adequate exposure is particularly important because it is essential that the entire abdomen be explored for extension of the abscess away from the pancreas, down either pericolic gutter, into the transverse mesocolon, or into the left and right upper quadrants. With the superb imaging with thin-section, three-dimensional CT scans today, when patients with pancreatic necrosis and abscess are explored, generally the extent of the disease has been clearly identified. Once the abdomen is entered, the omentum is taken off the transverse colon if possible and reflected cephalad. Sometimes the omentum is so adherent that this is not possible, and it is then divided below the level of the greater curvature of the stomach, and reflected cephalad. The entire lesser sac needs to be exposed (1). Rather than large collections of pus, the most frequent finding is of a grumous, necrotic material filling the lesser sac and surrounding the pancreas. This often is thought to be necrotic pancreas. More often, it is necrotic soft tissue and fat necrosis surrounding the inflamed pancreas. With the excellent preoperative imaging of three-dimensional CT scans, the areas of abscess extension out of the lesser sac are generally known.

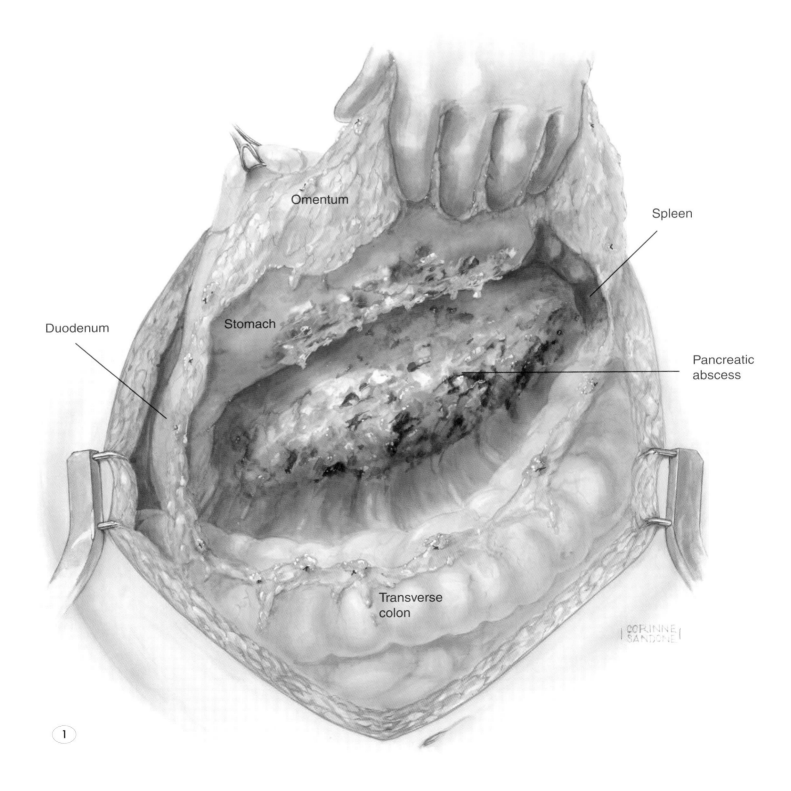

It is always important, however, that the transverse
colon be reflected cephalad to look for
extension of the abscess inferiorly in the
retroperitoneum and into the root
of the transverse mesocolon
(2). This is a frequent
route of extension.

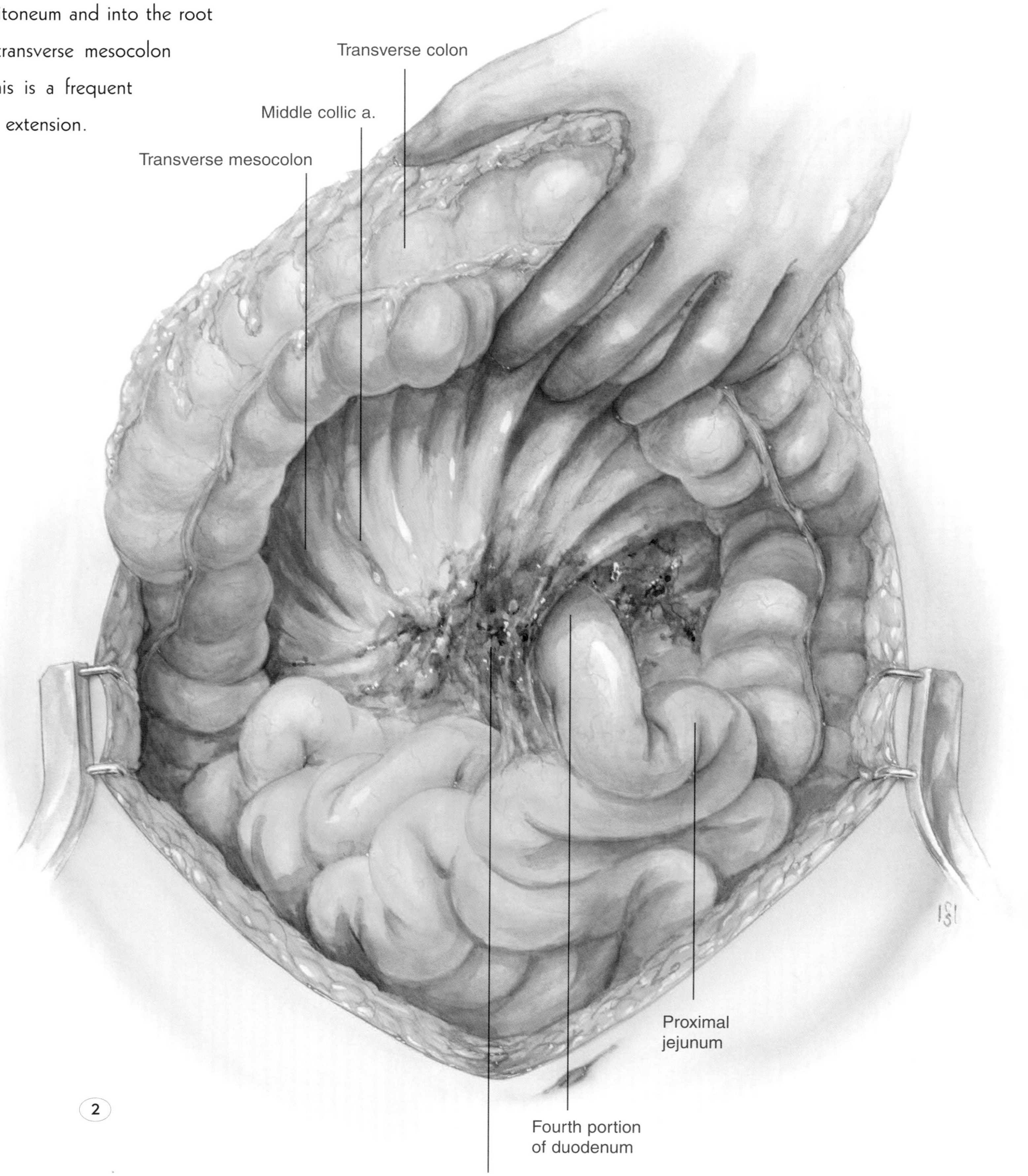

Transverse colon

Middle collic a.

Transverse mesocolon

Proximal
jejunum

Fourth portion
of duodenum

Retroperitoneal
extension of
abscess

2

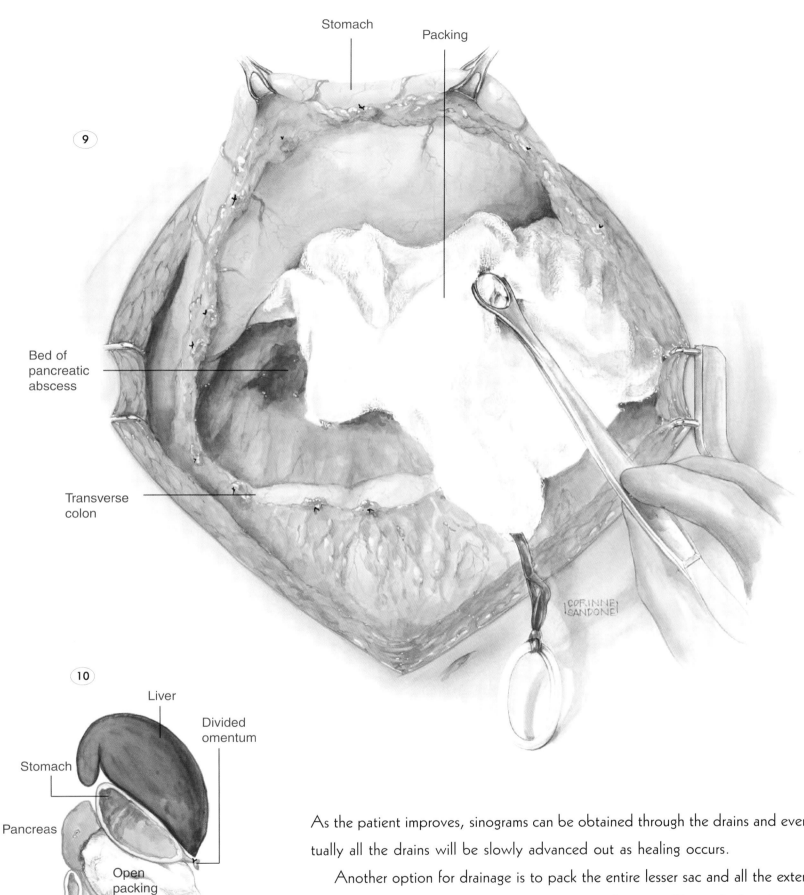

As the patient improves, sinograms can be obtained through the drains and eventually all the drains will be slowly advanced out as healing occurs.

Another option for drainage is to pack the entire lesser sac and all the extensions of the abscess with Mikulicz's pads, or soft gauze. The end of each packing needs to be brought out through the wound with a tag on the end (9, 10). These packs and pads are placed with the intention of changing them every 2 or 3 days, thereby continuing to mechanically débride the abscess cavities.

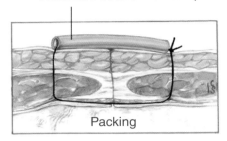

Retention suture with bumper

Packing

11

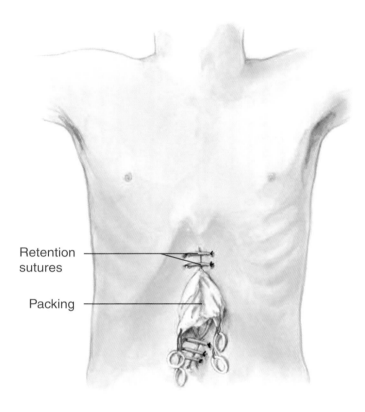

Retention sutures

Packing

12

This technique is particularly effective when complete débridement has not been possible with the initial exploration. The upper and lower portions of the wound are closed with large retention sutures of No. 2 nylon with rubber bumpers constructed from No. 16 French catheters (11, 12). The dressing can be periodically saturated postoperatively with antibiotic containing solutions. The initial repacking should be done under general anesthesia in the operating room in 48 to 72 hours. Eventually, however, the repacking may be performed under heavy sedation in the intensive care unit. The packing changes continue every 2 or 3 days until the abscess is clearly débrided and the cavity has started granulating. This often takes several packing changes. At this point, one can insert closed suction drains and close the abdominal wound. Another option is to continue the packing until granulation and wound contracture have progressed to the point where the cavity is actually closed. This option takes longer, but is perhaps safer.

THE SPLEEN

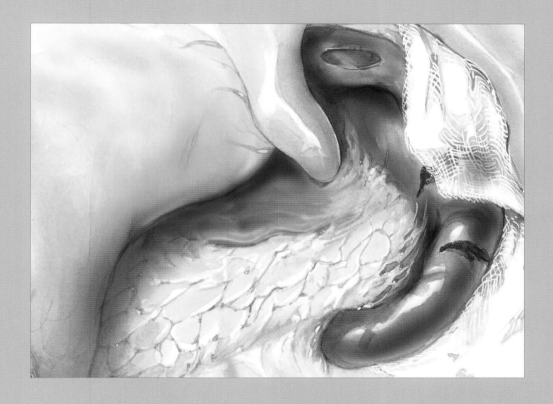

Splenectomy

Operative Indications:

Splenectomy is indicated for a wide spectrum of diseases. Perhaps the most common indication is trauma, either external or operative. A variety of hematologic disorders also require splenectomy. It may be a part of staging for a lymphoma. Finally, splenectomy may be performed as part of a cancer operation, either on the stomach, pancreas, or another left upper quadrant or retroperitoneal structure. A splenic abscess may also rarely be treated best by splenectomy.

Operative Technique:

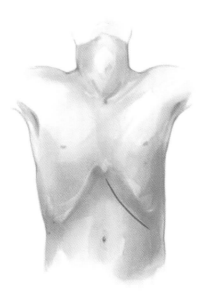

Splenectomy can be performed through either an upper midline or left subcostal incision. When the spleen is normal size, a left subcostal incision has some advantage over an upper midline incision. When the spleen is massive, a long midline incision should be used. Retraction of the left subcostal margin by a retractor fixed to a frame attached to the operating table is of great help. Initially, the areolar attachments to the spleen from the omentum are divided to avoid capsular tears and bleeding during the procedure (1).

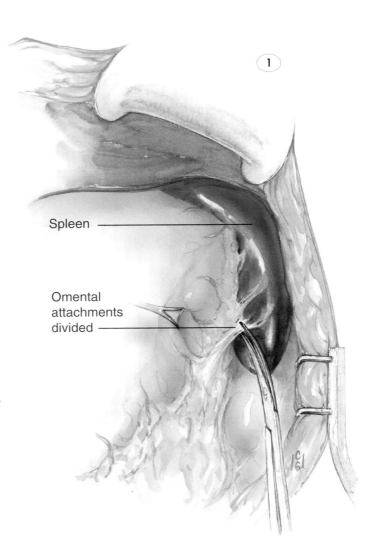

Spleen ——————

Omental
attachments
divided ——————

The lesser sac can be entered by going through the midportion of the omentum, but I prefer to take the omentum off of the transverse colon over towards the spleen, beginning in the mid-transverse colon (2). The junction of the omentum with the fat along the transverse colon is usually a relatively bloodless plane and can be divided with the electrocautery. This is carried out all the way over to the splenic flexure.

The splenic flexure of the colon is then mobilized by dividing the splenocolic ligament/attachments and retracting the splenic flexure inferiorly (3). Next the omentum anterior to the splenic hilum is divided between Kelly clamps and ligated with 2-0 silks (4). As one continues in a cephalad direction, the vasa brevia are encountered and can be divided along the greater curvature of the stomach (5). These vessels are clamped between Reinhoff clamps, divided, and ligated with 2-0 silks. As one divides the vasa brevia high on the stomach, long Reinhoff clamps can be helpful in a particularly deep-chested individual. The stomach can then be retracted medially either by using a thin Deaver retractor or by grasping the stomach with a Babcock clamp.

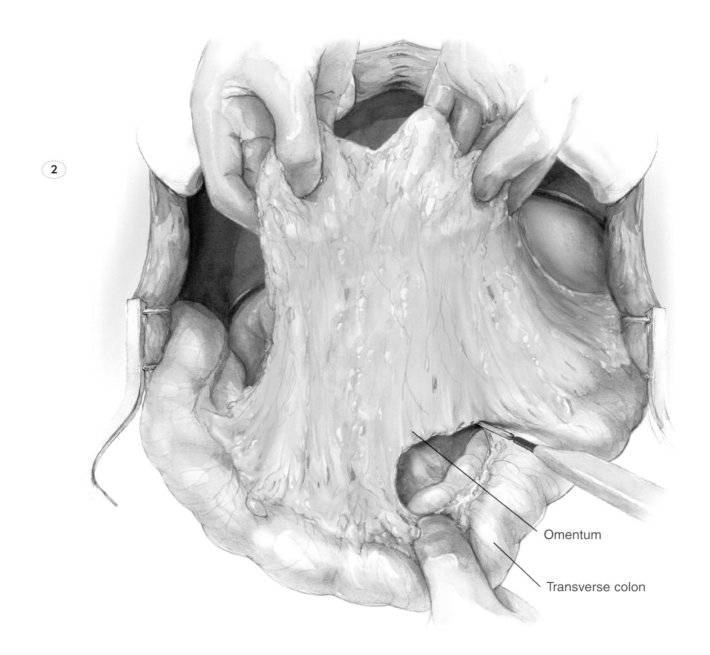

②

Omentum

Transverse colon

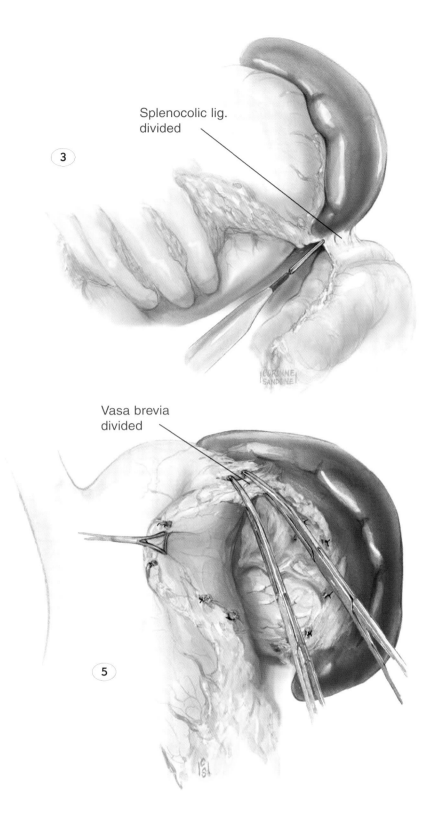

Splenocolic lig.
divided

3

Vasa brevia
divided

5

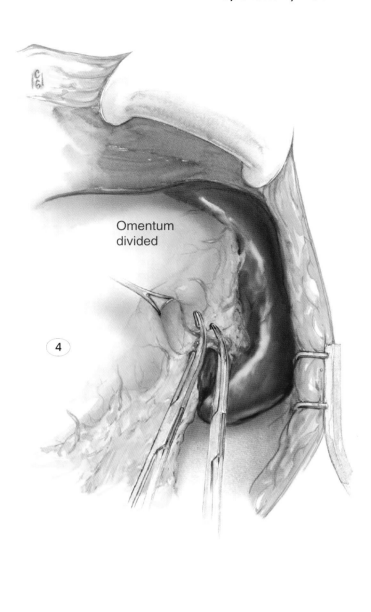

Omentum
divided

4

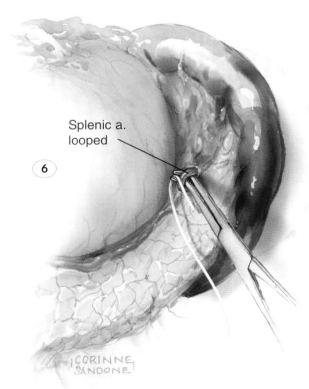

Splenic a.
looped

6

At this point, the body and tail of the pancreas are widely exposed in the lesser sac. It is often desirable to loop the splenic artery along the superior border of the mid-body of the pancreas. Generally, it is easily palpable and can be quickly mobilized and looped with a vessel loop (6). Subsequently, if one should get into troublesome bleeding during mobilization of the spleen, one can quickly clamp the splenic artery at this point with a DeBakey bulldog clamp.

Retroperitoneal
serosa divided

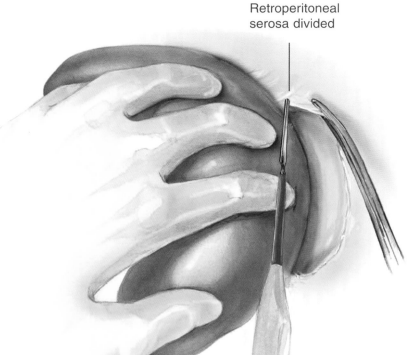

⑦

Next, the spleen can be mobilized out of the retroperitoneum. If the patient is obese or has an acute costal angle, and particularly if the patient has a deep thoracic cavity, this important part of the procedure can be very difficult. It is best accomplished by the surgeon placing the left hand on the spleen and retracting it medially, as if one is trying to compress it up against the spinal column. It is important not to retract anteriorly, as this can easily result in avulsing part of the splenic capsule. As the surgeon compresses the spleen medially, the assistant can lift up the retroperitoneal serosa with forceps, or with a long Reinhoff clamp, and the surgeon can incise the peritoneum close to the spleen with the electrocautery (7). An extension on the electrocautery often is helpful. This is obviously an important part of the procedure. If it is carried out along the entire length of the spleen, from the inferior border up to where the posterior aspect of the stomach is retroperitoneal, it will then allow free mobility of the entire spleen during the remainder of the procedure. At this point, the spleen and the tail of the pancreas can be elevated out of the retroperitoneum. This is a relatively bloodless plane. One has to be careful, however, not to injure the left adrenal gland, which is in close approximation to the superior aspect of the tail of the pancreas.

Once the spleen has been completely mobilized, the splenic vessels can then be divided. The splenic artery usually traverses along the superior aspect of the pancreas (8). One can either divide the main splenic artery at the splenic hilum, or separately ligate each of its branches. These are usually triply ligated with 2-0 silks and then divided. Occasionally, there is ample room between the tail of the pancreas and the splenic hilum so that vessel ligation can be easily carried out. Often, however, the tail of the pancreas seems to extend right into the splenic hilum, and one has to be very careful that the tail of the pancreas is not injured during this vessel ligation.

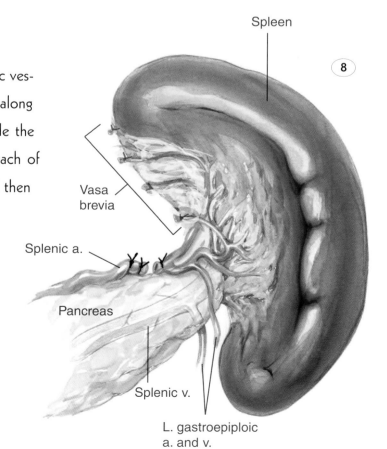

Spleen

⑧

Vasa
brevia

Splenic a.

Pancreas

Splenic v.

L. gastroepiploic
a. and v.

Division of the hilar vessels is the most challenging and potentially dangerous portion of the operation. Prior to this undertaking, blunt instruments should be used to ensure there is an adequate plane behind the splenic hilum. Then, sequential vascular load firings of a laparoscopic stapler are used to progressively divide the hilum adjacent to the spleen (5). Obviously, if untoward bleeding is encountered, rapid conversion to laparotomy may be necessary. If, however, less dramatic bleeding is encountered, a quick attempt can be made to control the bleeding by grasping a vessel with the laparoscopic instrument followed by control with either another stapler load or with another energy source. Care must be taken not to apply excessive heat or electrical energy to regions that already have clips. Doing so can affect those clips and precipitate post-operative bleeding.

5

Hilar vessels divided

6

Spleen

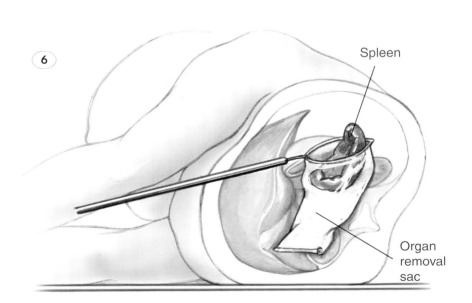

Organ removal sac

Once the splenic hilum is completely divided, it remains only for the surgeon to fully mobilize the spleen from the retroperitoneum and from the diaphragm. Once this is done, the spleen can be placed in an organ removal sac (6). The 12 mm auxiliary port is generally used for this purpose.

This incision is then enlarged to approximately one inch to allow removal of the spleen piecemeal with a ring forceps or other device (7). This wound is then closed, and the patient again undergoes laparoscopy. The surgical field is carefully examined for bleeding and for any sign of accessory spleens. If an accessory spleen is found, it should also be removed laparoscopically.

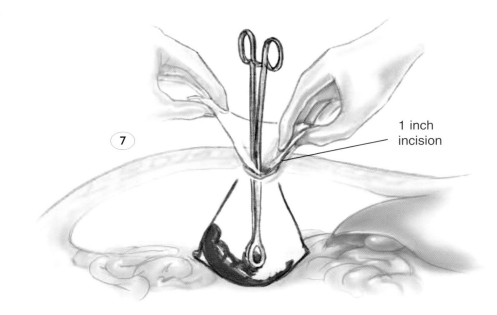

Spleen removed piecemeal from sac

Splenectomy for a Massive Spleen

Operative Indications:

There are a variety of situations when a splenectomy is required for a massively enlarged spleen. Myeloid metaplasia is perhaps the most notable. The potential for massive bleeding is much greater with a markedly enlarged spleen, but splenectomy may actually be easier than with a normal-sized spleen in a deep-chested or obese individual. Because of the massive enlargement, the spleen generally is no longer attached firmly to the retroperitoneum. It has become peritonealized. It can often be easily delivered out of the wound after opening the abdomen.

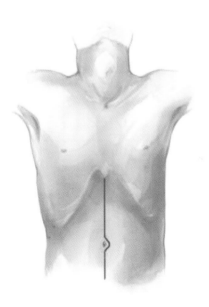

Operative Technique:

When performing a splenectomy in an individual with a normal-sized spleen, either an upper midline or left subcostal incision is appropriate. When performing a splenectomy for a massive spleen, a long midline incision should be used. It may be difficult to deliver the spleen through a shorter subcostal incision.

When the abdomen is entered, the spleen maybe mobile enough that it can be delivered up into the wound without the usual division of the retroperitoneum in the left upper quadrant (1).

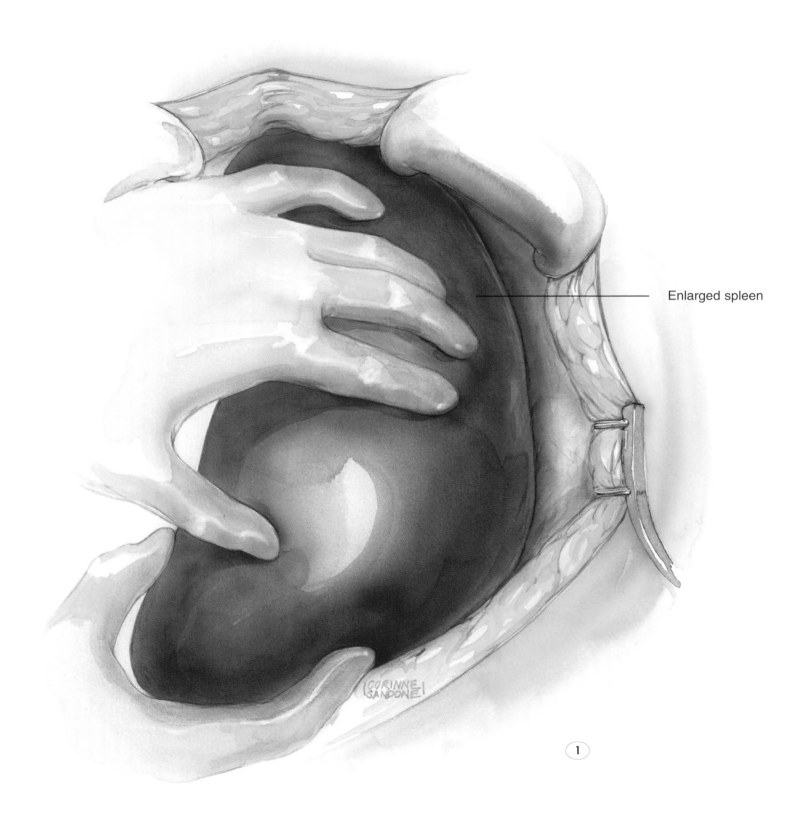

Enlarged spleen

1

If any bleeding continues, the argon beam coagulator is often helpful in further controlling such bleeding (9). A closed suction Silastic drain is left to this area (10), as much to protect against an unrecognized pancreatic tail injury as for drainage of the spleen.

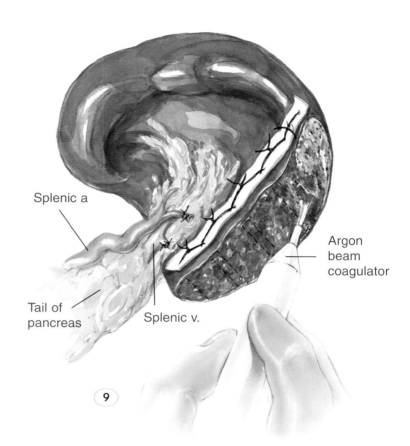

Splenic a

Tail of pancreas

Splenic v.

Argon beam coagulator

9

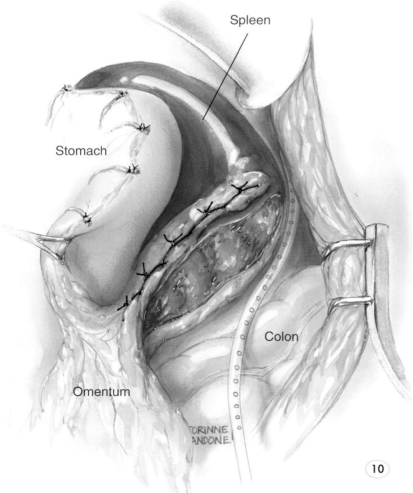

Spleen

Stomach

Colon

Omentum

10

Management of Splenic Trauma By Mesh Splenorrhaphy

Operative Indications:

Splenic salvage should be attempted when the splenic injury is isolated, and the patient is stable. If there are other organ injuries, or if the patient is unstable from blood loss from the splenic injury, splenic salvage generally should not be attempted. For many splenic injuries, hemostasis and salvage can be accomplished by a variety of hemostatic techniques or suture splenorrhaphy. In patients with lacerations that extend deep into the splenic hilum, a partial splenic resection may be required. A patient's spleen is rarely so macerated that the technique of using hemostatic agents, suture splenorrhaphy, or even partial resection are not sufficient to repair the badly injured spleen. A technique that is occasionally applicable to such patients is mesh splenorrhaphy. Since it is much more important to salvage a spleen in a young patient, this technique should only be applied when one is dealing with an otherwise young, healthy patient, who would be at risk for infections from encapsulated organisms if the spleen was removed.

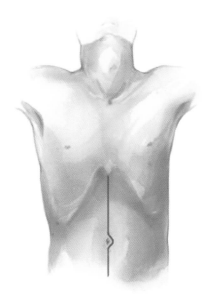

Operative Technique:

The patient is explored through a long midline incision. The entire abdomen is examined to rule out other injuries. If the only injury is to the spleen and the patient is relatively stable without evidence of great blood loss, splenic salvage can be attempted. In this instance, the spleen contains many lacerations through the capsule deep into the parenchyma, but the splenic hilum is intact. The lesser sac is entered by removing the omentum from the left transverse colon. The omentum is further divided anterior to the hilum of the spleen between Kelly clamps and is ligated with 2-0 silks. The splenic artery is then identified along the superior border of the body and the tail of the pancreas,

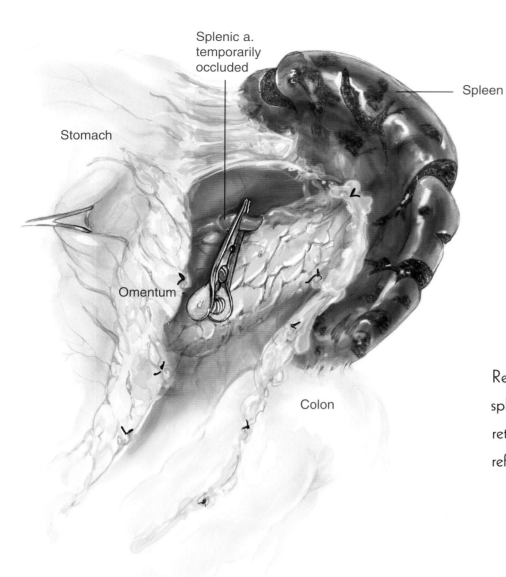

Splenic a.
temporarily
occluded

Spleen

Stomach

Omentum

Colon

mobilized, and clamped temporarily with a bulldog clamp (1). This, along with wrapping the spleen with a Mikulicz's pad and applying pressure with the hand, achieves adequate temporary hemostasis. The vasa brevia can then be further divided between Reinhoff clamps and ligated with 2-0 silks. The spleen is then completely mobilized out of the retroperitoneum by dividing the lateral peritoneal reflections (2).

1

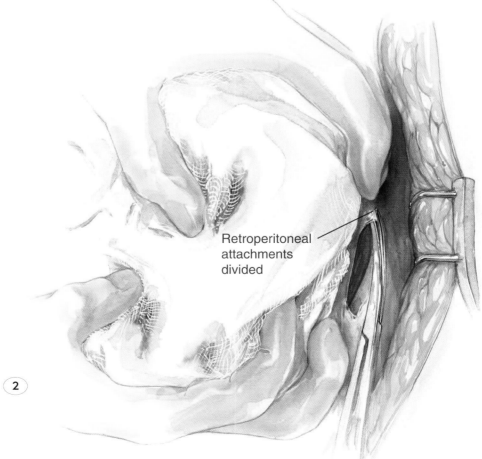

Retroperitoneal
attachments
divided

2

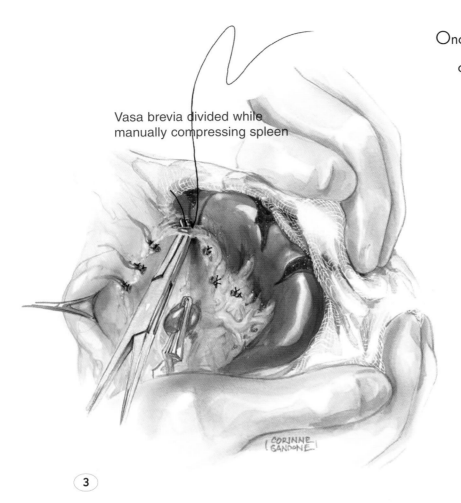

Vasa brevia divided while manually compressing spleen

CORINNE SANDONE

3

Once the spleen is completely mobilized so that it can be delivered up into the wound, the remaining vasa brevia are ligated and divided (3). At this point, the spleen is completely mobilized from all surrounding attachments and is connected only by its vessels in the splenic hilum to the tail of the pancreas.

A sheet of synthetic absorbable polyglycolic acid mesh is then wrapped around the spleen and gathered together at the splenic hilum (4). The mesh is elastic, and one can compress the splenic parenchyma evenly by placing a purse string around the splenic hilum, gathering all the mesh together under tension (5). This compression can be very effective in achieving hemostasis. One has to be certain, however, to not compress either the

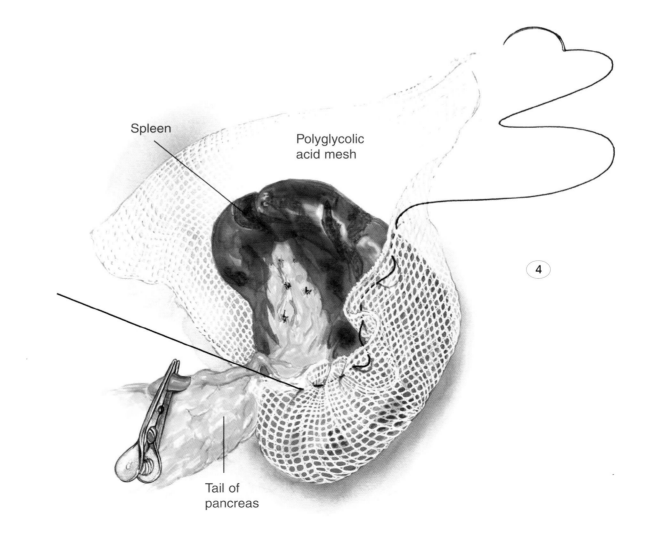

Spleen

Polyglycolic acid mesh

4

Tail of pancreas

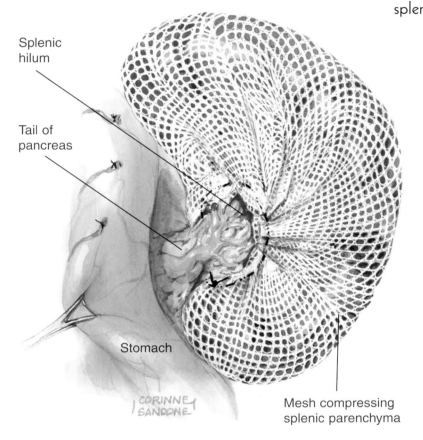

Splenic
hilum

Tail of
pancreas

Stomach

CORINNE
SANDONE

Mesh compressing
splenic parenchyma

splenic artery or splenic vein with the purse string. Before clos-
ing the patient, one has to remove the bulldog clamp from
the splenic artery and be absolutely certain that adequate hemostasis has been achieved. If this technique
is not effective, then one needs to proceed with
splenectomy which, at this point, will obviously
only take a few minutes as only the hilar vessels
remain. The patient needs to be watched carefully
postoperatively for evidence of bleeding. If hemostasis is achieved in the operating room, late bleeding is distinctly unusual, even with this technique.
Prior to discharge, the patient should be vaccinated
against the various encapsulated organisms.

Drainage of Splenic Abscess

Operative Indications:

Splenic abscesses are rare. They may be seen in patients with endocarditis or, perhaps more commonly today, intravenous drug abusers. They may, however, accompany a wide variety of disorders. If the splenic abscess is relatively small and the perisplenic inflammation not intense, the lesion should probably be treated by a splenectomy. In some instances, where the spleen is enlarged and there is substantial perisplenic inflammation with adhesions, splenectomy might be quite difficult in an ill patient. Under such circumstances, draining the splenic abscess is acceptable. Generally, this should be performed open rather than percutaneously to decrease the obvious risk of hemorrhage.

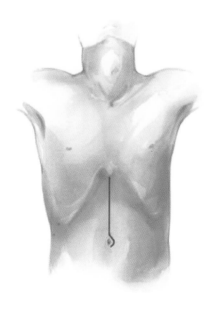

Operative Technique:

The patient is explored through either a midline or left subcostal incision. The abdomen is examined to rule out other pathology. The left upper quadrant is exposed, and the enlarged spleen palpated. Generally, the area of fluctuance is easily identified.

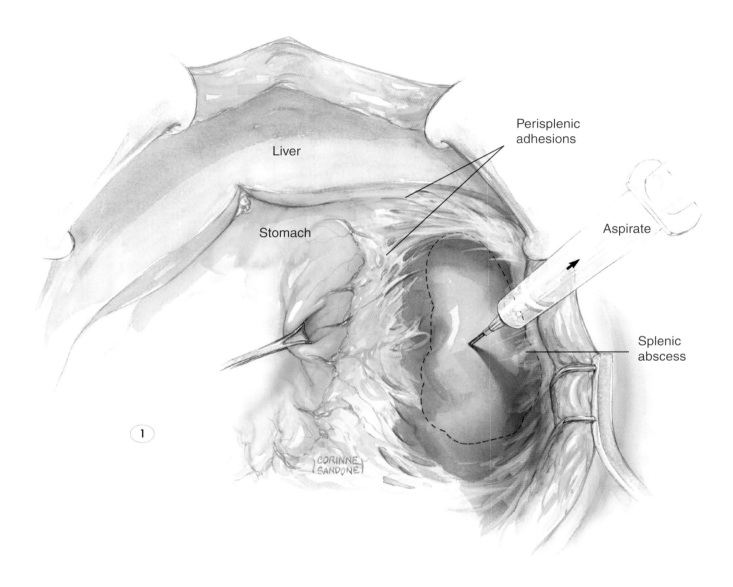

The location of the splenic abscess can be confirmed with intraoperative ultrasound or by aspirating with a 20-gauge needle on a 10-ml syringe (1).

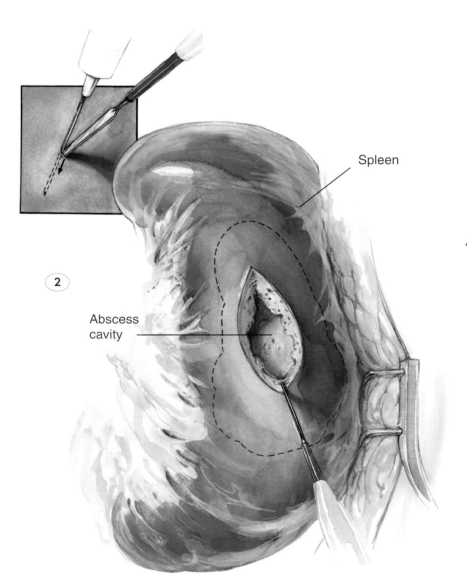

Spleen

2

Abscess
cavity

After its location has been identified, using an electrocautery and cutting down along the needle, the abscess cavity is entered (2). The splenic cavity is copiously irrigated with an antibiotic solution. Silastic closed suction drains are left in the abscess cavity and brought out through stab wounds in the left upper quadrant (3).

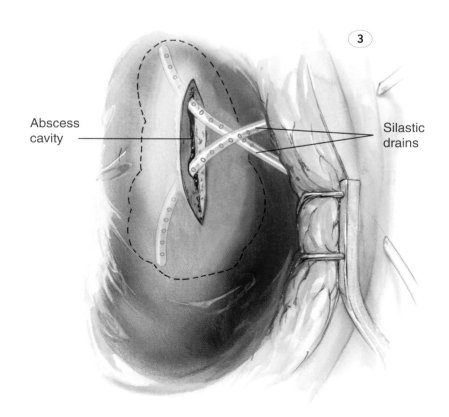

3

Abscess
cavity

Silastic
drains

THE ESOPHAGUS

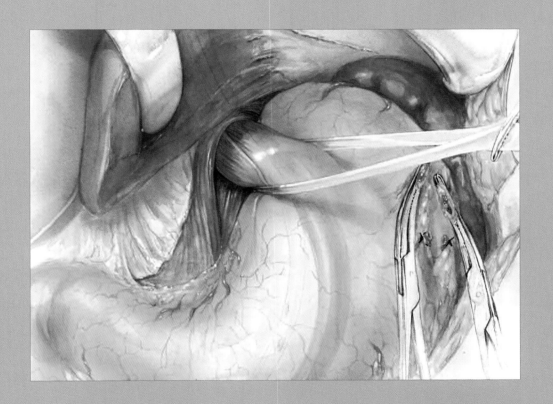

Antireflux Surgery—An Overview

The understanding and management of gastroesophageal reflux have evolved substantially over the past several decades. Symptoms previously associated with this entity were thought to be secondary to an anatomic defect, the hiatus hernia. The esophagus enters the abdomen through the esophageal hiatus, created by the crura of the right leaf of the diaphragm. The esophageal hiatus is anterior and slightly to the right of the aortic hiatus, and anterior and to the left of the inferior vena cava (1). Many factors can lead to the gastroesophageal junction sliding up into the mediastinum, pulling part of the peritoneum with it anteriorly. This translocation produces a sliding hiatal hernia (2), the posterior aspect of which is devoid of a peritoneal sac, and consists of the retroperitoneum. Patients with a hiatal hernia frequently have gastroesophageal reflux. The majority of patients with these hernias, however, do not have clinically significant reflux. In addition, many patients with gastroesophageal reflux do not have this anatomic abnormality. Although gastroesophageal reflux and a hiatal hernia are often associated, the correlation is not absolute. In addition, the clinical syndrome is caused by gastroesophageal reflux and the resulting esophagitis, and generally not by the anatomic abnormality. Gastroesophageal reflux is now known to result from an incompetent lower esophageal high-pressure zone or lower esophageal sphincter. When the sphincter is incompetent, gastric acid refluxes into the esophagus producing esophagitis and a variety of symptoms, including heartburn, retrosternal discomfort, regurgitation, and vomiting.

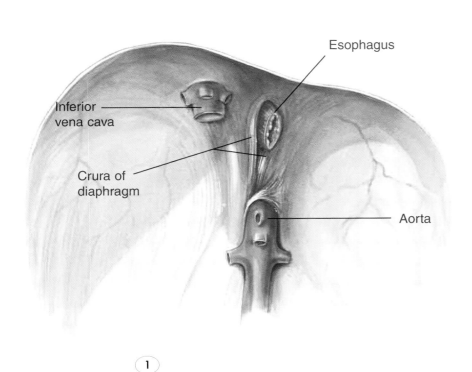

Esophagus

Inferior vena cava

Crura of diaphragm

Aorta

1

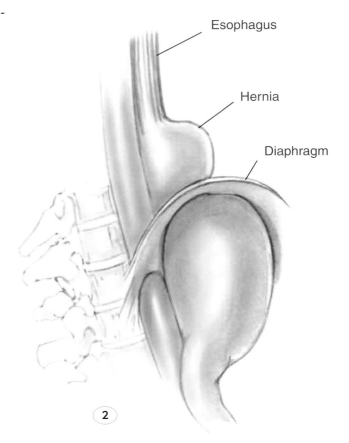

Esophagus

Hernia

Diaphragm

2

NISSEN

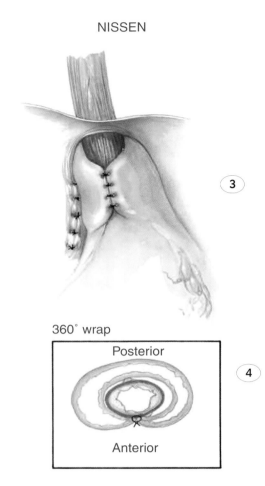

3

360° wrap

4

Three basic surgical repairs have gained popularity over the past three decades in treating symptoms of gastroesophageal reflux that are refractory to medical management. All three techniques correct the anatomic defect of the hiatal hernia (if present), but more importantly, all three are effective in creating a competent lower esophageal sphincter. The Nissen fundoplication (3) can be performed through either the abdomen or chest but is usually performed through the abdomen. The hernia is reduced, the crura are re-approximated, and the fundus is wrapped circumferentially around the intra-abdominal esophagus. This results in a 360° wrap of the intra-abdominal esophagus with the gastric fundus (4).

TOUPET

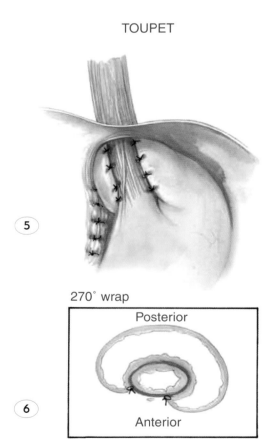

5

270° wrap

6

The Toupet procedure is a variant of the Nissen fundoplication, and differs in that the fundus is partially wrapped 270°s posteriorly around the esophagus (5, 6). This operation is also done through the abdomen. The Toupet procedure is usually reserved for those patients with altered esophageal motility.

Finally, the Belsey Mark IV procedure is performed through the chest. In this operation, the fundus is wrapped around the anterior and lateral aspects of the esophagus for approximately 270°, with the most posterior aspect of the esophagus remaining unwrapped (7, 8). All three repairs are similar in that the hernia is reduced, the crura are closed posterior to the esophagus, the distal segment of the esophagus is positioned intra-abdominally, and the air-filled gastric fundus with its positive pressure is positioned adjacent to the intra-abdominal portion of the esophagus to create a sphincter.

Classically, the Nissen and Toupet procedures have been performed through laparotomy incisions. More recently, these procedures have been performed using a laparoscopic or robotic approach. Though the Belsey Mark IV procedure can be performed using a thoracoscopic approach, this technique has not gained wide acceptance. The indications for laparoscopic treatment of gastroesophageal reflux are the same as those for the open procedures. This technique requires a well trained operating team familiar with the equipment, instruments and techniques of antireflux surgery. Minimally invasive techniques appear to be associated with shorter hospital stays and return to normal activities.

BELSEY

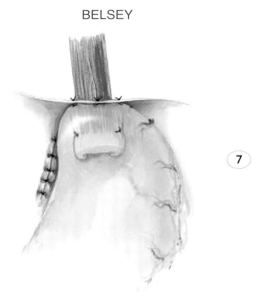

7

270° wrap

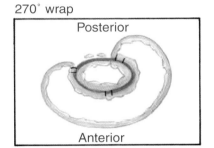

Posterior

Anterior

8

Nissen Fundoplication

Operative Indications

The Nissen fundoplication is the most commonly performed antireflux operation for patients with gastroesophageal reflux refractory to medical management. The majority of patients with symptomatic gastroesophageal reflux can be managed on a regimen of weight reduction, acid suppression, and elevation of the head of the bed. Some patients, however, continue to have symptoms after a trial of nonoperative management that are troubling enough to warrant surgical intervention. Other indications for fundoplication include complications of esophageal acid exposure such as a stricture or Barrett's esophagus.

Before considering surgical intervention, patients should have a thorough workup. Since gastroesophageal reflux can be easily confused with other disorders, one must be absolutely certain that the symptoms are secondary to reflux before performing an antireflux procedure. All patients should undergo acid reflux testing with a pH probe to be certain that gastroesophageal reflux is present. A Bernstein test is also helpful and is performed by instilling acid into the distal esophagus, thereby reproducing the patient's symptoms. This test clearly targets the distal esophagus as the source of the patient's symptoms. Most patients should also undergo endoscopy before having surgery. Barium studies are also frequently performed, more often to rule out other processes than to diagnose gastroesophageal reflux. A video esophagogram not only provides details of the anatomy of the esophagogastric junction, but also provides functional information on esophageal motility.

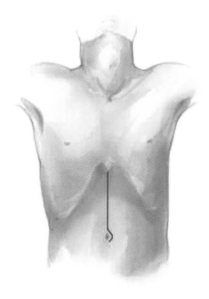

Operative Technique

The Nissen fundoplication can be performed either transthoracically or transabdominally. The transabdominal approach is utilized more frequently than the transthoracic approach. It is depicted here performed through an upper midline incision. Retraction of both costal margins by retractors suspended from a frame attached to the operating room table is particularly helpful. After the abdomen is entered, the peritoneal cavity is carefully explored. Since other diseases can be confused with gastroesophageal reflux, other abdominal pathology should be excluded. After that has been accomplished, the hiatal hernia is reduced and the esophagus is mobilized by opening up the peritoneum anterior to the esophagus. There is usually a variable amount of hernia sac that needs to be resected. Care is taken not to be too aggressive with the dissection above the esophageal hiatus to avoid entering the pleural spaces.

Using both blunt and sharp dissection, the esophagus is carefully mobilized and encircled with a Penrose drain. Both vagus nerves should be mobilized along with the esophagus. During this dissection, the two crura of the esophageal hiatus should be carefully dissected and defined. The gastrohepatic ligament is divided, and a portion of the lesser curvature next to the gastroesophageal junction is cleaned by dividing branches of the left gastric artery. The greater curvature of the stomach is mobilized by dividing a variable number of vasa brevia (1). The vasa brevia are divided beginning at a point high on the greater curvature and extending up to the gastroesophageal junction. The fundus of the stomach is then mobilized posteriorly out of the retroperitoneum. This dissection can often be done without mobilizing the left lobe of the liver, by merely retracting it in a cephalad direction. Occasionally, however, as depicted here, the triangular ligament and attachments of the lateral segment of the left lobe of the liver are mobilized, folded down, and retracted medially, to achieve optimal exposure of the hiatus.

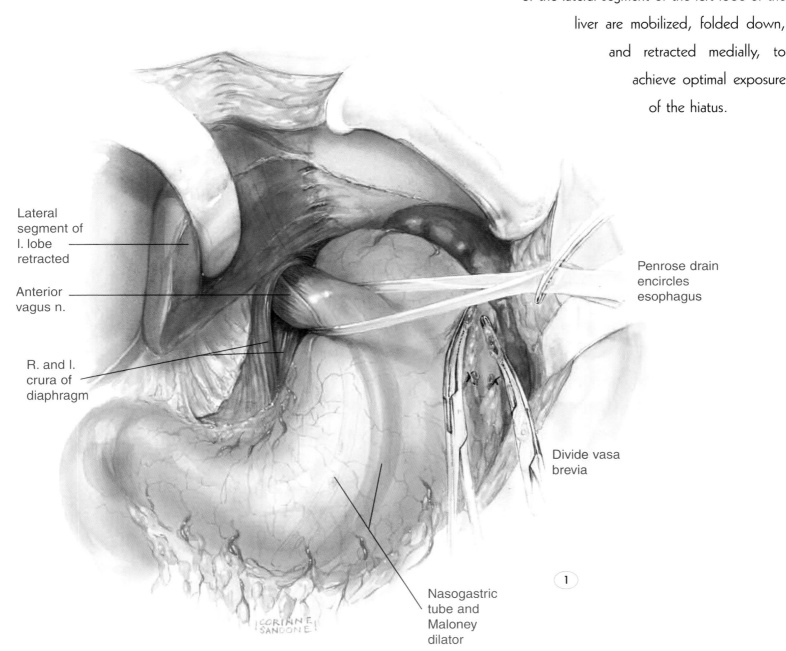

Lateral segment of l. lobe retracted

Anterior vagus n.

R. and l. crura of diaphragm

Penrose drain encircles esophagus

Divide vasa brevia

Nasogastric tube and Maloney dilator

1

A series of interrupted 0-silk sutures on large Ferguson needles are placed through the two crura of the diaphragm. A nasogastric tube is in place. Before the crural sutures are secured, a 46 French Maloney dilator is passed into the stomach. Generally five or six crural sutures are placed to snug the hiatus around the esophagus (2). They should be tied inferiorly, in a cephalad direction, so that the hiatus is snug around the esophagus containing the nasogastric tube and dilator.

Crura approximated

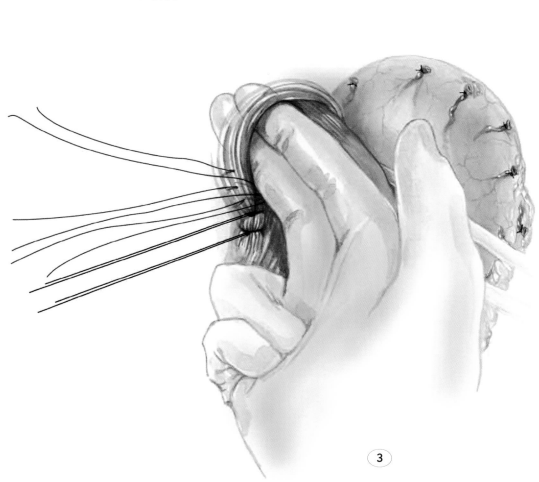

②

An alternate method, not using the Maloney dilator, is to be certain that two fingers can be accommodated in the hiatus after the crura are approximated (3).

③

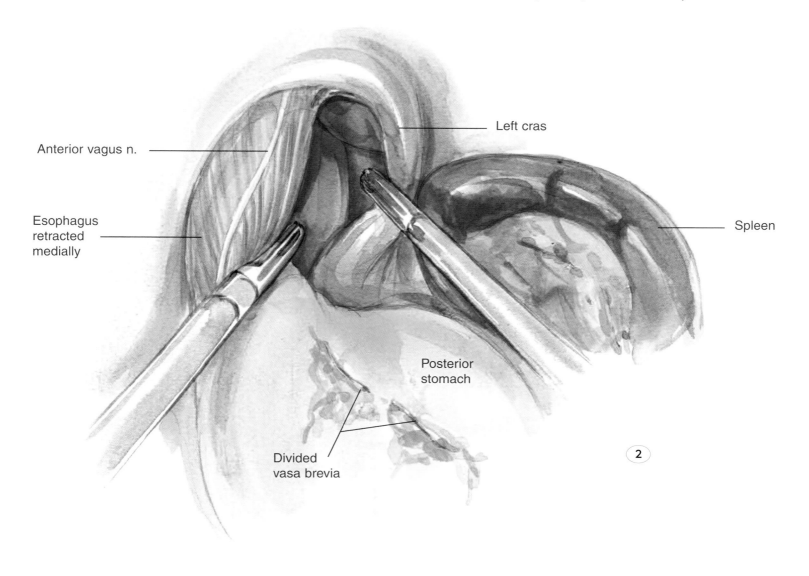

Anterior vagus n.

Left cras

Esophagus
retracted
medially

Spleen

Posterior
stomach

Divided
vasa brevia

(2)

At this point, the angle of His, the gastroesophageal junction, and the distal esophagus are
carefully dissected free. The surgeon begins this
retro-esophageal dissection from the left-hand side.
The more that can be safely accomplished from this
side during this portion of the procedure, the
easier the dissection will subsequently
be when dissecting from the right.

Next, the lesser sac is
opened from the right by dividing the filmy gastrohepatic ligament with the hook cautery
(3). This is initiated in a clear
spot where the tissue can be
safely divided.

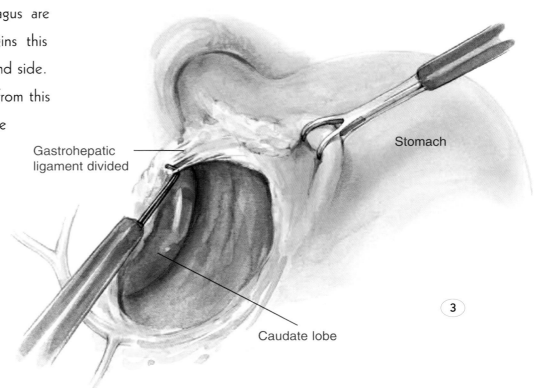

Gastrohepatic
ligament divided

Stomach

Caudate lobe

(3)

Retraction of the stomach to the left reveals the caudate lobe of the liver, the right crus of the diaphragm, and the posterior esophagus. The anterior (left) vagus nerve and its branches are often visible at this juncture. Care must be taken during this dissection to avoid inadvertent division of a replaced left hepatic artery. When this anomaly occurs (4), the primary arterial blood flow to the left lobe of the liver traverses this tissue.

The dissection is carried from this point anteriorly to release the anterior esophageal tissue from the arch of the crus. The anterior vagus nerve can be seen at this point, usually directly on the surface of the anterior esophagus. As the dissection is continued posteriorly (5), the stomach is lifted in an anterior direction. Dissecting only tissue that is filmy and safe, the surgeon can work posterior to the gastroesophageal junction and completely encircle it by connecting to the dissection previously performed along the left side of the esophagus.

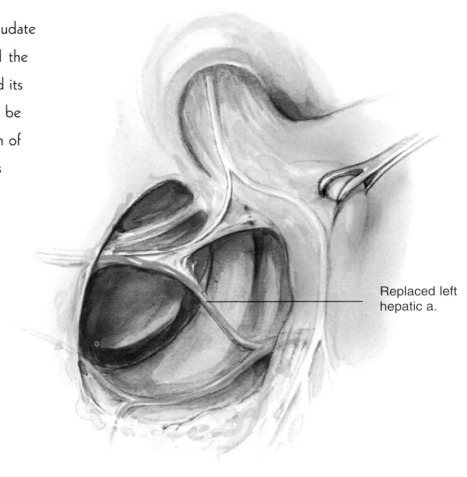

Replaced left
hepatic a.

4

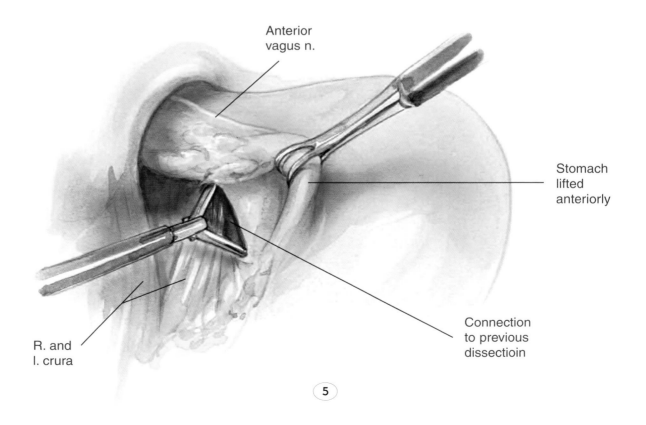

Anterior
vagus n.

Stomach
lifted
anteriorly

Connection
to previous
dissectioin

R. and
l. crura

5

An umbilical tape or Penrose drain is placed around the gastroesophageal junction (6) and locked with an endoloop. This provides a handle for retraction of the gastroesophageal junction in all directions (7). This dissection also allows the surgeon to clearly identify the anterior and posterior vagus nerves and to mobilize a significant length of intra-abdominal esophagus (5 to 7 cm).

With the gastroesophageal junction isolated and elevated, both the right and left crura should be visible behind the stomach, looking from the patient's right side toward the left. Tissue around the crura is carefully dissected away revealing the point where the crura come together. Care must be taken with this dissection, as the aorta is immediately deep to the crura. The gastroesophageal junction is then retracted to the patient's left, and the laparoscope moved to the patient's right. The angulation of the scope is adjusted so that the view is from the left. From this perspective, the left crus is further dissected away from the esophagus (7), creating additional intra-abdominal length.

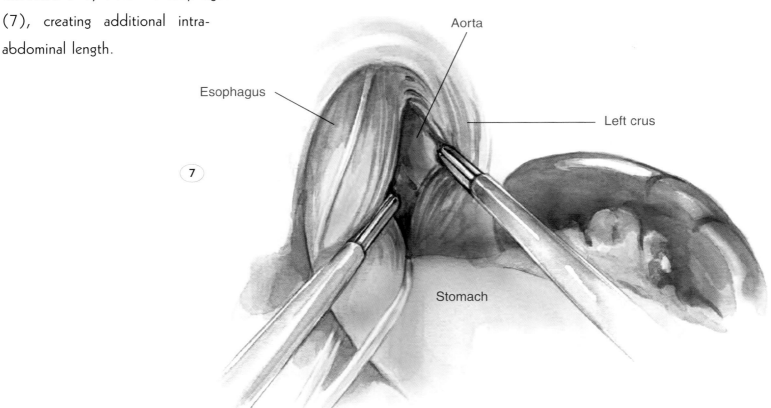

Esophagus encircled

R. and l. crura

⑥

Aorta

Esophagus

⑦

Left crus

Stomach

The next objective is closure of the crura. Many surgeons advocate the placement of a sizer passed by the anesthesiologist, either an inflatable orogastric tube or a Maloney dilator, within the esophagus to help judge how tightly the diaphragmatic crura should be closed. Teflon pledgets are usually used to buttress the crural closure (8). The sutures are placed laparoscopically and tied either intracorporeally or extracorporeally. With the sizer in place, the crura are approximated until closed snugly around the esophagus. One should check the adequacy of the crural closure by visualizing the amount of space anterior to the esophagus and the arch of the crura. If there is too much space, another stitch should be placed. If the anterior esophagus is impinged by the arch of the crura, the closure is too tight.

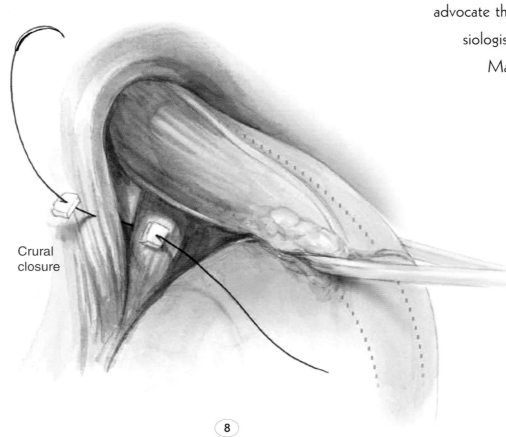

Crural closure

8

With the crural closure accomplished, the wrap is constructed. The gastroesophageal junction is once again retracted anteriorly and an atraumatic grasper is carefully placed behind the esophagus from left to right. The posterior fundus is then grasped, and pulled posterior to the esophagus (9). This should be carried out under direct vision by placing the angled telescope behind the gastroesophageal junction to view the posterior fundus. In some obese individuals, this can be very difficult. In these circumstances, the fundus can be "pushed" from the left side to the right side, or a suture can be placed in the

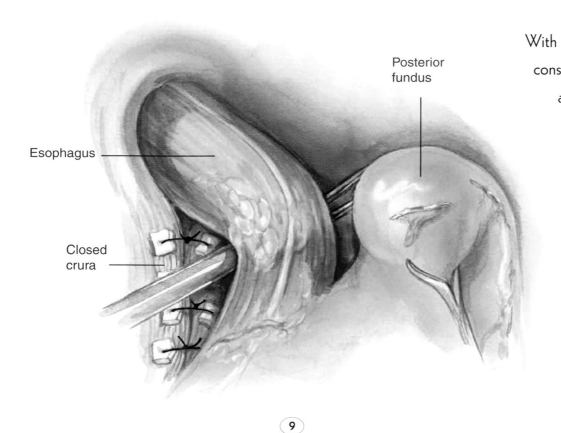

Esophagus

Closed crura

Posterior fundus

9

posterior fundus on the left side which is then passed posterior and used to pull the posterior fundus around to the patient's right side. With the posterior fundus in position, a spot on the anterior fundus on the patient's left is chosen, which will create an appropriately floppy esophageal wrap.

With the posterior fundus on the right of the esophagus and the anterior fundus on the left, each held by atraumatic graspers, the wrap is "rocked" back and forth to be sure it is not twisted, or too tight, or too loose.

The sutures are then placed, with pledgets. Each bite also includes a superficial bite of anterior esophagus to help avoid "slipping" of the fundoplication (10). Usually the fundoplication is constructed with three or four stitches, each approximately 1 cm apart, to create a wrap 3 to 5 cm in length (11). Following construction of the wrap, the sizer is removed from the esophagus. The abdomen is examined laparoscopically for bleeding, tissue injury, or other problems, prior to removal of trocars and closure of port sites.

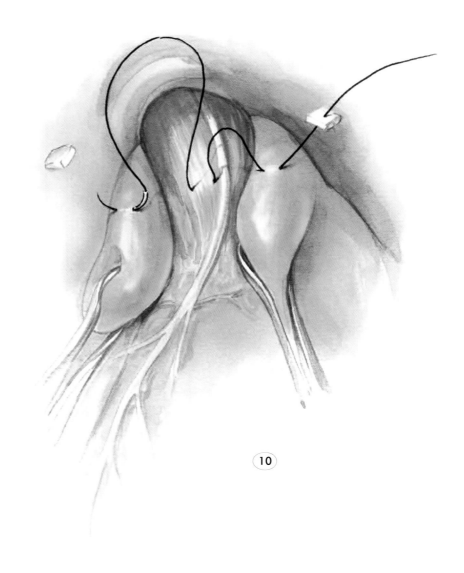

10

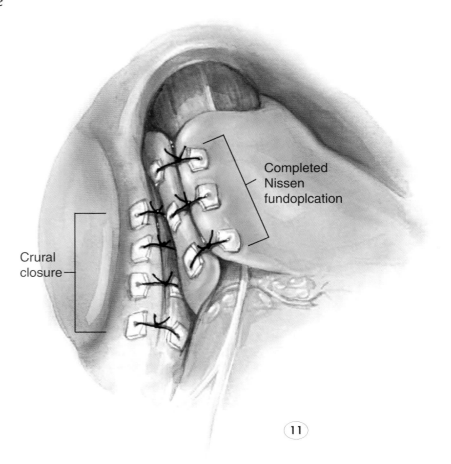

Completed
Nissen
fundoplcation

Crural
closure

11

Toupet Fundoplication: Open and Laparoscopic

Operative Indications

The Toupet procedure was proposed in 1963 when the Nissen fundoplication was emerging as the preferred approach for the surgical treatment of gastroesophageal reflux. Indications and evaluation are similar to that for any antireflux procedure, however, most feel that the Toupet method should be reserved for those patients with weak esophageal motility to avoid postoperative dysphagia since the wrap is only 270° rather than circumferential.

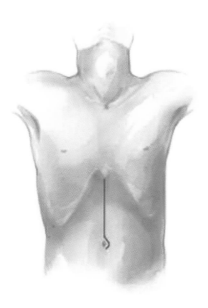

Operative Technique

Open Technique

The preparation, position and exposure are similar to that described previously for the Nissen fundoplication. The procedure is performed through an upper midline incision and can be broken down into three main steps. The first is reduction of the hiatal hernia and mobilization of the abdominal esophagus. Similar to the Nissen, the esophageal hiatus is exposed by dividing the left triangular ligament of the liver with electrocautery, and dividing the peritoneum overlying the esophagus. The diaphragmatic crura are mobilized away from the esophagus, and a long right-angle clamp is used to pass a Penrose drain around the back side of the distal esophagus to facilitate downward retraction. The esophagogastric junction is inspected and the two vagus nerves identified.

The second step involves mobilization of the posterior fundus. This is performed in the same fashion as for the Nissen fundoplication. The important maneuver is to expose the inferior aspect of both diaphragmatic crura. The mobilization is completed by dividing the phrenogastric ligament. The preaortic adhesions between the peritoneal fold of the left gastric artery and the inferior aspect of the esophageal hiatus fixing the fundus are divided with great care. By doing so, the posterior aspect of the fundus can be pulled behind the esophagus.

The final step is the esophagogastroplasty with phrenogastropexy. The posterior aspect of the fundus is pulled behind the esophagus carefully with a Babcock clamp or pushed manually from the patient's left to right. The vagus nerves are identified, taking care not to incorporate them in the sutures. The fundus is fixed first to the right border of the esophagus with interrupted 2-0 silk sutures (1). The fundus is then fixed to the right crus of the diaphragm with four or five sutures. The superior suture incorporates the esophagus, the fundus, and the crus. The lowest suture fixes the fundus to the aortic fibrous orifice and should be placed without tension (2).

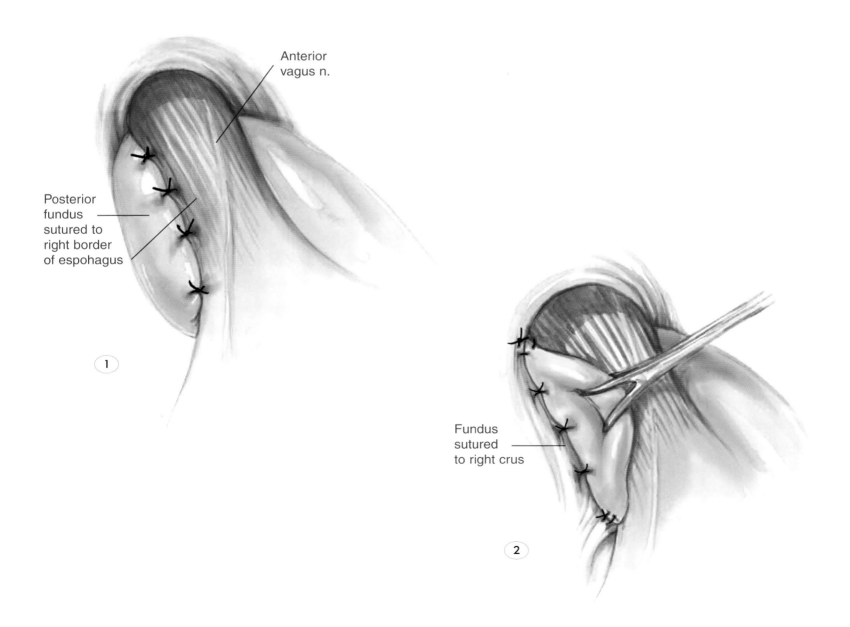

Anterior
vagus n.

Posterior
fundus
sutured to
right border
of espohagus

1

Fundus
sutured
to right crus

2

This same technique is used on the left side with the same number of sutures approximating the fundus to the left crus of the diaphragm (3), starting with the inferior suture. Then the left border of the esophagus is attached to the fundus (4). The procedure is completed by suturing the superior aspect of the fundus to the phrenoesophageal membrane. The enlarged esophageal hiatus can be closed with O-silk sutures on a large Ferguson needle over a 46 French Maloney dilator and nasogastric tube, as with the Nissen fundoplication.

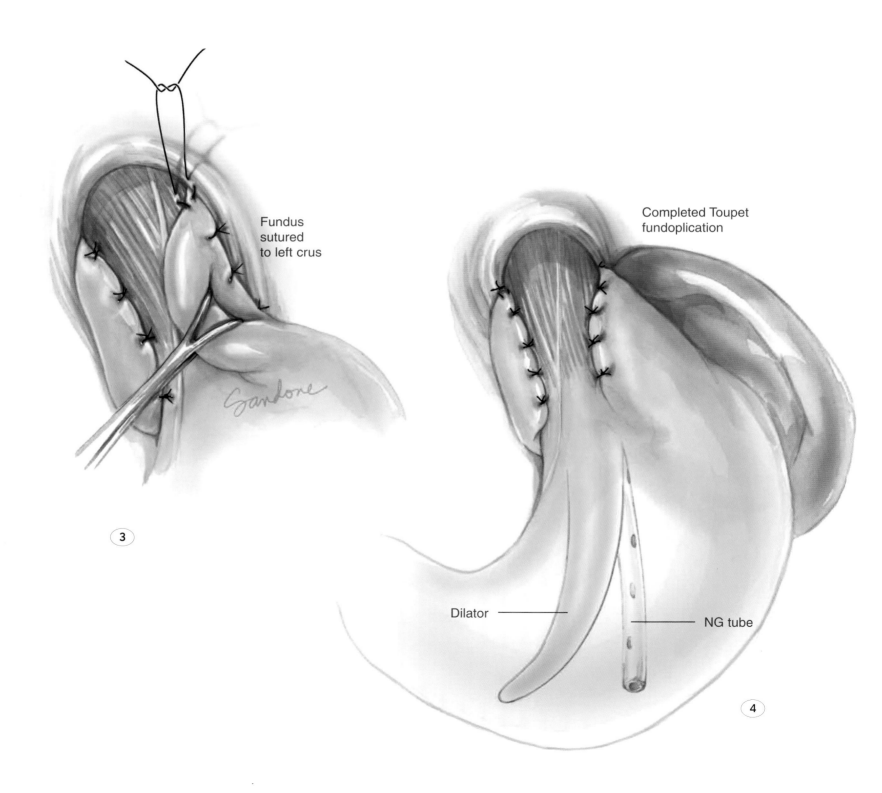

Fundus
sutured
to left crus

Completed Toupet
fundoplication

Dilator

NG tube

3

4

Laparoscopic Technique

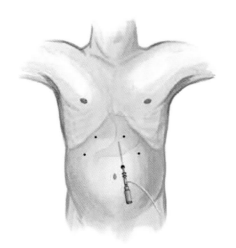

The patient is placed in the prone position with arms on arm boards. The appropriate site for the camera port is approximately 16 cm caudal to the xiphoid process and 3 to 4 cm to the left of the patient's midline. With a 30° angled laparoscope, this position affords the best opportunity to view the esophagus from both sides and from behind when necessary. In order to obtain such a position, the site can be accessed directly using the Hasson technique. Alternatively, a simple stab just above the umbilicus can be used to place a Veress needle carefully at the umbilicus, which is the safest spot for blind placement of the Veress needle. Once the abdomen is insufflated, the patient is placed in a fairly steep reverse Trendelenburg's position. It is important to make the appropriate measurements and mark potential port sites after this has been accomplished because the abdominal dimensions change, and the surface anatomy is altered relative to bony structures.

A measurement is made 16 cm caudal to the xiphoid process and 3 to 4 cm to the left of midline for insertion of the laparoscope. An auxiliary 5-mm port for retraction of the left lateral segment of the liver is generally placed in the anterior axillary line at the right costal margin. Two prime operative ports are placed fairly high along each costal margin on the right and left side. Finally, an additional working laparoscopic port is placed in the anterior axillary line slightly below the left costal margin.

Initially, the abdomen is explored for other pathology. The left lobe of the liver is lifted anteriorly to expose the esophageal hiatus. The gastrohepatic ligament is divided using electrocautery. Any hiatal hernia is reduced with downward traction after incising the peritoneal covering. The right crus of the diaphragm is identified and dissected down to its confluence with the left crus. Using blunt dissection, a space posterior to the esophagus is created. The esophagus is encircled with a Penrose drain, retracted downward and further mobilized to allow a 3- to 4-cm segment of intra-abdominal esophagus.

The enlarged esophageal hiatus can be closed with 0 silk. A 46 French Maloney dilator and nasogastric tube within the esophagus help judge how tightly the diaphragmatic crura should be closed. Teflon pledgets are usually used to buttress the crural closure. The sutures are placed laparoscopically and tied either intracorporeally or extracorporeally.

The 270° posterior wrap is constructed by pulling the posterior fundus of the stomach around behind the esophagus with an atraumatic grasper. The fundus is then sutured laparoscopically to the crus on the right, using pledgets (5). Similarly, the anterior fundus of the stomach is sutured to the left crus, using pledgets (6). Once these are secured, each side of the fundus of the stomach is sutured to the anterolateral aspect of the esophagus (7). In combination, these sutures anchor the 270° wrap (8).

The nasogastric tube is left in place and the abdomen is examined laparoscopically for bleeding, tissue injury, or other problems, prior to removal of trocars and closure of port sites.

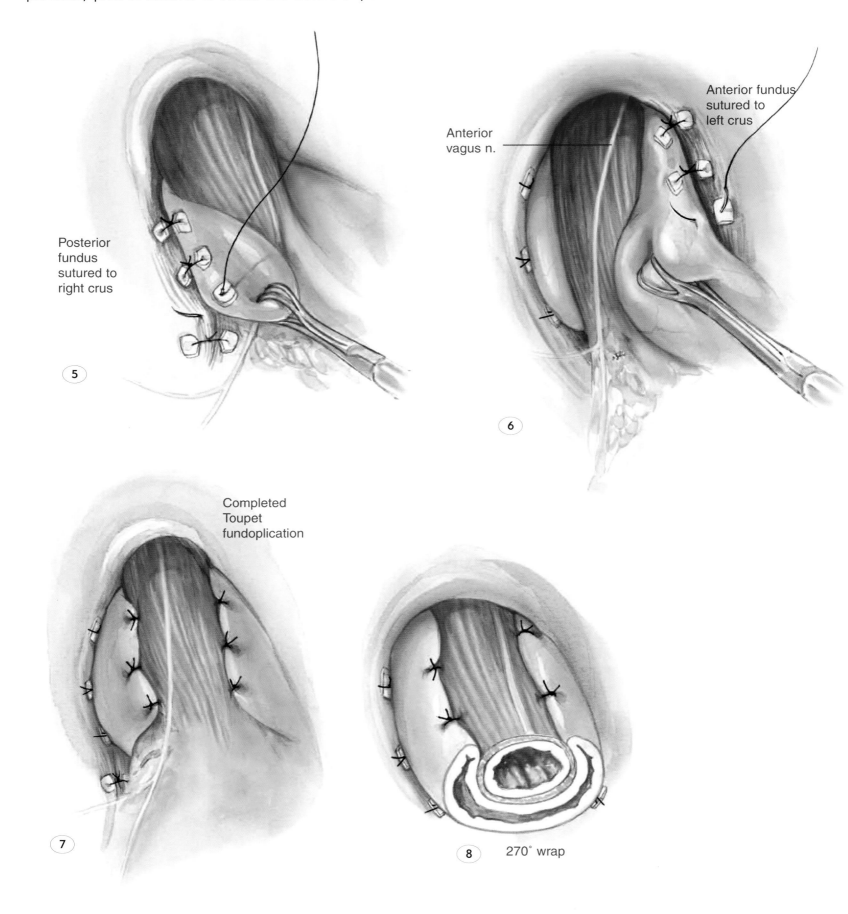

Posterior fundus sutured to right crus

5

Anterior vagus n.

Anterior fundus sutured to left crus

6

Completed Toupet fundoplication

7

8   270° wrap

Belsey Mark IV Antireflux Procedure

Operative Indications

The Belsey Mark IV antireflux procedure is a surgical option for patients with gastroesophageal reflux refractory to medical management. The majority of patients with symptomatic gastroesophageal reflux can be managed with antacids, weight reduction, and elevation of the head of the bed. However, some patients even with this regimen continue to have bothersome symptoms warranting surgical intervention. Because gastroesophageal reflux can mimic other disorders, patients should have a thorough workup to be certain that their symptoms are secondary to reflux. All patients should undergo acid reflux testing with an esophageal pH probe, the Bernstein test infusing acid into the distal esophagus, and endoscopy. Barium studies are also generally indicated; if video esophagography is available, it can often reveal the functional quality of the esophagus. A circumferential wrap should be avoided in the presence of abnormal esophageal function.

Since this procedure is performed through the chest, one should be certain that no abdominal pathology is present that requires management at the same time as the antireflux procedure is performed. Such a finding would preclude a transthoracic approach. However, a transthoracic approach may be the preferred option for several reasons. In patients who have had prior antireflux surgery through an abdominal approach, often the gastric fundus is fixed in the mediastinum with adhesions and thus direct visualization is necessary to release them. Another concern is shortening of the esophagus such that the gastroesophageal junction will not reduce easily into the abdomen; in this situation, the esophagus needs to be visualized so it can be mobilized up to the level of the aortic arch. Finally, patients who have undergone partial gastric resections are not good candidates for other antireflux procedures performed through the abdomen; the Belsey Mark IV antireflux procedure is appropriate for this situation.

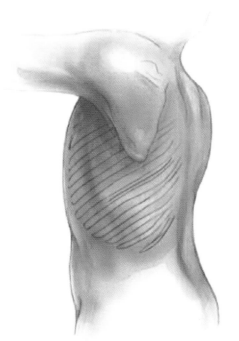

Operative Technique

A left lateral thoracotomy is performed through the seventh or eighth intercostal space.

The intercostal muscles are divided along the anterior surface of the rib (1). The ribs are separated with a self-retaining retractor. The inferior pulmonary ligament is mobilized up to the inferior pulmonary vein. The mediastinal pleura is opened (2) and the esophagus and hiatus hernia, if present, are identified by palpating for the previously placed nasogastric tube. It is often difficult to distinguish the mediastinal pleura and the hernia sac, especially if a prior fundoplication was performed.

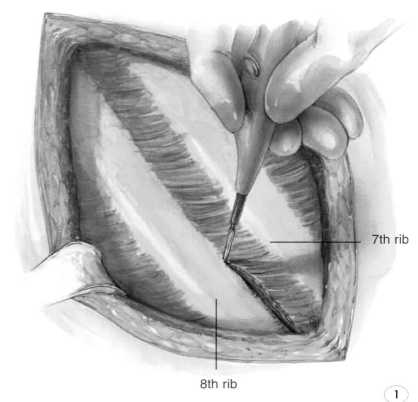

7th rib

8th rib

①

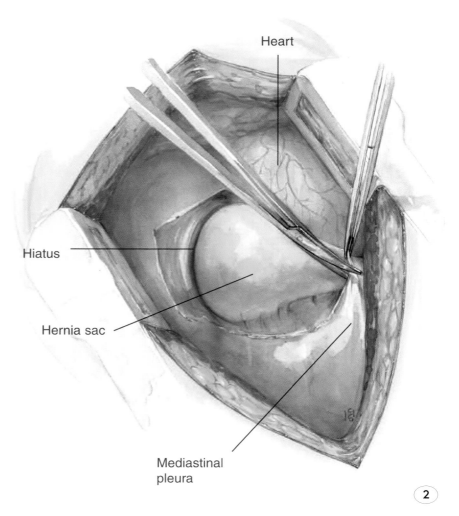

Heart

Hiatus

Hernia sac

Mediastinal pleura

②

Once the true hernia sac is identified, it is opened widely (3) and most of it resected. The esophagus is mobilized, taking care to keep the vagus nerves adjacent to the esophagus. The esophagus is encircled with a small Penrose drain. It is very important to mobilize the fundus of the stomach and the gastroesophageal junction circumferentially and adequately. This step requires division of branches of the left gastric artery along the lesser curvature of the stomach and division of several vasa brevia along the greater curvature (4). That portion of the distal esophagus and cardia of the stomach that is ordinarily retroperitoneal is mobilized.

It is important that enough fundus be freed up so that it can be easily delivered into the chest through the widened hiatus. Classically, enough of the stomach is mobilized so that when the crura are retracted, the caudate lobe of the liver can be visualized. To achieve close approximation between the fundus of the stomach and the distal esophagus, it is necessary to completely remove the fat pad that is invariably present at the gastroesophageal junction (5).

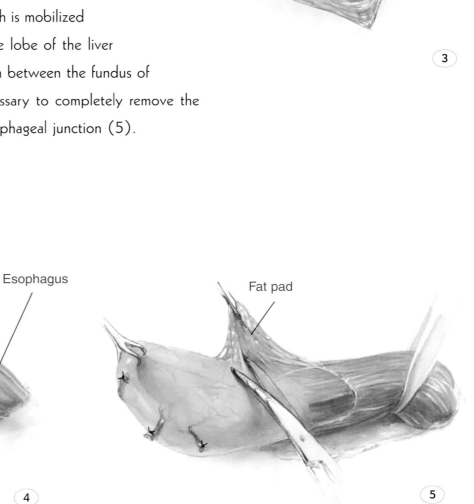

Hernia sac

Esophagus

(3)

Fundus

Vasa brevia

Esophagus

Left vagus n.

(4)

Fat pad

(5)

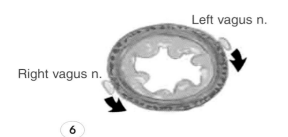

(6)

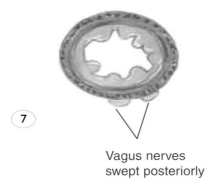

(7)

Vagus nerves
swept posteriorly

This is done sharply but often requires the clamping of small vessels that will bleed if not secured. During mobilization and dissection of the distal esophagus and proximal stomach, both vagus nerves are swept posteriorly (6), so that they come to reside side by side (7).

Once the distal esophagus and proximal stomach have been completely mobilized, the posterior crural sutures are placed, but not secured (8). The definition of the two crura of the diaphragm is aided by placing a Babcock clamp anteriorly on the hiatus and creating tension. This step often is very helpful in defining the tendinous portions of the two crura. Interrupted crural sutures of heavy silk or No. 2 polypropylene are placed advancing 1 cm at a time (8). The sutures are tagged with hemostats and brought out posteriorly in an organized fashion.

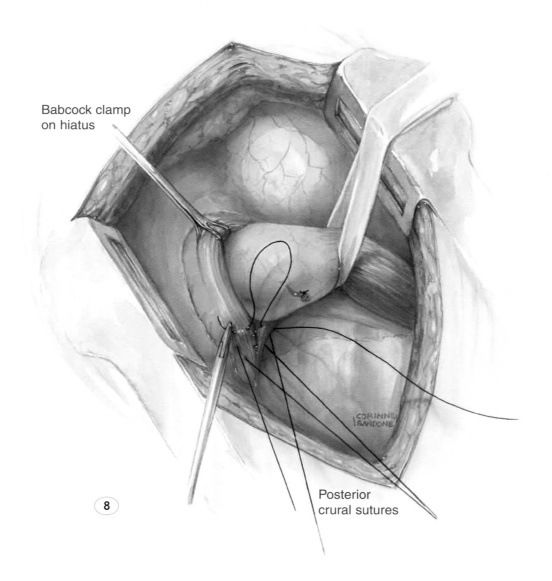

Babcock clamp
on hiatus

(8)

Posterior
crural sutures

The Belsey Mark IV antireflux procedure is performed by placing two rows of sutures between the stomach and esophagus, with three sutures in each row. These two rows of sutures effectively intussuscept the anterior and lateral aspects of the distal esophagus into the stomach.

The two rows of sutures ensure approximation of the fundus of the stomach for 270° of the circumference of the esophagus and fix it below the diaphragm. The first row of sutures is started on the gastric side 2 cm from the gastroesophageal junction. The sutures are 2-0 silk on cardiovascular needles. After a seromuscular bite of stomach (including the submucosa) 2 cm from the gastroesophageal junction, the suture is passed longitudinally through the esophagus, also 2 cm above the gastroesophageal junction. The suture is then passed back down through the esophagus, in a horizontal mattress fashion, and the suture is completed by passing it through the fundus of the stomach, adjacent to the first gastric suture (9). Three such sutures are placed so that approximately 270° of the esophagus are encompassed. Those two sutures close to the left and right vagus nerves are placed just anterior to them, taking care not to incorporate the nerve into the wrap. Traction is first placed on all three sutures simultaneously to take tension off while the sutures are tied. It is important to snug the sutures down firmly but not so hard that the sutures cut through the esophagus (10).

A second row of the same sutures is then placed, identical to the first row. Three horizontal mattress sutures are placed 2 cm below the first row on the stomach and 2 cm above the first row on the esophagus (11). These three sutures are

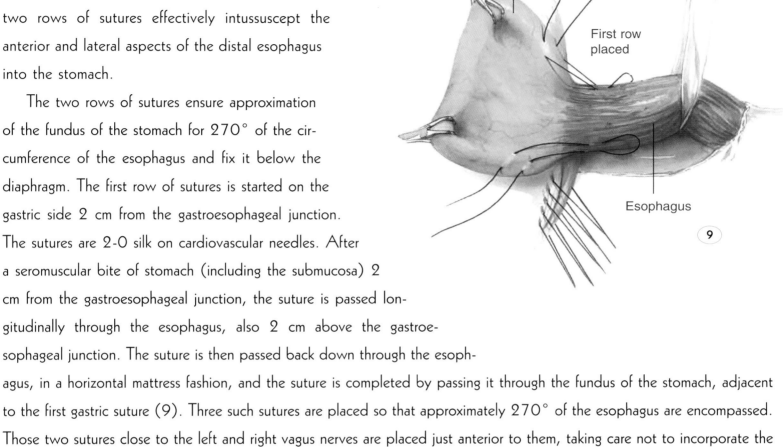

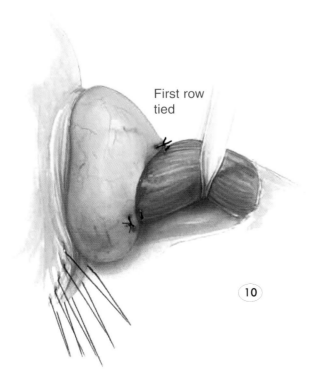

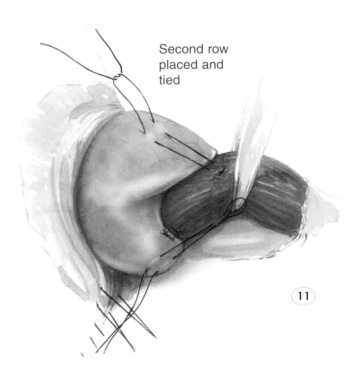

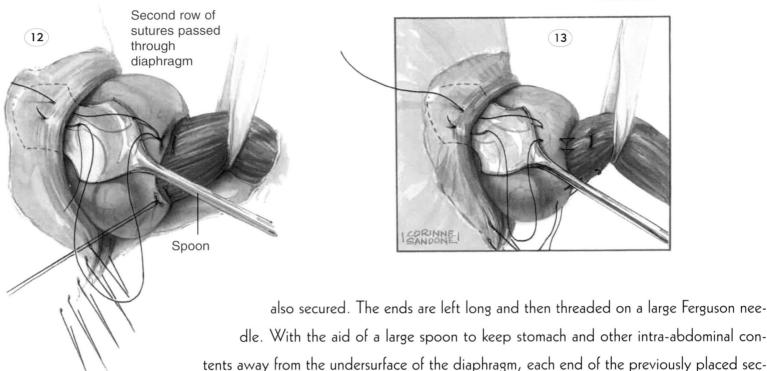

also secured. The ends are left long and then threaded on a large Ferguson needle. With the aid of a large spoon to keep stomach and other intra-abdominal contents away from the undersurface of the diaphragm, each end of the previously placed second row of sutures is passed through the hiatus and then up through the diaphragm from the peritoneal side (12).

An alternative method of placing the second row of sutures is depicted (13). As described initially by Belsey, the second row of sutures is started by passing the suture through the diaphragm from the thoracic to the peritoneal surface, again with the aid of a large sterilized spoon. The suture then passes through the gastric fundus 2 cm below the first row of sutures, and through the esophagus 2 cm above the first row of sutures. The stitch is brought back through the esophagus, stomach, and diaphragm in a horizontal mattress fashion. This method of placement of the second row of sutures is probably used by the majority of surgeons performing this repair. However, we prefer to secure the esophageal and gastric part of the suture before passing it through the diaphragm. It is exceedingly important to be able to place the appropriate amount of tension while tying the esophageal and gastric portions of the suture. The esophagus is obviously the weak part of this repair; if the sutures are tied too tightly, they can easily rip out through the esophagus, leading to a recurrence or, perhaps worse, to an esophageal leak.

Regardless of how the second row of sutures is placed, the fundus of the stomach and the gastroesophageal junction are reduced at this point into the peritoneal cavity, and the three sutures comprising the second row of stitches are secured (14).

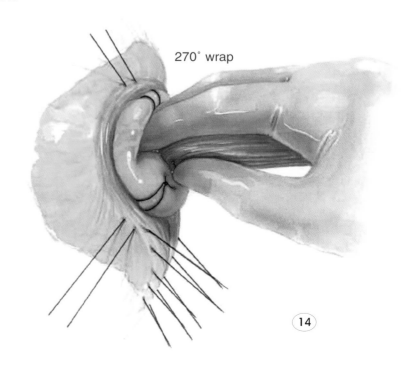

The securing of this second row of sutures ensures that a 4 cm segment of esophagus will remain intra-abdominally and intimately in contact for 270° of its circumference with gastric fundus. Once these three sutures have been secured, the previously placed crural sutures are tied. A 46 French Maloney dilator is placed orally into the stomach by the anesthesiologist before tying the crural sutures. If a Maloney dilator is in place, the crural sutures should be secured snugly against the esophagus allowing passage of the surgeon's fingertip (15). If only a nasogastric tube is in place, one should be able to admit more of the surgeon's finger between the last crural suture and the esophagus. Many recurrences appear posteriorly in this space; it is important that the crura sutures are placed appropriately, ensuring that this space is kept to a minimum.

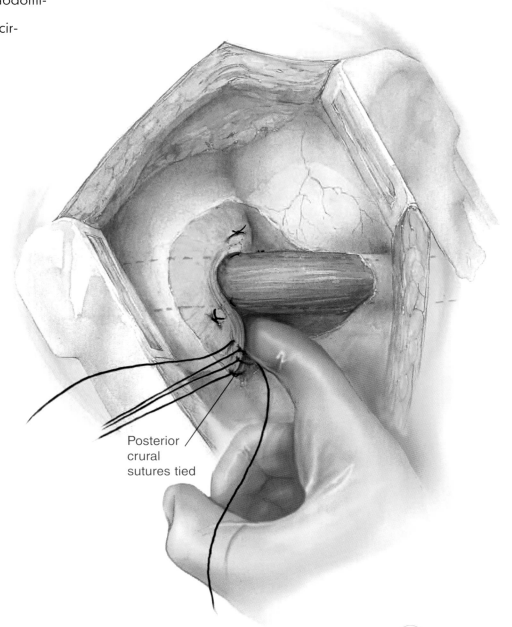

Posterior crural sutures tied

15

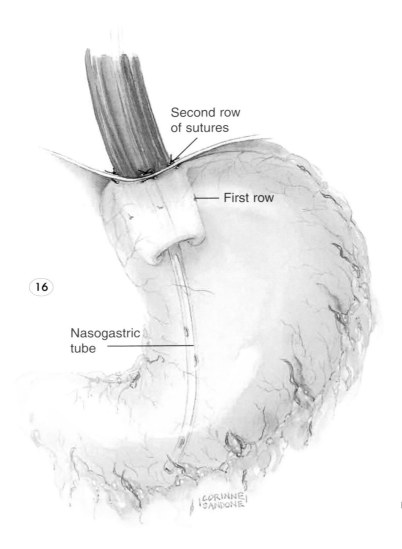

Second row of sutures

First row

Nasogastric tube

16

When the two rows of repair sutures are appropriately placed, approximately 270° of the esophagus are wrapped with gastric fundus with 4 cm of esophagus being placed in the abdominal position (16). The two vagus nerves are swept posteriorly and are not included in the wrap (17, 18). A chest tube is inserted, and the thoracotomy incision is closed.

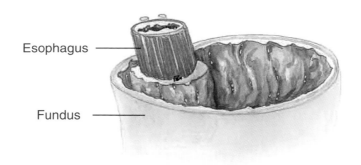

Esophagus

Fundus

17

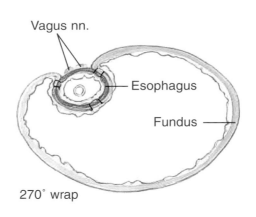

Vagus nn.

Esophagus

Fundus

270° wrap

18

Collis-Nissen Repair for Esophageal Stricture and Shortened Esophagus

Operative Indications

Most patients who develop an esophageal stricture secondary to gastroesophageal reflux require an operative intervention. Many of these strictures are dilatable with a variety of esophageal bougies or dilators. An antireflux procedure is needed to eliminate gastroesophageal reflux and allow healing of the stricture. Some patients, however, also have a shortened esophagus, usually those with long-standing symptoms of chronic gastroesophageal reflux, and develop the stricture due to chronic inflammation and scarring (1). In these patients, the stricture may be dilatable, but they are not candidates for the traditional antireflux

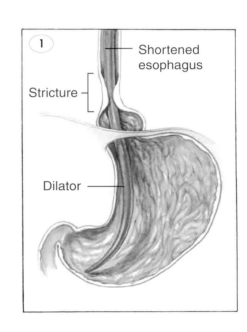

procedures that require an abdominal segment of esophagus. In these patients, the esophagus must be lengthened for a successful antireflux procedure. The Collis gastroplasty, in which a neoesophagus is created, thus lengthening the true esophagus, allows a tension-free Nissen fundoplication and is uniquely applicable to such situations.

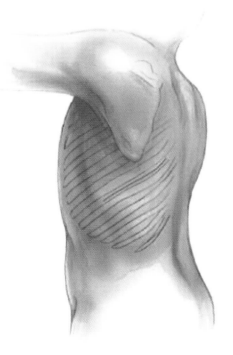

Operative Technique

The patient is placed in the posterolateral thoracotomy position with the left chest up. The pleural cavity is entered through the sixth or seventh interspace. The mediastinal pleura is opened, the esophagus is identified and mobilized, and a small Penrose drain is passed around it. The initial part of the operative procedure is identical to that of the Belsey antireflux procedure. The esophagus is mobilized up to the aortic arch to gain maximum length. During dissection of the gastroesophageal junction and subsequent fundoplication, both vagus nerves have to be carefully identified and preserved. With chronic inflammation and frequently associated prior surgery in the region, these nerves can be easily injured. In addition, the cardia of the stomach is mobilized circumferentially. This requires division of branches of the left gastric vessels along the lesser curvature, and mobilization of the retroperitoneal posterior aspect of the cardia and fundus. The fundus of the stomach is mobilized by ligating and dividing all of the vasa brevia; approximately 50% of the stomach should be deliverable into the chest.

For most patients with gastroesophageal reflux and a benign stricture, with mobilization of the esophagus up to the aortic arch, a standard Belsey or Nissen antireflux procedure can be performed, placing the repair below the diaphragm. However, in those few individuals with a truly shortened esophagus, such that the stomach cannot be placed below the diaphragm, a Collis gastroplasty is required. In most of these patients, the stricture will have been successfully dilated preoperatively. If it has not, however, with the surgeon's hands on the distal esophagus and stricture, the stricture is dilated from above by the passing of progressively larger Maloney dilators. Once the stricture has been dilated, a 50 French Maloney dilator is passed into the stomach. The dilator is positioned along the lesser curvature of the stomach. The fundus and greater curvature of the stomach are stretched laterally with a Babcock clamp.

Using a gastrointestinal anastomosis (GIA) stapler, the surgeon lengthens the esophagus by firing the stapler parallel to the Maloney dilator (2). A 50 French Maloney dilator is used to ensure an adequate lumen in the neoesophagus. Generally, enough lengthening is obtained by firing the GIA stapler just once. If need be, however, the amount of esophagus converted from the lesser curvature of the stomach can be extended to any length.

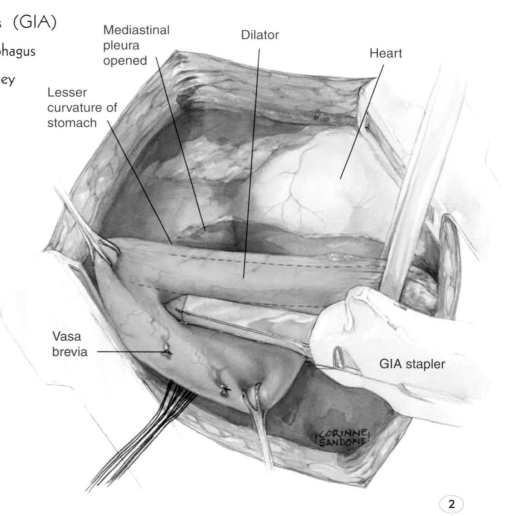

The staple line is reinforced with an interrupted layer of 3-0 silk Lembert sutures (3). Care is taken particularly in reinforcing the staple line at its apex. The diverticulum of fundus thus created is then grasped with a Babcock clamp and encircled posteriorly around the esophagus in preparation for a Nissen fundoplication. Sutures of 0 silk or polypropylene are placed in the two leaves of the right crux of the diaphragm to narrow the hiatus (4).

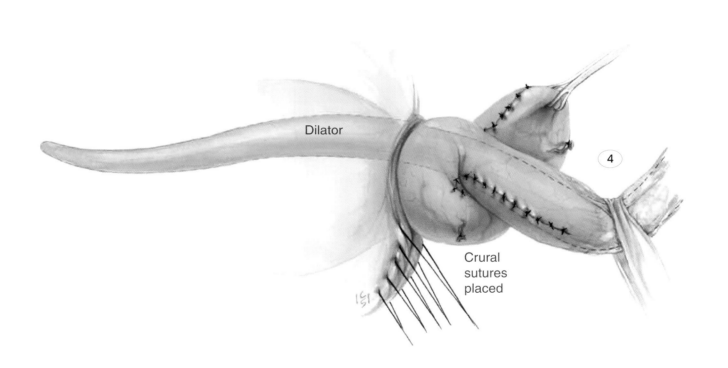

The Nissen fundoplication is completed by suturing the diverticulum of the stomach created by the stapler to the fundus of the stomach to the left of the new "gastroesophageal" junction. Effectively, the neoesophagus, which is in fact the lesser curvature of the stomach, is wrapped with fundus of the stomach to create a new esophageal sphincter. The wrap is performed with three 2-0 silk sutures placed from the fundus of the stomach, to the neoesophagus, and through the opposite side of the fundus (5). Thus, there is essentially a 2-cm wrap. Once the wrap is completed, it is reduced into the peritoneal cavity (6), so that the new gastroesophageal junction lies below the diaphragm.

The crural sutures are then tied and secured over a 50 French Maloney dilator. The surgeon should be able to insert a finger alongside the esophagus through the hiatus (7). A chest tube is inserted, and the thoracotomy incision is closed.

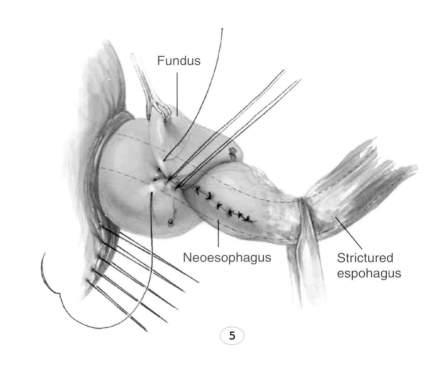

Fundus

Neoesophagus   Strictured espohagus

5

Diaphragm   360° wrap

6

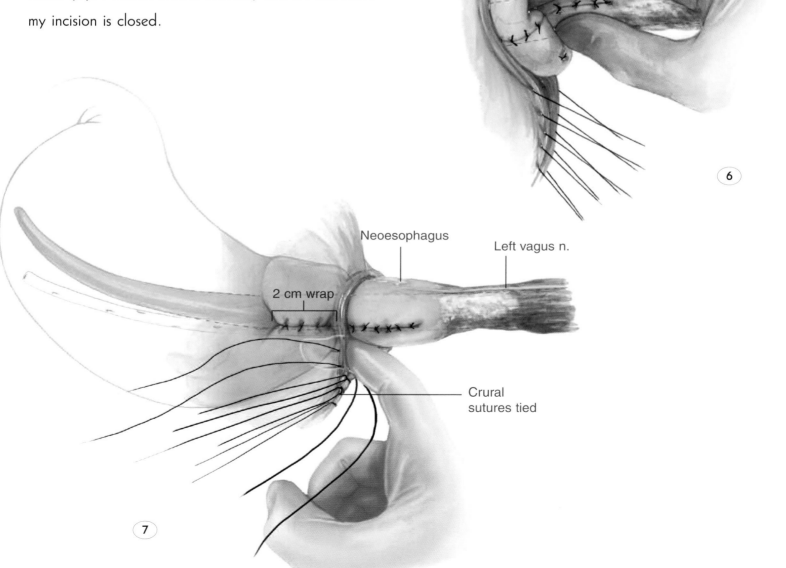

Neoesophagus   Left vagus n.

2 cm wrap

Crural sutures tied

7

Short Segment Colon Interposition for Benign Esophageal Stricture

Operative Indications

Most patients with gastroesophageal reflux can be managed medically. Those with symptoms refractory to medical management can be cared for with a variety of antireflux procedures performed surgically. If gastroesophageal reflux has produced an esophageal stricture, most can be managed with dilatation and the performance of an antireflux procedure. If the inflammation and stricture have resulted in a shortened esophagus (1), the esophagus can be lengthened by the Collis gastroplasty, and a Nissen fundoplication performed. The vast majority of patients with gastroesophageal reflux can be managed in this fashion. There remains a small number of patients who need to have their distal esophagus

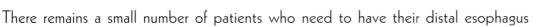

Stricture

(1)

replaced. In these patients, the gastroesophageal reflux has resulted in such severe fibrosis and scarring that the stricture cannot be dilated, or, if it is dilated, the esophagus may split. Many of these patients have had prior antireflux procedures, such as a Belsey Mark IV or Nissen fundoplication. For these patients, resection of the distal esophagus including the stricture and replacement with a short segment of colon is the appropriate operative procedure.

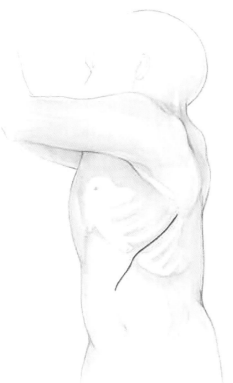

Operative Technique

This operative procedure is best performed through a left thoracoabdominal incision. The patient is placed in the right lateral decubitus position with the left chest up. The hips are rotated back toward the table at a 45° angle, to allow

Diaphragm viewed from above

Radial
incision

Circumferential
incision

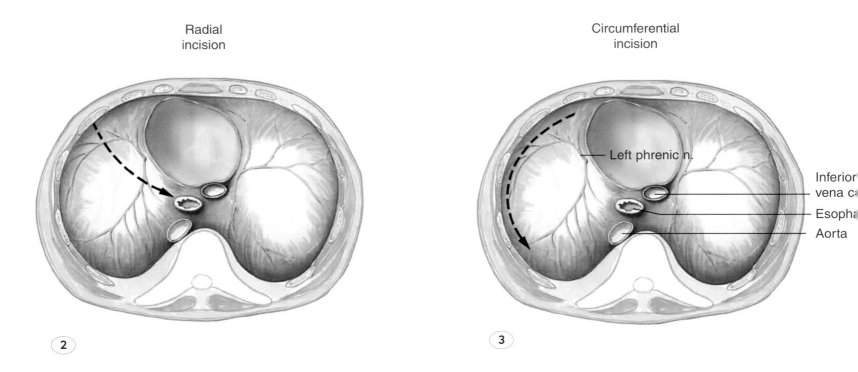

Left phrenic n.

Inferior
vena ca

Esopha

Aorta

2

3

better abdominal exposure. The left pleural cavity is entered through the seventh or eighth interspace; the incision is carried onto the abdomen to a point midway between the xiphoid and umbilicus, and generally extended to the midline of the abdomen. The costal cartilage is divided, removing a section of cartilage so that chondritis is not a problem when the ribs are subsequently re-approximated. It is necessary to divide the diaphragm in order to provide appropriate exposure to mobilize the colon. Whereas many surgeons divide the diaphragm radially (2), extending the incision toward but not through the esophageal hiatus, fewer branches of the phrenic nerve are divided if the diaphragm is opened circumferentially (3). When the latter is done, it is important to leave at least 3 cm of diaphragm attached to the chest wall, to facilitate approximation during closure.

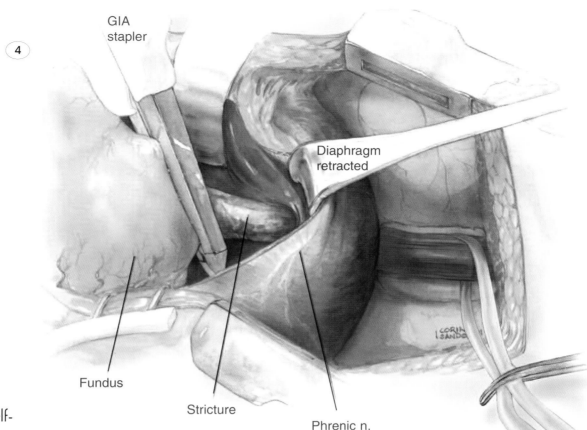

④

GIA
stapler

Diaphragm
retracted

Fundus

Stricture

Phrenic n.

After the incision is made, the ribs are spread with a self-retaining rib retractor, and the abdomen is exposed with an abdominal wall retractor. The mediastinal pleura is opened, and the distal esophagus mobilized. A great deal of edema, scarring, and fibrosis may exist in the distal esophagus, due to prior inflammation or surgery, making mobilization of the esophagus and stomach tedious and difficult. If the esophagus is difficult to find, a 46 French Maloney dilator can be inserted early to locate the esophagus. Often, it is difficult to identify the vagus nerves. Since they will be sacrificed during the procedure, little attention has to be paid to this detail. The diaphragm having been opened circumferentially allows excellent exposure of the upper abdomen. Through the abdominal portion of the incision, the fundus of the stomach is mobilized. Branches of the left gastric vessels in the gastrohepatic ligament are ligated and divided. Several vasa brevia along the fundus close to the gastroesophageal junction are also ligated and divided. The distal esophagus, gastroesophageal junction, and fundus of the stomach are mobilized, and the hiatus is dissected free. The gastroesophageal junction on the gastric side is divided with a GIA stapler (4). The gastric staple line is reinforced with a row of interrupted 3-0 silk Lembert sutures (5).

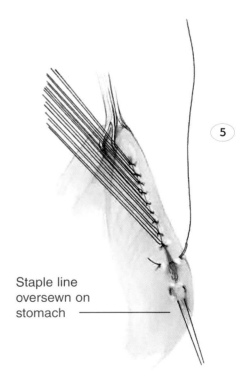

⑤

Staple line
oversewn on
stomach

The short segment of colon (6) used as the interposition graft consists of the splenic flexure based on the ascending branch of the left colic artery. The greater omentum is removed from the left transverse colon. The splenic flexure is separated carefully from the spleen, dividing the splenocolic ligament. The left colon is mobilized out of the retroperitoneum, completely freeing up the splenic flexure. This short segment colon graft is vascularized by the marginal artery, fed by the ascending branch of the left colic artery (7). Before the marginal artery is divided proximally and distally, Bulldog clamps can be applied to be certain there is sufficient vascular supply to the graft. The descending colon is then cleaned, the marginal artery ligated and divided, and the colon divided with a GIA stapler. The left transverse colon is cleaned, the mar-

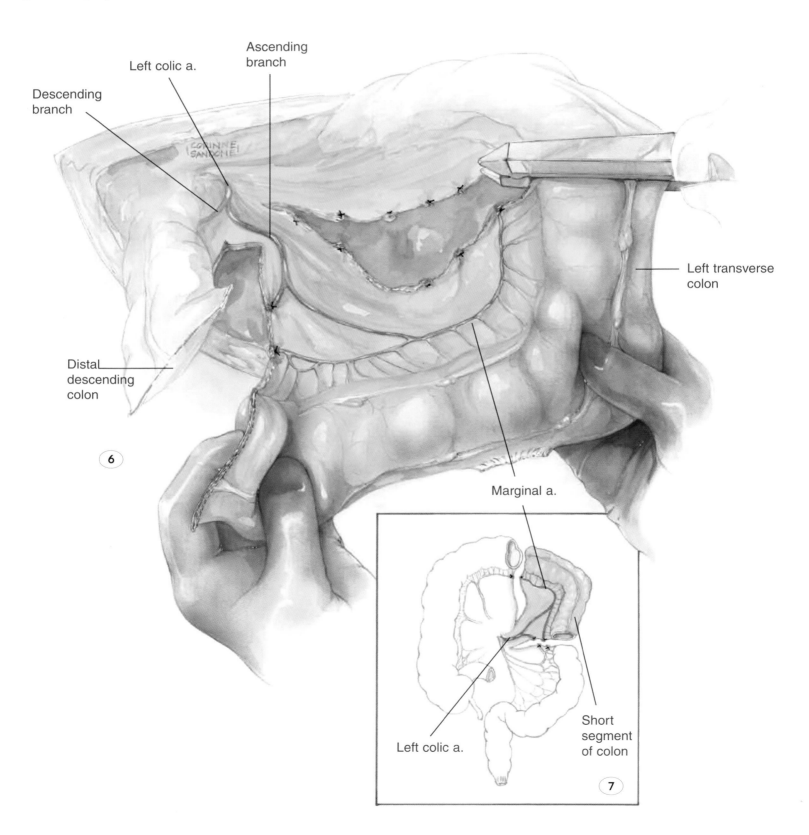

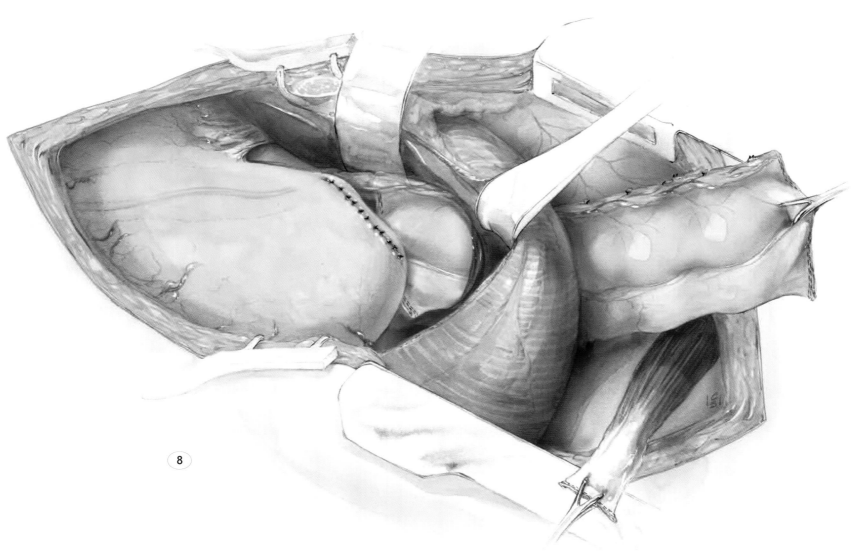

8

ginal artery is ligated and divided, and the colon is divided with a GIA stapler (6). The total length of the short segment colon graft should be approximately 8 inches.

The proximal end of the short segment of colon is then advanced through the esophageal hiatus, passing posterior to the stomach (8). Positioning is critical, since it allows the vascular pedicle to take the shortest and most direct route through the hiatus, and minimizes the danger of being compressed by a dilated stomach. The hiatus will have already been enlarged somewhat by the extensive dissection necessary to remove the scarred and strictured distal esophagus. Most surgeons prefer to place the graft onto the posterior aspect of the stomach body (9a), though some place it on the anterior surface of the stomach (9b).

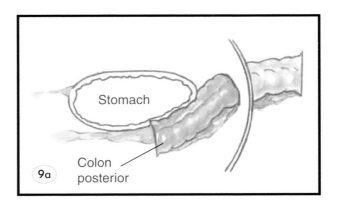

Stomach

Colon posterior

9a

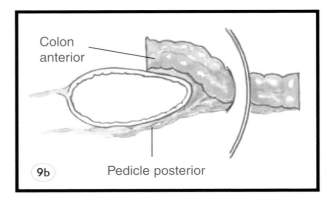

Colon anterior

Pedicle posterior

9b

The first anastomosis is done in the chest, where an end-to-end esophagocolostomy is performed between the normal esophagus, well above the strictured fibrotic area, to the proximal end of the colon graft. An outer posterior layer of interrupted 3-0 silk Lembert sutures is placed first. After placement of this posterior row, the staple line is removed from the colon using electrocautery (10). On the esophageal side, the posterior aspect of the esophagus is partially opened, and the inner layer of the posterior row of sutures is placed, again using interrupted through-and-through sutures of 3-0 silk (11). The remaining esophagus is then divided and removed from the operative field. The inner layer of the anterior row is placed using an inverting suture that passes from inside out on the esophagus and outside in on the colon, taking full thickness of both layers (12). Prior to finishing the anterior inner layer, a nasogastric tube is passed into the esophagus, carefully through the proximal anastomosis, as well as through the short segment colon interposition, and into the stomach.

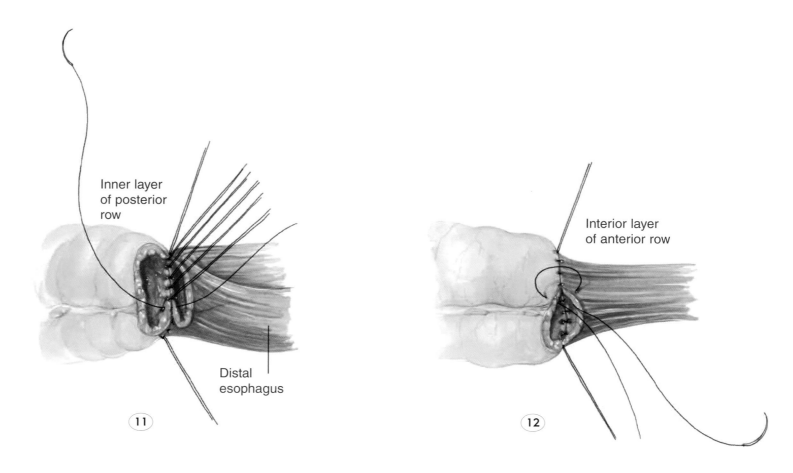

Outer layer of posterior row

Staple line removed from colon

Proximal colon

Strictured distal esophagus

10

Inner layer of posterior row

Distal esophagus

11

Interior layer of anterior row

12

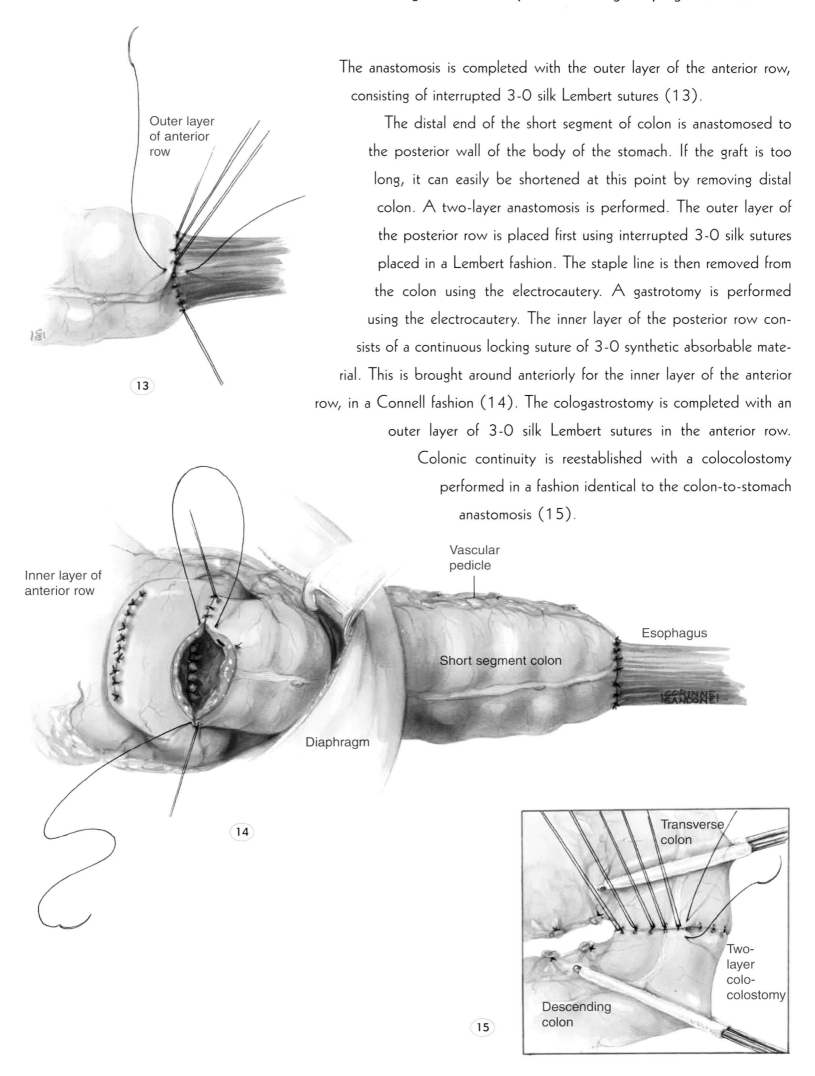

Outer layer
of anterior
row

13

Inner layer of
anterior row

14

Vascular
pedicle

Esophagus

Short segment colon

Diaphragm

Transverse
colon

Two-
layer
colo-
colostomy

Descending
colon

15

The anastomosis is completed with the outer layer of the anterior row, consisting of interrupted 3-0 silk Lembert sutures (13).

The distal end of the short segment of colon is anastomosed to the posterior wall of the body of the stomach. If the graft is too long, it can easily be shortened at this point by removing distal colon. A two-layer anastomosis is performed. The outer layer of the posterior row is placed first using interrupted 3-0 silk sutures placed in a Lembert fashion. The staple line is then removed from the colon using the electrocautery. A gastrotomy is performed using the electrocautery. The inner layer of the posterior row consists of a continuous locking suture of 3-0 synthetic absorbable material. This is brought around anteriorly for the inner layer of the anterior row, in a Connell fashion (14). The cologastrostomy is completed with an outer layer of 3-0 silk Lembert sutures in the anterior row. Colonic continuity is reestablished with a colocolostomy performed in a fashion identical to the colon-to-stomach anastomosis (15).

Since a bilateral vagotomy is performed in resecting the distal esophagus, either a pyloroplasty or a pyloromyotomy is required. A pyloromyotomy is often preferred, to minimize entrance into the gastrointestinal lumen. For this method, the seromuscular layers of the distal stomach, pylorus, and proximal duodenum are divided carefully with the electrocautery on low voltage, being certain not to open the mucosal layer (16). A fine right angle clamp is used not only to gently lift the circular muscular layers off the mucosa, but also to gently spread them; this allows the mucosal layer to bulge out (17). Once the pyloromyotomy is completed, it is covered with a piece of omentum and the sutures marked with metal clips so that, if dysphagia due to pyloric stenosis develops postoperatively, this site can be found radiographically and used to guide endoscopic dilatation (18).

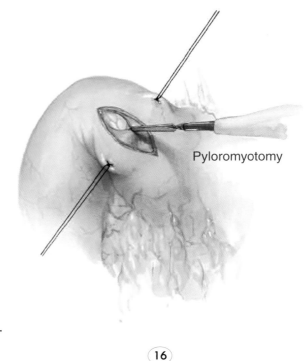

Pyloromyotomy

(16)

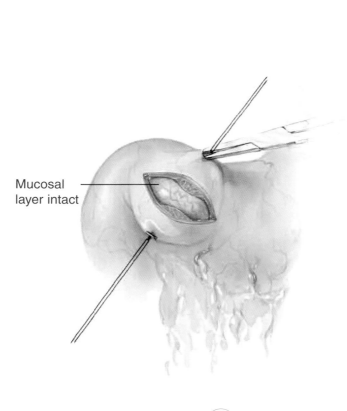

Mucosal
layer intact

(17)

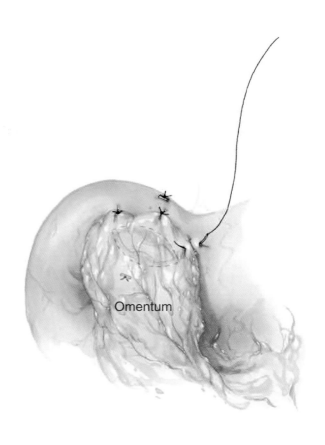

Omentum

(18)

If the mucosa is inadvertently opened, it should be converted to a pyloroplasty by opening the mucosal layer the length of the seromuscular defect. If
a Heineke-Mikulicz pyloroplasty is performed, the pylorus is opened in a
horizontal fashion and closed vertically (19). The Gambee stitch is used,
passing through and through the stomach, then back up through gastric
mucosa only. The suture is then passed through mucosa only into the
duodenal lumen on the duodenal side, and then back full thickness
through the duodenum. This suture ensures good approximation of the
stomach and duodenum, without narrowing of the pyloric channel.
Similarly, a piece of omentum with metal clips is sutured over the site.

The short segment of colon replaces the strictured distal esophagus
and effectively prevents subsequent gastroesophageal reflux up into the
mid-esophagus. With the cologastric anastomosis in the posterior position, this
shorter distance places the vascular pedicle away from potential tension if the
stomach becomes dilated (20, 21).

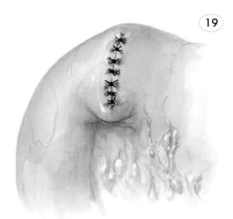

(19)

Heineke-Mikuliz
pyloroplasty

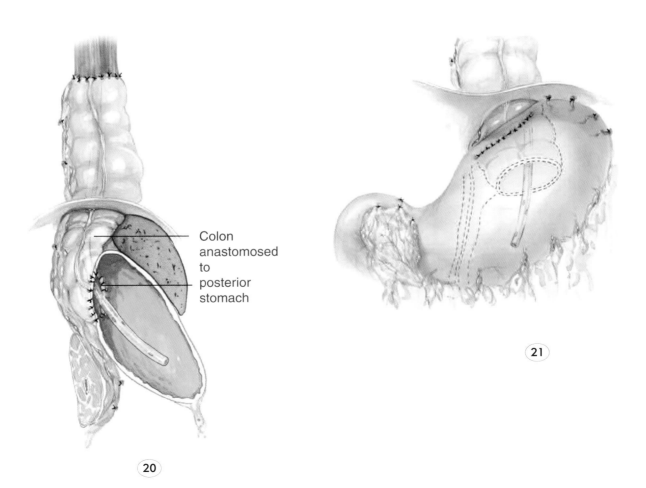

Colon
anastomosed
to
posterior
stomach

(20)

(21)

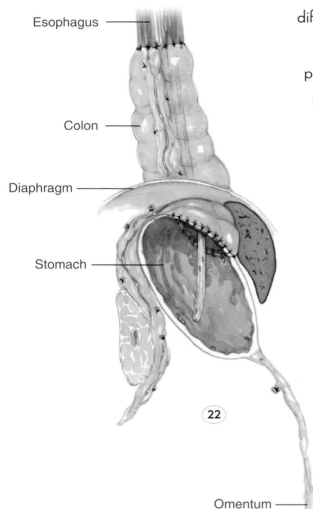

Esophagus

Colon

Diaphragm

Stomach

22

Omentum

Alternatively, this anastomosis can be done anteriorly (22, 23), particularly if it is difficult to do posteriorly.

The transverse and descending colon are easily re-approximated anterior to the pedicle supplying the colon interposition, either by a two-layer hand-sewn technique or using stapling devices. Occasionally, the hiatus will be somewhat larger than the colon conduit, so that tacking it circumferentially to the colon interposition with interrupted sutures of 4-0 silk is required to prevent herniation of abdominal content through it. The abdominal and thoracic retractors are removed, and the diaphragm re-approximated with 0 synthetic non-absorbable suture in a horizontal mattress fashion. This step is usually best done from the thoracic side. A single chest tube is left in place. The thoracoabdominal incision is closed in layers.

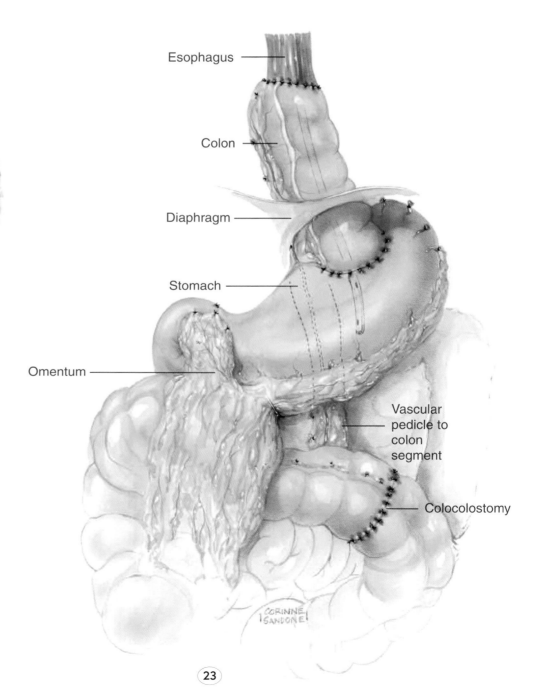

Esophagus

Colon

Diaphragm

Stomach

Omentum

Vascular pedicle to colon segment

Colocolostomy

23

Repair of Paraesophageal Hernia

Operative Indications

Paraesophageal hernias are relatively uncommon and are generally seen in the older patient. A true paraesophageal hernia, Type I, is defined without a sliding component where the gastroesophageal junction remains in the abdomen, and a large peritoneal hernia sac develops around the esophagus, usually anteriorly and/or to the left (1). The hiatus is usually very enlarged. The hernia sac in the anterior mediastinum generally contains the fundus of the stomach. More commonly, in the Type II hernia, the esophagogastric junction and the upper stomach herniate as one unit into the chest (2). Rarely, if the hiatal opening and sac become very large, most of the stomach will flip anteriorly into the mediastinum in a Type III hernia (3). With an upside down stomach, virtually all of the stomach can be in the chest (3).

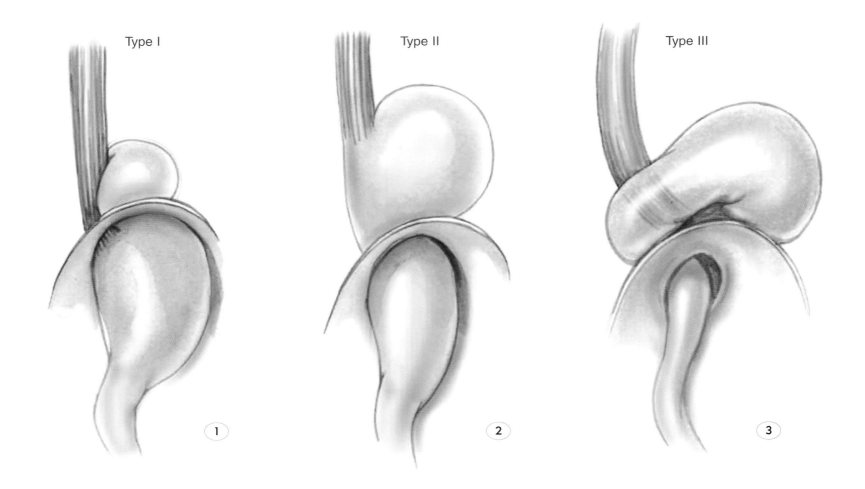

Type I   Type II   Type III

1   2   3

Most paraesophageal hernias have a sliding component, with the gastroesophageal junction actually residing in the chest. Because gastroesophageal reflux is not a frequent symptom in these patients, they may be asymptomatic or have mild nonspecific symptoms of belching, early satiety, or a sense of fullness in the chest. Currently, it is thought that if patients are asymptomatic repair is not necessary. However, if significant symptoms are present a substantial risk of incarceration, bleeding, and/or perforation is believed to exist. Gastric stasis can lead to ulceration and gastritis in the herniated portion of the stomach. The most serious complication is incarceration and strangulation, which presents as a catastrophic event with an exceedingly high mortality.

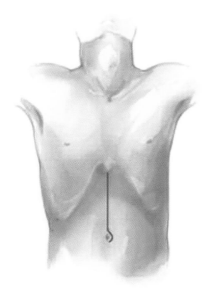

Operative Technique

The patient can be explored through either the chest or the abdomen. The latter approach is usually favored because of lower morbidity from the incision. An upper midline incision is made and both costal margins are retracted using retractors suspended from a frame fixed to the operating room table. In addition to the stomach, the spleen and colon are components that can be found herniated into the mediastinum, Type IV. The stomach can almost always easily be reduced by gentle downward traction (4). Exposure is often aided if the triangular ligament is taken down, retracting the left lobe of the liver to the right.

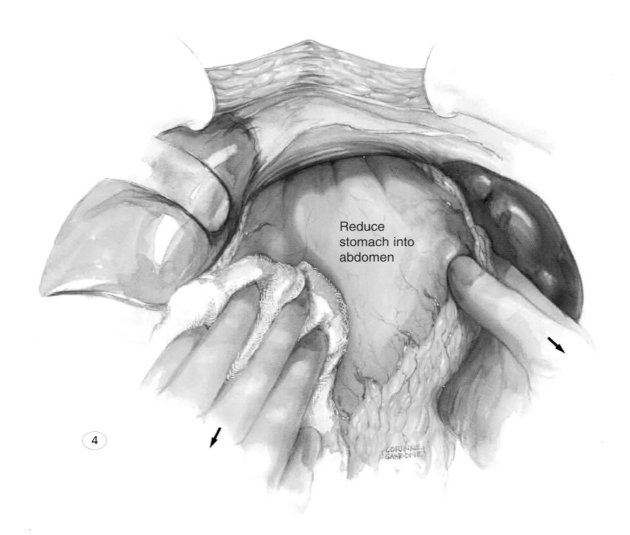

Reduce stomach into abdomen

4

Removing the large peritoneal sac, which invariably accompanies the paraesophageal hernia, from the mediastinum is not essential. However, if it is removed it helps facilitate identification of proper tissue planes when the repair is performed (5). One has to be careful while excising the sac posteriorly that the posterior (right) vagal trunk is not injured. In the process of excising the sac, the esophagus is completely mobilized, and both vagal nerves are identified and kept adjacent to the esophagus.

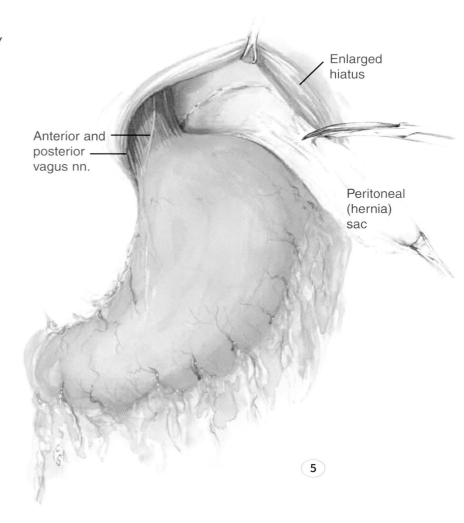

Enlarged hiatus

Anterior and posterior vagus nn.

Peritoneal (hernia) sac

5

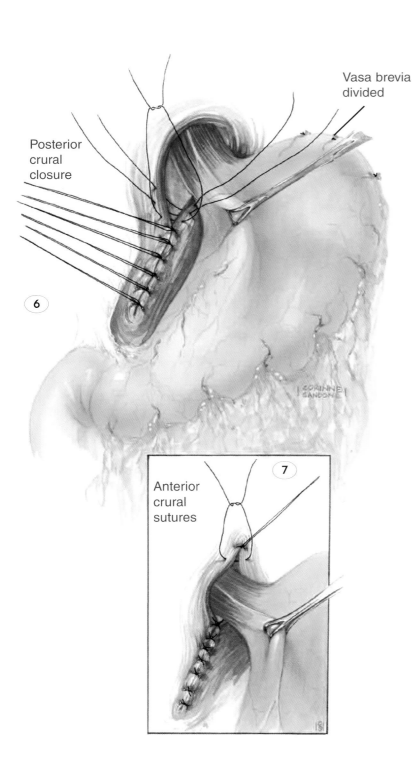

Vasa brevia divided

Posterior crural closure

6

Anterior crural sutures

7

After the hernia has been reduced, the sac excised, and the abdominal esophagus and fundus completely mobilized, the large hiatal opening is closed. It is preferable to close the hiatus from posterior to anterior, thereby displacing the esophagus anteriorly (6). As with the previously described diaphragm repairs, the crural sutures of No. 2 silk or polypropylene are placed first, prior to tying them. The crural leaves should be approximated with a 46 French Maloney dilator in place, making the hiatus snug. Some favor anterior crural sutures (7), thereby avoiding the marked anterior displacement of the esophagus. In addition, some surgeons feel that the closure fo the hiatus should be reinforced with a synthetic or biologic mesh.

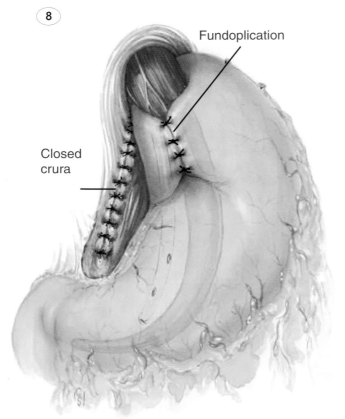

During mobilization of the cardia, the gastrohepatic ligament is divided, along with branches of the left gastric vessels. In addition, several vasa brevia are divided so that a fundoplication can be performed. Because of the herniation of the stomach, the vasa brevia are elongated and easily divided. A fundoplication is performed by wrapping the very mobile fundic portion of the stomach around the esophagus posteriorly and suturing it to adjacent fundus and esophagus with a series of four 2-0 silk sutures (8). Many of these hernias actually have a sliding component. Even if a sliding component is not present, the gastroesophageal junction is completely mobilized and its posterior attachments are taken down during the dissection. A fundoplication is important because it adds bulk to the fundic portion of the stomach, which makes a recurrence of the hernia less likely. The abdomen is closed without drains.

Alternatively, the stomach can be simply tacked to the anterior abdominal wall and held in place with a gastrostomy tube after the hernia is reduced and the crura closed, without doing a formal fundoplication. This procedure can be considered in the older patient or when a quicker operation is desired because of comorbid patient factors, or when extensive adhesions are encountered precluding mobilization of the fundus for wrapping.

Resection of Zenker's Diverticulum

Operative Indications

 Zenker's diverticulum is a herniation of esophageal mucosa that occurs posteriorly below the inferior pharyngeal constrictor muscles and just above the cricopharyngeus (1). Discoordination of the cricopharyngeus, or upper esophageal sphincter, is thought to be responsible for the high pressure that is generated above the sphincter, and thus the herniation of mucosa (inset). Zenker's diverticulum can be seen in any age group but is more common in the older patient. It generally presents with dysphagia, and an associated sensation of gurgling or bubbling in the neck. Occasionally, undigested food that was ingested days earlier will be regurgitated.

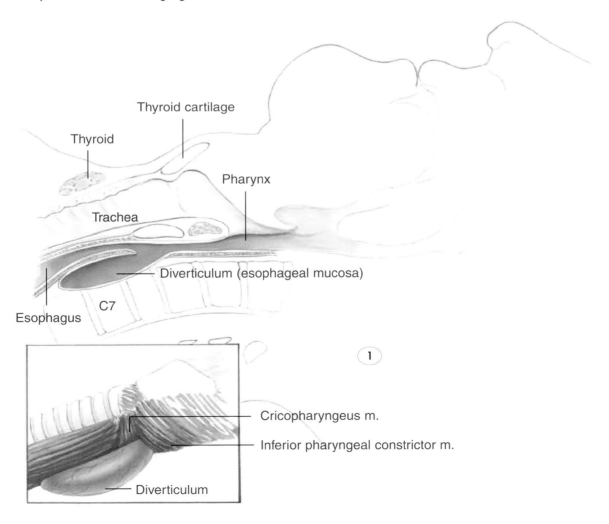

Thyroid cartilage

Thyroid

Pharynx

Trachea

Diverticulum (esophageal mucosa)

Esophagus

C7

1

Cricopharyngeus m.

Inferior pharyngeal constrictor m.

Diverticulum

Particularly in the elderly, recurrent bouts of aspiration or awakening at night with coughing spells is common. When a patient with a Zenker's diverticulum swallows, the liquid or solid bolus takes the path of least resistance. Since the cricopharyngeus muscle is not coordinated with a swallow, food preferentially enters the diverticulum, compressing the esophagus, and leading to dysphagia. Virtually all patients with symptomatic Zenker's diverticulum should be treated surgically. There is no medical management.

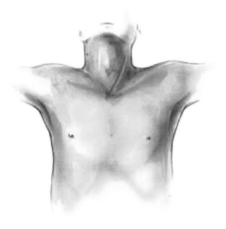

Operative Technique

It is advised that the patient be on a clear liquid diet for several days prior to surgery. The patient is placed supine on the operating room table with the head rotated to the right. The diverticulum arises from the midline posteriorly but is often deviated somewhat to the left side of the neck. Thus, approaching these lesions from the left neck is preferred. An incision is made along the anterior border of the left sternocleidomastoid muscle, usually at the midportion of the neck. The platysma is divided, and the sternocleidomastoid muscle retracted laterally. The trachea and the thyroid gland are retracted medially by the assistant using only fingers. Retractors should not be placed on the trachea for fear of injury to the recurrent laryngeal nerve, which resides in the groove between the trachea and esophagus. The omohyoid muscle can be retracted but, depending on its size and orientation, is usually in the way and is best divided. The esophagus is easily identified. At this point, the anesthesiologist gently passes the tip of a 46 French Maloney dilator, which invariably enters the diverticulum, making identification of the tip of the diverticulum easy. The diverticulum is grasped with a small Babcock clamp and mobilized by sharp and blunt dissection (2).

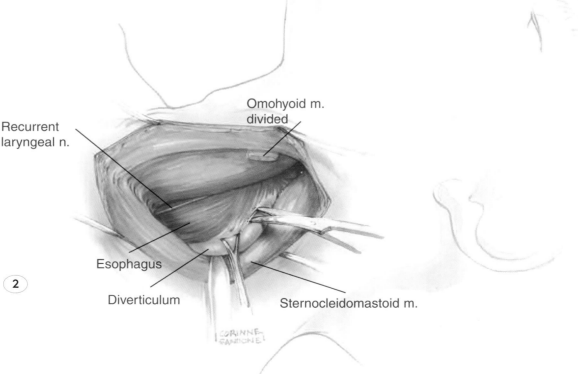

Recurrent
laryngeal n.

Omohyoid m.
divided

Esophagus

Sternocleidomastoid m.

Diverticulum

(2)

Using sharp and blunt dissection, the diverticulum is easily mobilized until it is attached to the esophagus only by its neck (3). If the diverticulum is not treated gently, bleeding and hematomas quickly result. When the diverticulum has been completely mobilized, the anesthesiologist can reposition the Maloney dilator into the esophagus proper beyond the opening of the diverticulum and into the stomach; this is facilitated by pinching the neck of the diverticulum between the surgeon's fingers.

The diverticulum can then be excised and closed with a layer of interrupted 4-0 synthetic absorbable suture material. Alternatively, it can be divided with a thoracoabdominal (TA) stapler (4). In dividing the diverticulum, one has to be careful to divide it flush with the esophagus and to not pull normal esophageal mucosa into the stapler, thus narrowing the esophageal lumen. This is avoided with the Maloney dilator in place. In addition, it is advised to open up the tip of the diverticulum prior to firing the stapler to ensure that all solid food debris has been removed so it is not caught in the staple line.

Once the diverticulum has been resected, the dilator is removed, and the staple line is covered posteriorly by reapproximating the inferior constrictor muscles with a layer of interrupted 3-0 synthetic absorbable suture material (5).

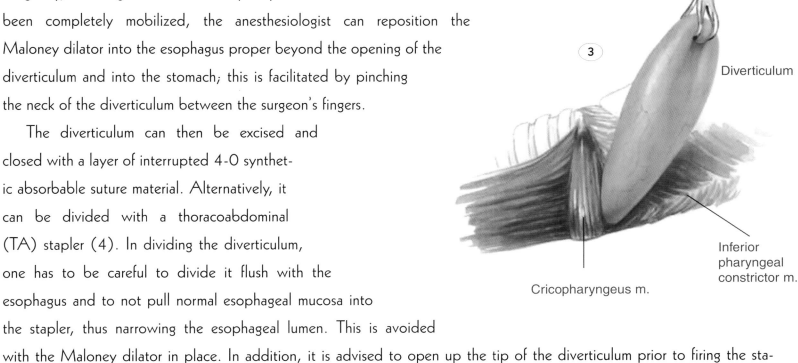

3

Diverticulum

Inferior pharyngeal constrictor m.

Cricopharyngeus m.

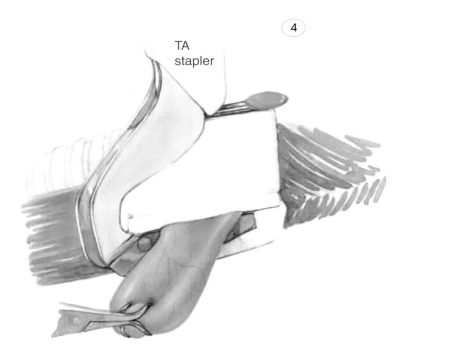

4

TA stapler

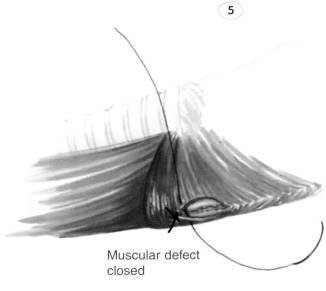

5

Muscular defect closed

Most patients will do well in the long term with just a diverticulectomy. Recurrences do occur, however; to prevent these, an esophagomyotomy should be performed (6). The myotomy is performed along the lateral esophageal wall, to avoid the area previously closed at the site of the diverticulectomy (7, 8). The muscle layer of the esophagus is easily separated from the underlying mucosa with a fine right angle clamp and divided with the electrocautery on low voltage. The myotomy should extend approximately 3 to 4 cm, being certain that it is brought cephalad to the point where the cricopharyngeus muscle is completely divided. A small Penrose or closed-suction drain is left around the area of the diverticulectomy and is brought out inferior to the operative site. The wound is closed in layers.

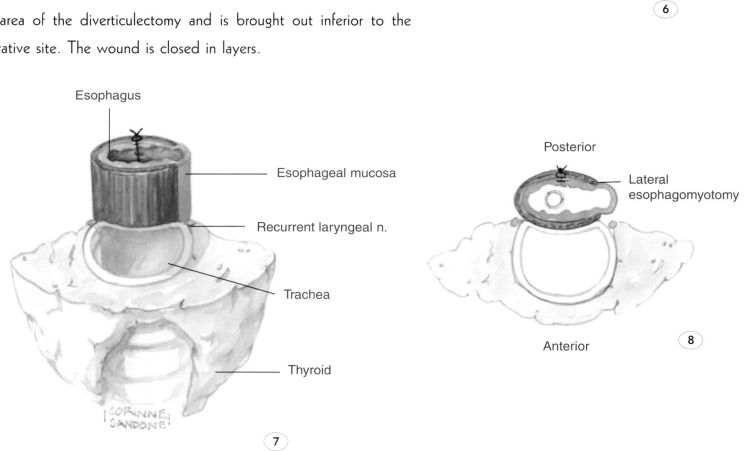

Lateral esophagomyotomy

Cricopharyngeal m.

6

Esophagus

Esophageal mucosa

Recurrent laryngeal n.

Trachea

Thyroid

7

Posterior

Lateral esophagomyotomy

Anterior

8

Suspension of Zenker's Diverticulum

Operative Indications

For patients who present with symptoms of a Zenker's diverticulum and in whom the Zenker's diverticulum is small (< 3 cm), one has the option of not resecting the diverticulum but merely suspending it. This may also be a useful approach in the high-risk surgical patient, and thus could be done under sedation with local anesthesia. An esophagomyotomy is added below the diverticulum. In several small series, this has proven to be entirely satisfactory. If one tries to suspend a large diverticulum, however, symptoms may persist or recur, and reoperation becomes necessary. Therefore, the operation of suspension of the diverticulum should be performed only for small diverticula. The advantage of this operative procedure over diverticulectomy is that the esophagus is not opened. This is only a small advantage because leakage at the site of the diverticulectomy is uncommon. Nevertheless, some esophageal surgeons favor this operative procedure.

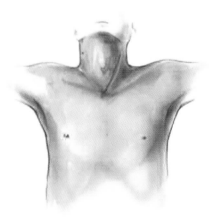

Operative Technique

The patient is placed in the supine position, with the head rotated to the right. An incision is made along the anterior border of the left sternocleidomastoid muscle. The initial part of the operative procedure is identical to that for diverticulectomy.

The omohyoid muscle is divided, the middle thyroid vein is divided, and the carotid sheath is retracted laterally along with the sternocleidomastoid muscle. The trachea and thyroid are gently retracted medially. The diverticulum is identified and dissected free. An esophagomyotomy is performed beginning at the defect in the muscular layer at the neck of the diverticulum, and extended inferiorly for approximately 4 cm, thus ensuring that the entire cricopharyngeus muscle is divided. The esophagomyotomy is performed by dissecting the muscle layer from the mucosa with a right angle clamp and dividing it with the electrocautery (1). When the myotomy is completed, the diverticulum is gently stretched in a cephalad direction and fixed to the prevertebral fascia with two or three 3-0 silk sutures (2, 3). Since the esophagus has not been entered, the wound is not drained.

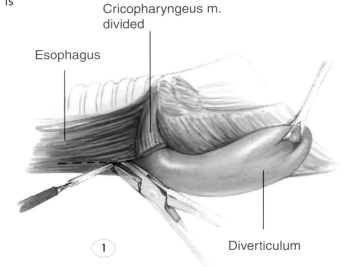

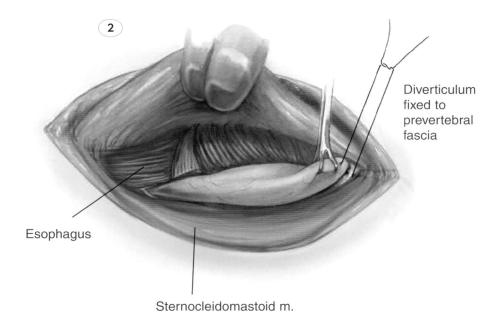

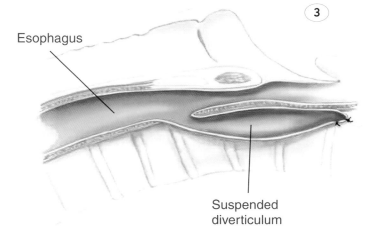

Resection of Epiphrenic Esophageal Diverticulum with Esophagomyotomy and Belsey Repair

Operative Indications

Epiphrenic diverticula are pulsion pseudodiverticula that are secondary to discoordination of the lower esophageal high-pressure zone. The underlying pathophysiology of this motor disorder is not entirely clear. Epiphrenic diverticula invariably arise above the lower esophageal sphincter, and generally present to the right (1). They can become quite large over time if left untreated. Patients generally present with mild dysphagia, with occasional regurgitation of previously ingested food. Recurrent bouts of aspiration can occur but are less frequently seen than with a Zenker's diverticulum. Symptoms of dysphagia may be relatively mild; if a patient is elderly and frail, surgical intervention may not be mandatory. However, for most patients who present with symptomatic epiphrenic diverticula, surgical management is indicated. There is no medical management for this disorder.

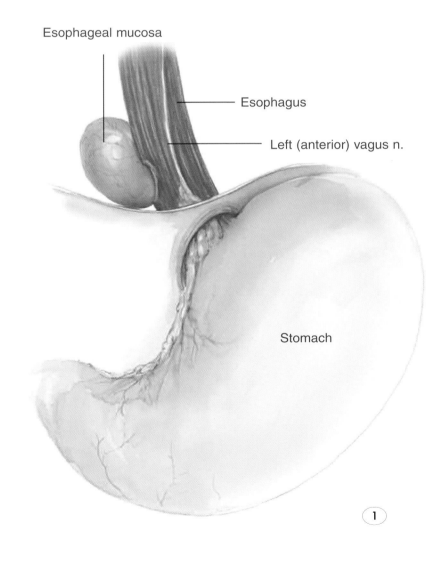

Esophageal mucosa

Esophagus

Left (anterior) vagus n.

Stomach

1

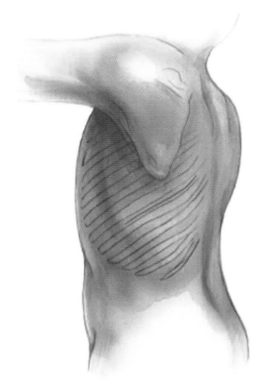

Operative Technique

The patient is placed in the lateral thoracotomy position with the left chest up. The left pleural cavity is entered through the sixth or seventh intercostal space. The mediastinal pleura is opened and the esophagus is identified. Identification of the esophagus is aided by having a nasogastric tube in place. The nasogastric tube, however, will generally enter the diverticulum and therefore has to be inserted with care to avoid perforation. The esophagus is identified and mobilized. It is looped with a small Penrose drain for gentle traction (2). As the esophagus is mobilized, the pulsion diverticulum will be identified arising from the right lateral aspect of the distal esophagus, residing in the mediastinum to the right of the midline. Despite the fact that these generally present to the right, they are easily accessed from a left posterolateral thoracotomy. The diverticulum is mobilized with both blunt and sharp dissection, aided by grasping it with a small Babcock clamp. These are generally imbedded in soft areolar tissue and easily dissected free.

When the diverticulum has been completely mobilized, the esophagus is rotated to expose the muscular defect. The nasogastric tube is then advanced into the stomach. The diverticulum is excised using a thoracoabdominal (TA) stapler (3). As previously described for Zenker's diverticulum, one has to be certain that mucosa from the esophagus is not tented out and removed, thus narrowing the esophageal lumen. A 46 French Maloney dilator is inserted to avoid this problem. The diverticulum should be opened at the apex if residual food debris is palpated so it is not incorporated in the staple line. The muscular layer is closed over the staple line with a series of interrupted 3-0 silk sutures (4, inset).

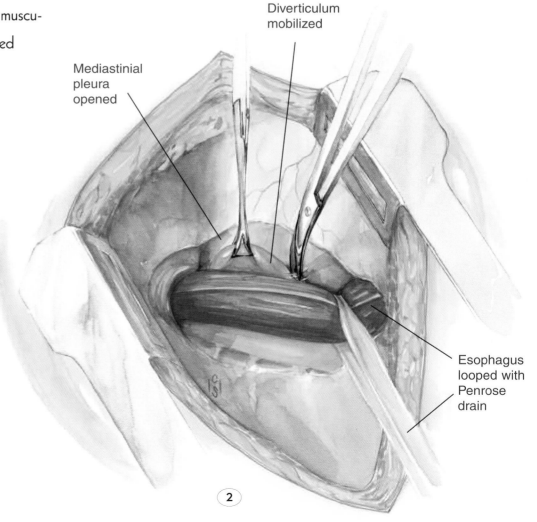

Mediastinial pleura opened

Diverticulum mobilized

Esophagus looped with Penrose drain

2

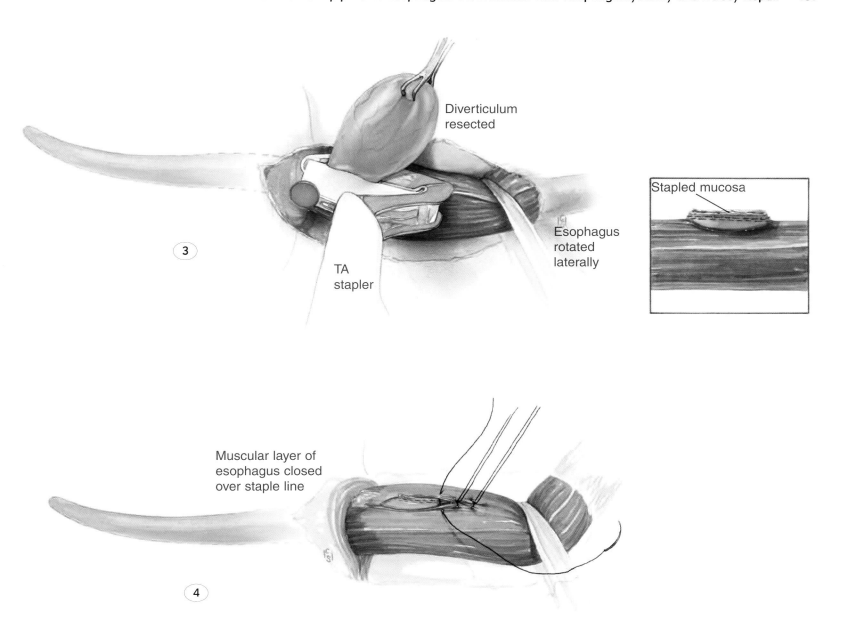

With the diverticulum completely excised, attention is turned toward the esophageal motility disorder commonly associated with these diverticula. This is managed with a distal esophagomyotomy. Once the esophagomyotomy is performed and the lower esophageal sphincter destroyed, a new sphincter needs to be created by performing a loose Belsey Mark IV antireflux repair. To accomplish this, the distal esophagus and hiatus are further mobilized, bringing the fundus of the stomach up into the chest. This mobilization includes division of branches of the left gastric vessels along the lesser curvature of the stomach and the upper vasa brevia along the greater curvature, with removal of the fat pad along the esophagogastric junction anteriorly (5).

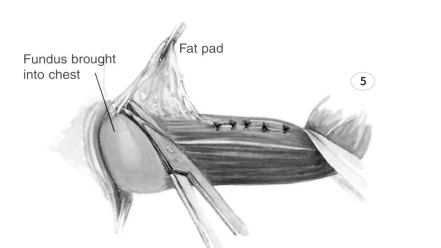

Once the distal esophagus and fundus of the stomach have been mobilized sufficiently, an esophagomyotomy is performed that involves the distal 5 cm of the esophagus and extends onto the gastric wall for at least 1 cm. The muscle layer of the esophagus is elevated from the mucosa with a right angle clamp and is divided with either scissors or the electrocautery (6).

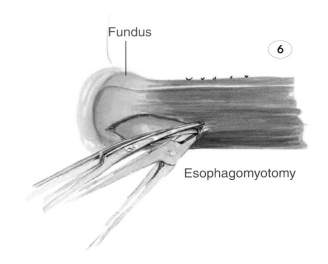

The muscle layer is then dissected free from the esophageal mucosa for at least 50% of the circumference of the esophagus (7). This dissection is easily accomplished with scissors using both sharp and blunt dissection.

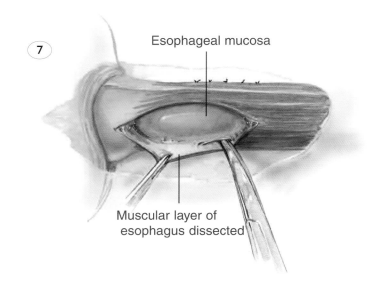

The fundus of the stomach is further mobilized in preparation for performing a Belsey Mark IV antireflux procedure. Because the esophageal hiatus has been stretched to dissect the fundus and deliver it into the chest, interrupted crural sutures of No. 2 silk are placed posteriorly. A modified Belsey procedure is then performed (8).

Instead of the usual two rows of three sutures, two rows of only two sutures are placed. One horizontal mattress suture is placed on either side of the myotomy in each row. For the first row, a suture of 2-0 silk is placed through gastric fundus 2 cm from the gas-

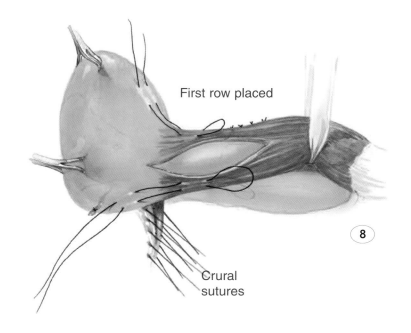

troesophageal junction, then longitudinally through the esophagus lateral to the esophagomyotomy, 2 cm above the gastroesophageal junction. The mattress suture is brought back down through the esophagus and stomach. A similar suture is placed on the other side of the esophagomyotomy (8).

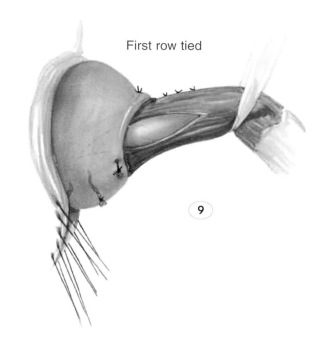

First row tied

9

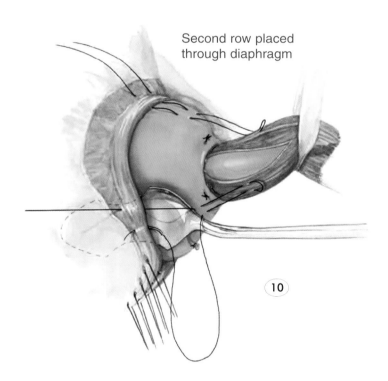

Second row placed through diaphragm

10

After tying both sutures (9), a second row of two sutures is then placed by first passing the 2-0 silk through the diaphragm (from the chest to the abdominal side), through fundus of the stomach 2 cm below the first row of repair sutures, and then longitudinally through the esophagus 2 cm above the first row. The mattress suture is brought back down through the esophagus and fundus and out through the diaphragm. Two such sutures are placed, one on either side of the myotomy. The placement of the diaphragmatic portions of the sutures is aided by retraction with a large spoon (10).

Once both sutures of the second row have been placed, the fundus of the stomach is reduced below the diaphragm, and the two sutures are secured. The previously placed diaphragmatic crural sutures are secured (11). When securing these crural sutures, one should have in place an indwelling 46 French Maloney dilator and a nasogastric tube, leaving only enough space between the esophagus and the crural sutures to admit a fingertip.

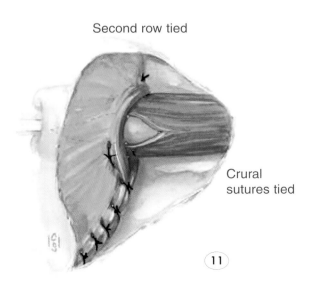

Second row tied

Crural sutures tied

11

Thus, the procedure has resulted in resection of the diverticulum, destruction of the discoordinated lower esophageal sphincter, and construction of a new sphincter with a Belsey Mark IV procedure (12, 13, 14). The integrity of the esophageal mucosa can be checked by exchanging the Maloney dilator with a flexible esophagoscope, submerging the area under saline, and insufflating the esophagus while holding distal pressure on the lumen. Any leaks should be repaired with a 4-0 absorbable suture. A chest tube is inserted, and the thoracotomy incision closed.

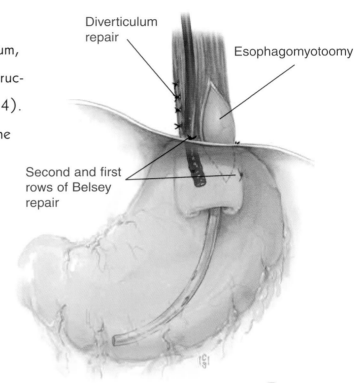

Diverticulum repair

Esophagomyotoomy

Second and first rows of Belsey repair

12

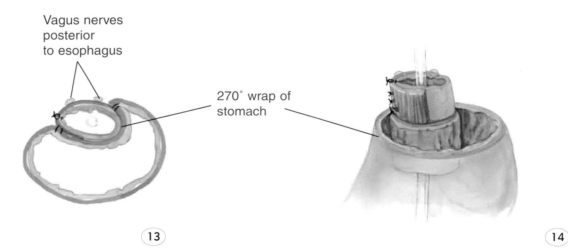

Vagus nerves posterior to esophagus

270° wrap of stomach

13

14

Achalasia: Heller Esophagomyotomy and Belsey Repair

Operative Indications

Achalasia is an esophageal disorder that presents as dysphagia and is secondary to failure of relaxation of the lower esophageal sphincter and the absence of progressive peristalsis in the esophagus. Failure of the sphincter to relax with swallowing, along with a higher resting pressure, are characteristics of this disorder. It presents insidiously over a long period. Since the symptoms of dysphagia are gradual and may not be appreciated initially, when achalasia is finally diagnosed, a very large dilated esophagus may be present (1). In many institutions, the initial management of achalasia is with either balloon dilatation, or by local injection of the lower esophageal sphincter with botulinum toxin. Each of these may require two or more treatments. In at least half of the patients, these treatments are eventually ineffective. For patients who fail these two options, or who subsequently have a recurrence, surgically destroying the lower esophageal sphincter by Heller esophagomyotomy and then creating a new sphincter with a Belsey Mark IV operation is the procedure of choice.

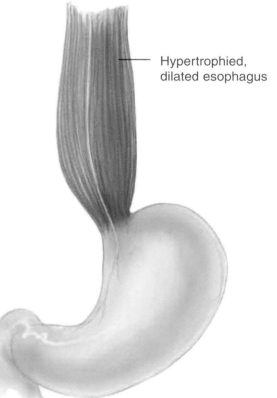

Hypertrophied, dilated esophagus

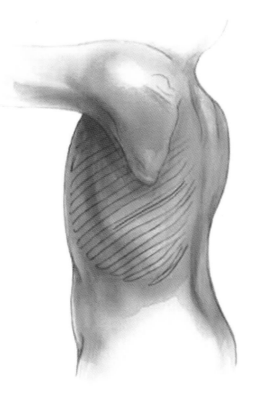

Operative Technique

The patient is placed in the lateral thoracotomy position with the left chest up. The left pleural cavity is entered through the sixth or seventh interspace. The mediastinal pleura is opened, and the markedly dilated and hypertrophied esophagus is easily identified. It is mobilized out of the mediastinum with both sharp and blunt dissection. The esophagus is looped with a Penrose drain (2). The hiatus is enlarged so that the fundus of the stomach may be delivered up into the chest. To do this, it is necessary to divide the branches of the left gastric vessels along the lesser curvature of the stomach and the vasa brevia along the greater curvature. The distal esophagus, cardia, and fundus are dissected out of the retroperitoneum.

Once the esophagus and stomach have been appropriately mobilized, the fat pad is dissected free from the gastroesophageal junction. The vagus nerves are identified and carefully preserved, and both are swept posteriorly (inset). An esophagomyotomy is performed that extends up onto the esophagus for approximately 10 cm and onto the stomach for approximately 1 cm.

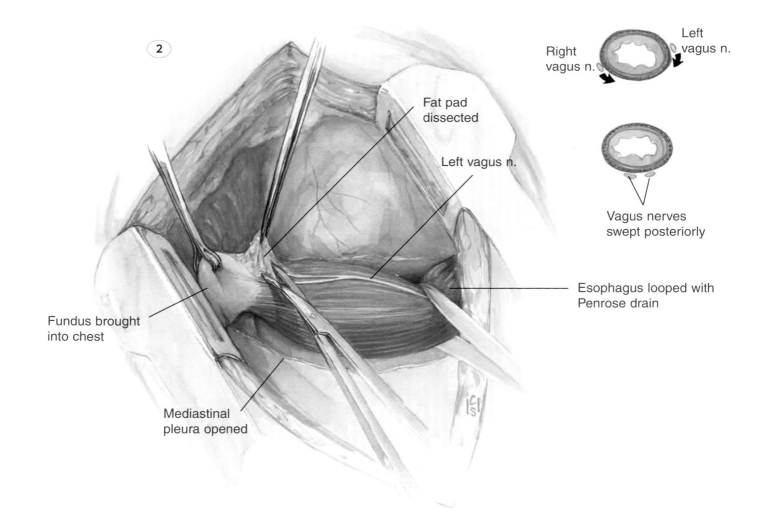

2

Fat pad
dissected

Left vagus n.

Fundus brought
into chest

Mediastinal
pleura opened

Right
vagus n.

Left
vagus n.

Vagus nerves
swept posteriorly

Esophagus looped with
Penrose drain

This is best done by separating the muscular layer of the esophagus from the mucosa with a right angle clamp and then dividing the muscle with the electrocautery on low voltage (3). The muscular layer of the esophagus is easily separated from the mucosal tube, and should be freed for at least 50% of the circumference of the esophagus (4). However, in a small number of cases where repetitive dilatation or toxin injection have taken place preoperatively, there may be scarring between the muscle and mucosal layers. The integrity of the esophageal mucosa can be checked by inserting a flexible esophagoscope, submerging the area under saline, and insufflating the esophagus while holding distal pressure on the lumen. Any leaks should be repaired with 4-0 absorbable suture prior to the fundoplication.

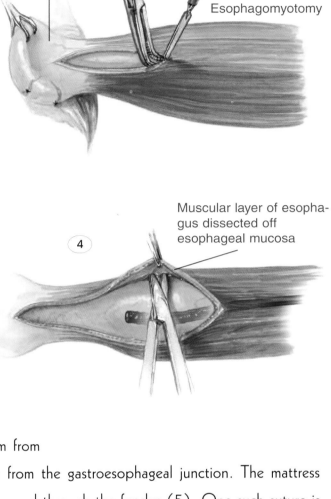

Fundus

Esophagomyotomy

Once the esophagomyotomy has been performed and the distal esophageal sphincter destroyed, a new sphincter is created by a modified Belsey Mark IV procedure. Crural sutures of No. 2 silk are placed, but not tied. In the presence of the esophagomyotomy, it is only possible to place two sutures in each of the two rows of stitches used in the Belsey

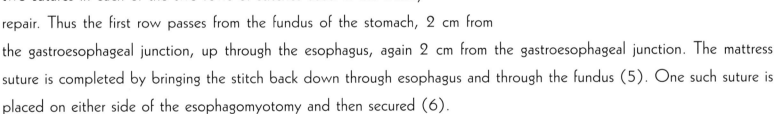

Muscular layer of esophagus dissected off esophageal mucosa

repair. Thus the first row passes from the fundus of the stomach, 2 cm from the gastroesophageal junction, up through the esophagus, again 2 cm from the gastroesophageal junction. The mattress suture is completed by bringing the stitch back down through esophagus and through the fundus (5). One such suture is placed on either side of the esophagomyotomy and then secured (6).

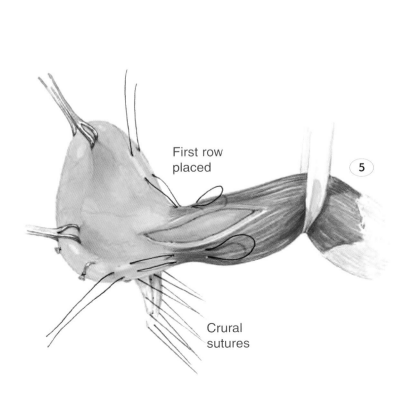

First row placed

Crural sutures

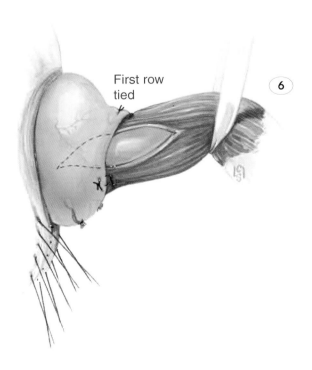

First row tied

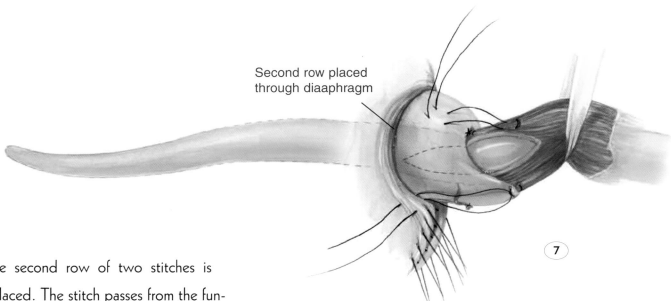

Second row placed
through diaaphragm

7

The second row of two stitches is
then placed. The stitch passes from the fundus of the stomach, through the esophagus,
back down through esophagus and fundus, each
being placed 2 cm from the first row of sutures.
These are secured, and the two ends then rethreaded
on large Ferguson needles and passed through the
diaphragm, from the abdominal to the thoracic side
(7). The fundus is then reduced below the
diaphragm, and the sutures are secured.

The previously placed crural sutures
are tied (8) with a 46 French
Maloney dilator in place. Since the
esophagus is aperistaltic, a Nissen
fundoplication should not be used to
create a new lower esophageal sphincter,
for it may lead to partial obstruction.

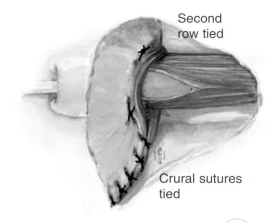

Second
row tied

Crural sutures
tied

8

As with the Nissen fundoplication, the crura are approximated by suturing posterior to the gastroesophageal junction using Teflon pledgets, as described for the laparoscopic Nissen fundoplication.

Then, the 270° posterior wrap is constructed by pulling the posterior fundus of the stomach around behind the esophagus with an atraumatic grasper. The fundus is then sutured laparoscopically to the crus on the right, using pledgets (5). Similarly, the anterior fundus of the stomach is sutured to the left crus using pledgets (6).

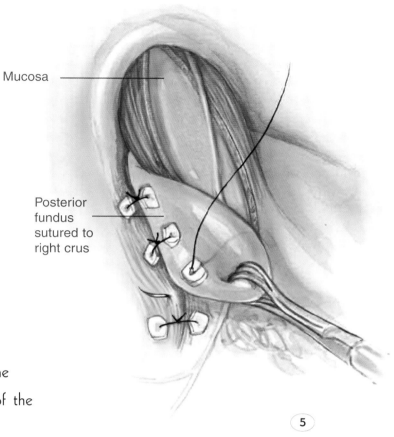

Mucosa

Posterior fundus sutured to right crus

5

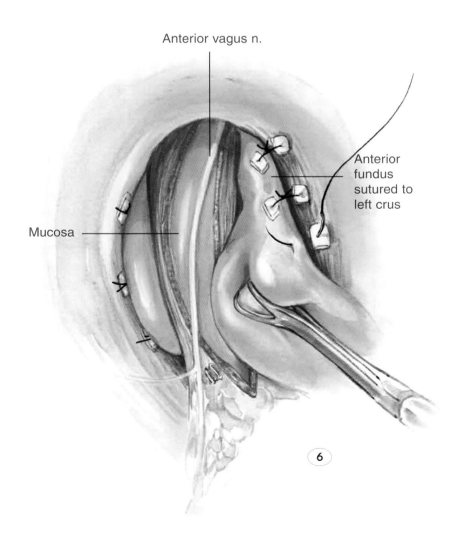

Anterior vagus n.

Anterior fundus sutured to left crus

Mucosa

6

Once these are secured, each side of the fundus of the stomach is sutured to the divided edge of the esophageal muscle layers (7). In combination, these sutures anchor the 270° wrap and keep the myotomized edges of the muscle separated.

The abdomen is then surveyed laparoscopically to ensure that there is no unexpected bleeding or injury. Then, an endoscope is passed orally to examine the construction from within the esophagus (8). If the myotomy is adequate, the scope will pass easily from the esophagus into the stomach. To ensure that there is no defect in the mucosa, some irrigation fluid is dripped onto the anterior esophagus while the scope insufflates air. The scope is then withdrawn, and the port sites closed.

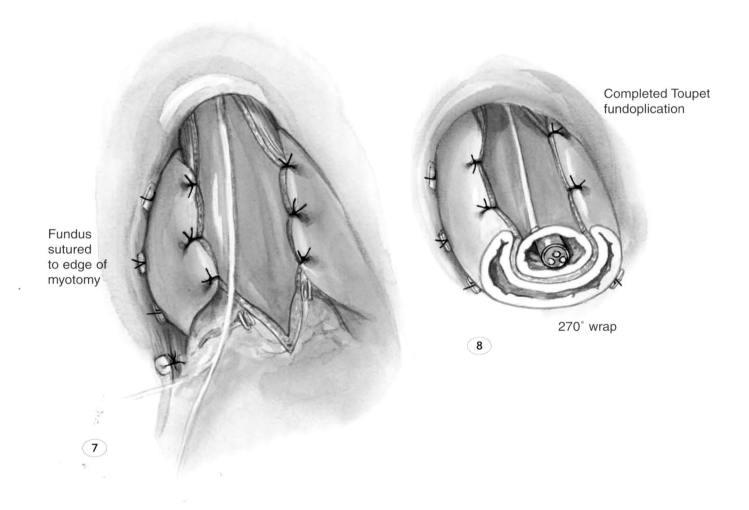

Fundus sutured to edge of myotomy

Completed Toupet fundoplication

270° wrap

7

8

Esophageal Spasm: Long Esophagomyotomy and Belsey Repair

Operative Indications

Diffuse esophageal spasm is a disorder characterized by chest pain, secondary to marked uncoordinated contractions of the thoracic esophagus. Esophageal manometrics demonstrate uncoordinated, nonprogressive, high-amplitude contractions in the esophagus. This disorder may initially be confused with coronary artery disease and angina pectoris. Some of these patients undergo extensive cardiac testing, and only when it is normal does the diagnostic workup lead to the esophagus. It is not clear what triggers the spasm in many of these patients, but in up to half of them, emotional stress is associated. Dysphagia, gastroesophageal reflux, and a hiatal hernia are usually absent. Interestingly, patients may initially receive some benefit from the administration of nitroglycerin and calcium channel blockers, further delaying recognition of the entity. If the management of this disorder with smooth muscle relaxants is unsuccessful, surgical intervention is indicated.

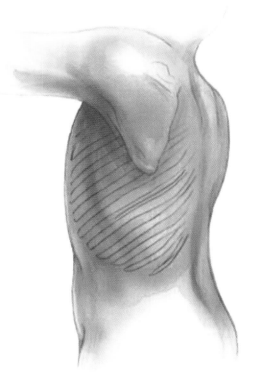

Operative Technique

The patient is placed in the lateral thoracotomy position with the left chest up. The left pleural cavity is entered through the sixth or seventh interspace. The mediastinal pleura is opened and the esophagus identified. The esophagus is often markedly thickened and hypertrophied and is easily palpated in the mediastinum. Preoperative manometrics can map out the section of esophagus that is involved with the uncoordinated high-amplitude contractions. Generally, it is the distal two-thirds of the esophagus, so an esophagomyotomy that extends up to the aortic arch encompasses all of the involved esophagus. The myotomy should also extend down onto the stomach.

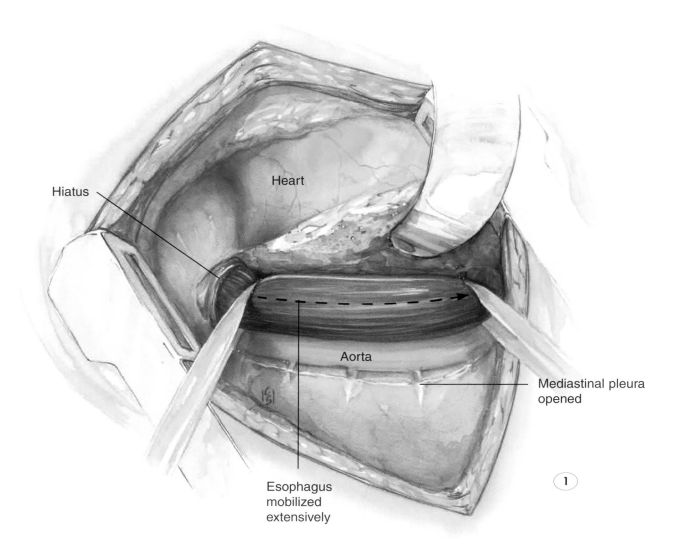

Hiatus

Heart

Aorta

Mediastinal pleura
opened

Esophagus
mobilized
extensively

The esophagus is mobilized
extensively up to and even under the aortic arch
(1). The hiatus is stretched, and the fundus of the stomach mobilized and delivered into
the chest. This maneuver may require division of branches of the left gastric vessels along the
lesser curvature and the vasa brevia along the greater curvature.

Open Resection of Esophageal Leiomyoma

Operative Indications

Leiomyomas arise from the muscular layer of the esophageal wall (1). The mucosa is not involved and remains intact over the benign tumor, resulting in the characteristic smooth appearance on barium swallow. The defect seen radiographically is smooth and usually protrudes in a semicircular fashion into the esophageal lumen. These lesions are easily differentiated from the more common malignant mucosal lesions. If these leimyomas are large, they may be seen on a plain chest x-ray or a computed tomography (CT) scan. If the tumors are large enough to result in dysphagia, the characteristic appearance on barium swallow makes the diagnosis almost a certainty. If endoscopy is carried out, one can see an intact mucosa over the lesion protruding into the esophageal lumen. One should not perform a biopsy of the mucosa overlying the lesion, because an opening into the esophageal lumen at the time of surgical resection will result. If the radiographic appearance is pathognomonic and symptoms are minimal or absent, some surgeons have advocated following the patient and not removing the tumor surgically unless symptoms increase. Most, however, think these lesions should be excised when they are found to prevent or alleviate symptoms and to do so while they are smaller and more manageable. Esophageal resection is rarely indicated.

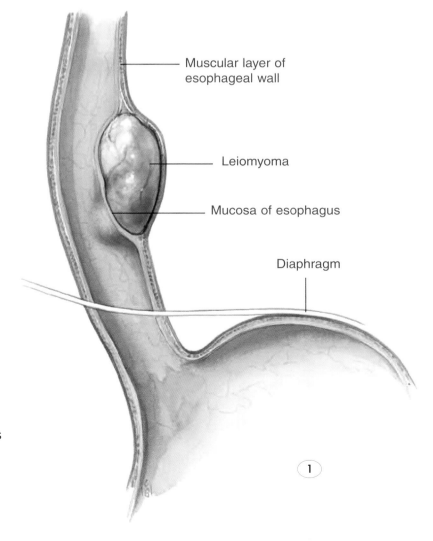

Muscular layer of esophageal wall

Leiomyoma

Mucosa of esophagus

Diaphragm

1

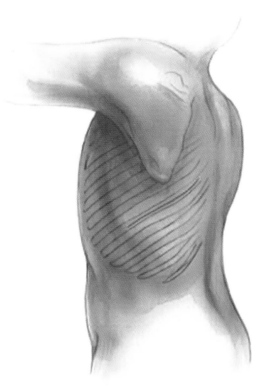

Operative Technique

Flexible esophagoscopy should be performed after induction of anesthesia to localize the tumor and again, after resection, to check for mucosal leaks. The patient is positioned in the lateral thoracotomy position. Most esophageal leiomyomas can be approached via the right chest, but those approaching the esophagogastric junction should be resected from the left side; the illustrations depict the latter. The thoracic cavity is entered through the sixth intercostal space.

The mediastinal pleura is opened, and the esophagus identified and dissected free. The lesion is easily palpated in the esophageal wall. It has a firm, rubbery consistency and is easily differentiated from a malignant neoplasm. Occasionally, the flexible esophagoscope can be used to help localize it. Once the esophagus has been mobilized and encircled with a Penrose drain, the outer longitudinal muscle layer is opened with the scalpel (2).

The incision in the esophageal wall is deepened until the whitish, rubbery, benign smooth muscle neoplasm is identified. It can be gently grasped with a Babcock clamp or Ring forceps.

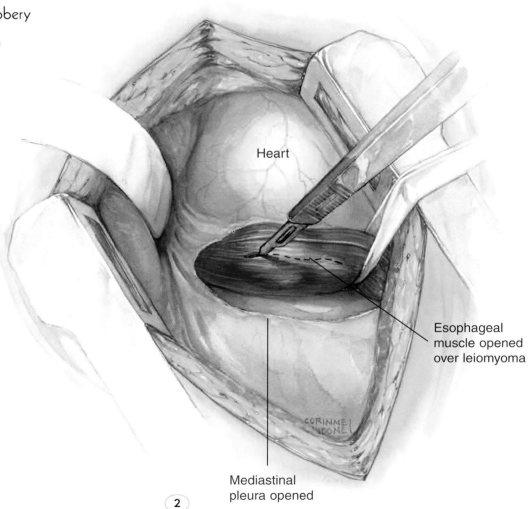

Heart

Esophageal muscle opened over leiomyoma

Mediastinal pleura opened

2

(10)

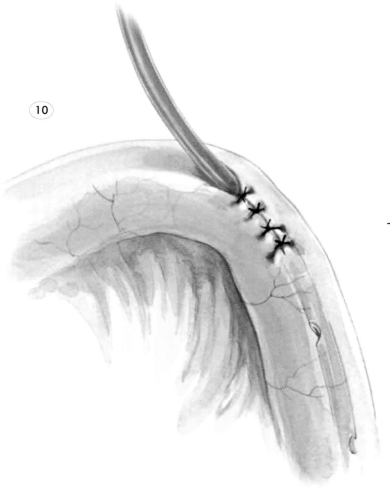

The enterotomy site is imbricated with several interrupted 3-0 silk Lembert sutures. (10, 11). The jejunostomy tube is then brought out in the left upper quadrant; the jejunal site is tacked up to the anterior abdominal wall with interrupted 3-0 silk sutures. The abdomen is irrigated and closed.

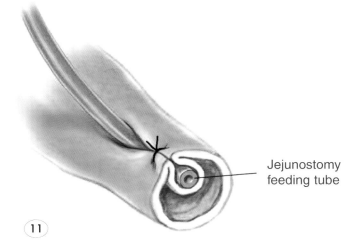

Jejunostomy feeding tube

(11)

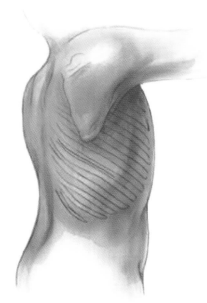

The patient is repositioned in preparation for a right lateral thoracotomy. The right pleural cavity is entered through the fifth intercostal space. A short segment of the fifth rib posteriorly can be removed to improve exposure if needed. The ribs are spread with a self-retaining retractor. The mediastinal pleura is opened over the entire length of the thoracic esophagus (12).

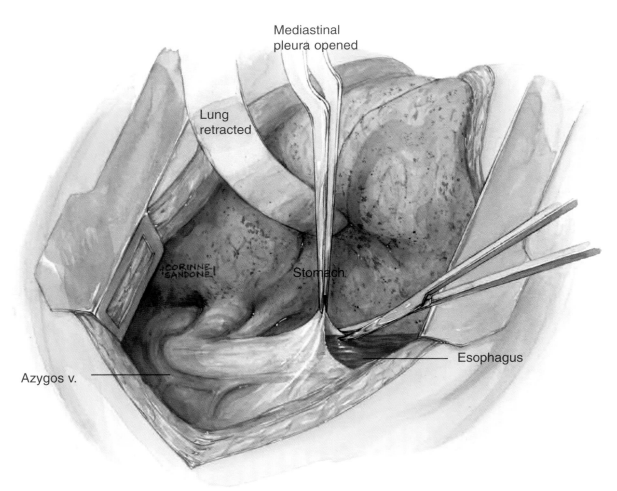

12

The distal portion of the esophagus, including the tumor, has been dissected free through the abdominal incision. The esophagus is further mobilized up to the azygos vein through the thoracotomy incision using both sharp and blunt dissection (13). The azygos vein is ligated and divided to aid in the most cephalad portion of the dissection. When the entire thoracic esophagus has been mobilized, the stomach is pulled up through the widened hiatus into the chest.

Using the linear stapler and starting at the greater curvature, a gastric tube is created. Two or three firings of the linear stapler are required to reach the point previously cleaned along the lesser curvature (14, 15).

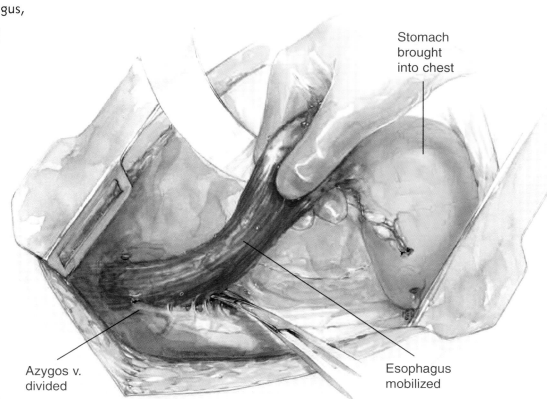

Stomach brought into chest

Azygos v. divided

Esophagus mobilized

(13)

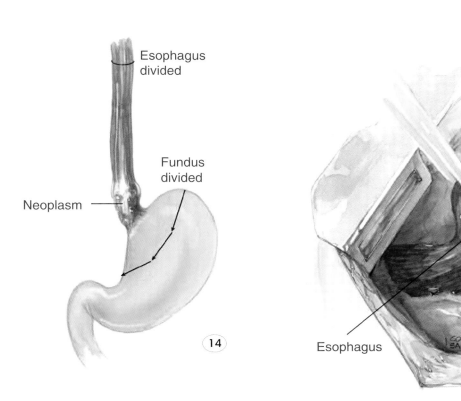

Esophagus divided

Fundus divided

Neoplasm

(14)

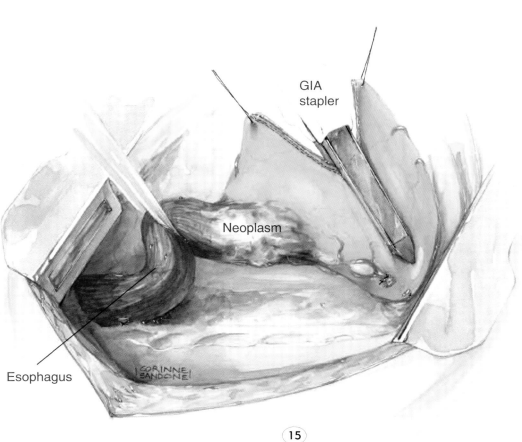

GIA stapler

Neoplasm

Esophagus

(15)

This usually requires three firings of the stapler. Care is taken not to make the gastric tube too wide. The points of division along the greater and lesser curvatures of the stomach are chosen to provide an adequate distal tumor margin of at least 5 cm from the gastroesophageal junction. The staple line on the stomach is reinforced with an interrupted layer of 3-0 silk Lembert sutures (16).

The esophagogastrostomy is performed with two layers of interrupted 3-0 silk sutures. The site of the anastomosis on the stomach is placed down from the most cephalad portion of the fundus and midway between the staple line and the greater curvature on the anterior wall. The posterior outer layer of interrupted 3-0 silk sutures is placed first (17). A gastrotomy is performed cutting out a 1- to 1.5-cm elliptical button of the stomach using electrocautery on low voltage. The posterior wall of the esophagus is divided, preserving as much of the mucosal layer as possible (18). The sutures of the inner layer of the posterior row pass through and through the full thickness of both the gastric and esophageal walls (19).

Once the inner layer of the posterior row has been placed, the remaining esophagus is divided and the specimen removed from the operative field. At this point, frozen sections can be performed on both the proximal and distal margins. The nasogastric tube is passed into the stomach. The inner layer of the ante-

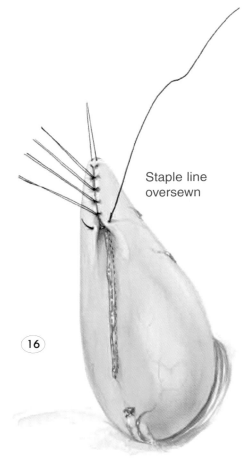

Staple line oversewn

(16)

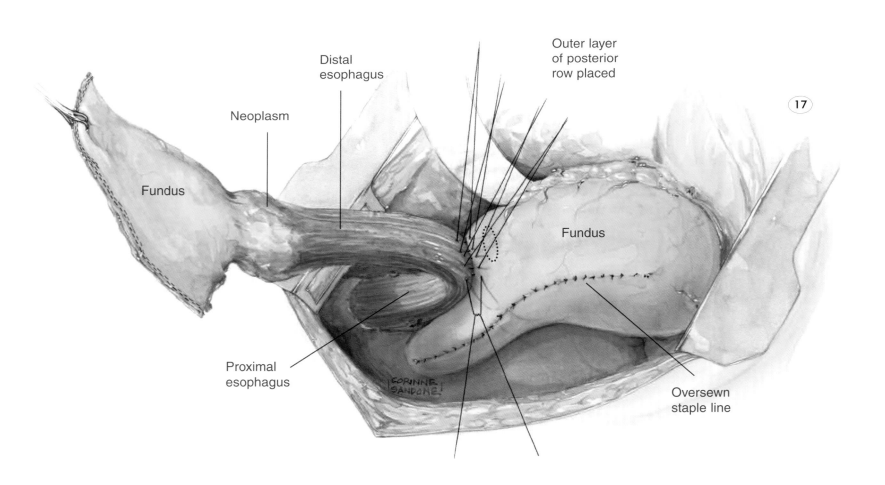

Distal esophagus

Neoplasm

Outer layer of posterior row placed

(17)

Fundus

Fundus

Proximal esophagus

Oversewn staple line

rior row is performed with an interrupted inverting suture that passes from inside out on the esophageal wall, and then outside in on the gastric wall (20). The anastomosis is completed by placing the outer layer of the anterior row with interrupted 3-0 silk Lembert sutures (21). The tip of the fundus is the most ischemic part of the conduit. To help minimize leaks in this area, a purse-string suture is placed circumferentially (22), and once tied, the tip is inverted and the purse-string is secured (23).

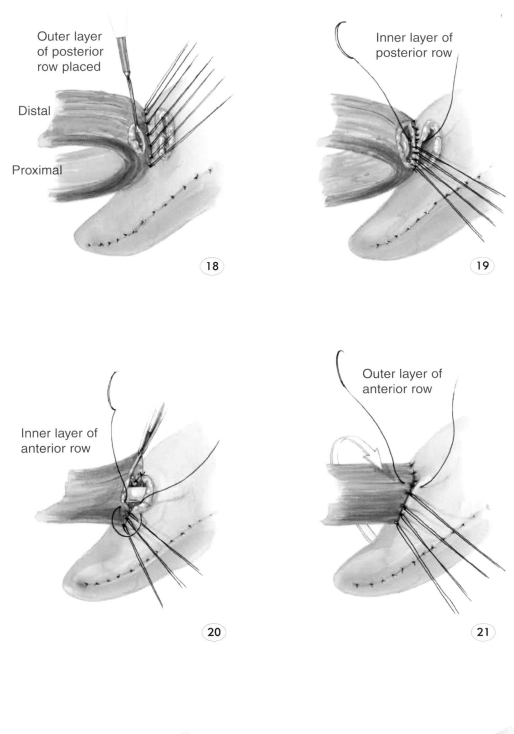

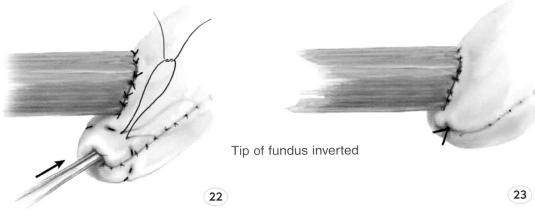

The anastomosis can be wrapped either with a piece of parietal pleura based on a long pedicle or, alternatively, with any redundant stomach, like a Nissen fundoplication (24). Mediastinal lymph nodes are either sampled or a complete dissection performed. The stomach is sutured to the enlarged hiatus with interrupted 3-0 silk. A chest tube is inserted, and the incision closed in layers.

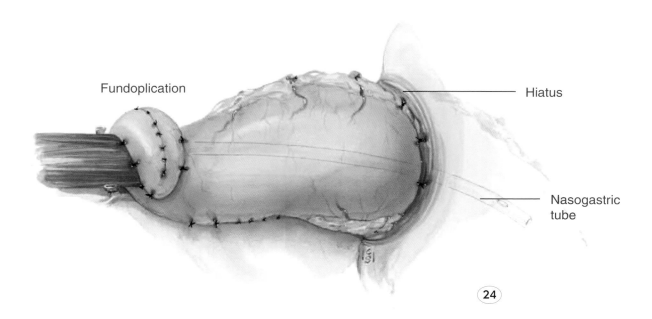

Fundoplication   Hiatus

Nasogastric tube

24

Esophagogastrectomy through a Left Thoracoabdominal Incision

Operative Indications

In contrast to the esophagogastrectomy (described in the previous section) performed through separate abdominal and thoracic incisions, an esophagogastrectomy can be performed through one incision utilizing the thoracoabdominal approach. One has to be certain that the malignancy is confined to the area of the gastroesophageal junction. With this approach, the proximal extent of the esophageal resection is restricted by the aortic arch. If, however, after radiographic studies and endoscopic biopsies, it is certain that the neoplasm is confined to the distal esophagus without submucosal spread and without Barrett's mucosa extending proximally, the thoracoabdominal incision can be used. This approach is perhaps best suited for gastric cancers near the gastroesophageal junction that extend up into the distal esophagus.

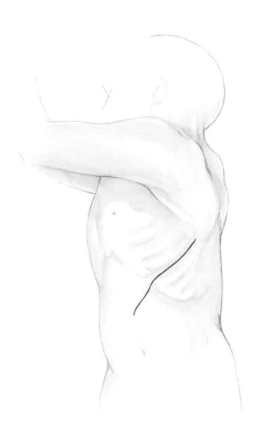

Operative Technique

The patient is placed in a left thoracotomy position, with the hips rotated back toward the table at a 45° angle, to provide access to the abdomen. The left pleural cavity is entered through the seventh or eighth interspace; the incision extends across the abdomen to a point midway between the xiphoid and umbilicus. If preoperative staging has left some uncertainty as to the resectability of the lesion, the abdominal portion of the incision can be made first; the abdomen is explored with the hand before deciding whether to open the entire thoracoabdominal incision.

The costal cartilage is divided, removing a section of cartilage so that chondritis is not a problem when the ribs are subsequently re-approximated.

Diaphragm viewed from above

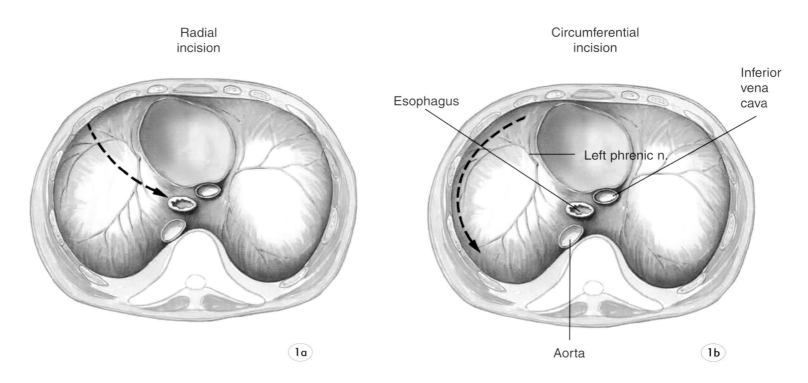

Radial
incision

Circumferential
incision

Esophagus

Left phrenic n.

Inferior
vena
cava

Aorta

1a   1b

Once the chest and abdomen have been opened, it is necessary to divide the diaphragm in order to provide appropriate exposure to mobilize the colon. Whereas many surgeons divide the diaphragm radially (1a), extending the incision toward but not through the esophageal hiatus, fewer branches of the phrenic nerve are divided if the diaphragm is opened circumferentially (1b). When the latter is done, it is important to leave at least 3 cm of diaphragm attached to the chest wall, to facilitate approximation during closure.

Once the abdomen and chest have been opened, the esophagus in the chest is mobilized and encircled with a Penrose drain. The esophageal hiatus is dissected and widened, and the gastroesophageal junction, distal esophagus, and tumor are extensively mobilized. The left gastric vessels along the lesser curvature and the vasa brevia along the greater curvature are divided. The retroperitoneal portion of the fundus of the stomach and distal esophagus is mobilized. Through the abdominal incision the greater omentum is divided, leaving the right gastroepiploic vessels intact. The fundus is divided using the linear stapler, taking several applications. The line of division is chosen to ensure an adequate distal tumor margin of at least 5 cm. The staple line in the distal stomach is reinforced with an interrupted layer of 3-0 silk Lembert sutures (2). A pyloromyotomy or pyloroplasty is performed, as described in "Short Segment Colon Interposition for Benign Esophageal Stricture" above.

The proximal fundus, gastroesophageal junction, distal esophagus, and tumor are retracted up through the hiatus into the chest. The proximal stomach is also pulled through the hiatus into the chest (3).

Operative Technique

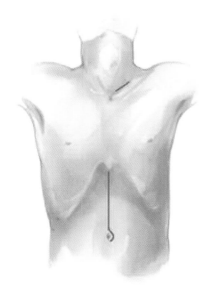

The patient is placed in the supine position. The abdomen, anterior chest, and left neck are prepped and draped appropriately, with the head turned to the right. The abdomen is opened first through an upper midline incision. The initial part of this procedure is identical to that of esophagogastrectomy done through separate abdominal and chest incisions. The abdomen is explored to be certain that widely disseminated tumor is not present, thus obviating the indication for esophagectomy.

The intra-abdominal esophagus is mobilized, and the esophageal hiatus dilated. The vasa brevia are ligated and divided (2). Clips are avoided on the stomach because they may come off when the stomach is subsequently advanced through the posterior mediastinum. The greater omentum is divided, carefully preserving the right gastroepiploic vessels and the entire gastroepiploic arch. The gastrohepatic ligament is divided, and the left gastric vessels are dissected free both anteriorly and posteriorly through the lesser sac. The left gastric vessels are ligated close to their takeoff from the celiac axis and divided (3).

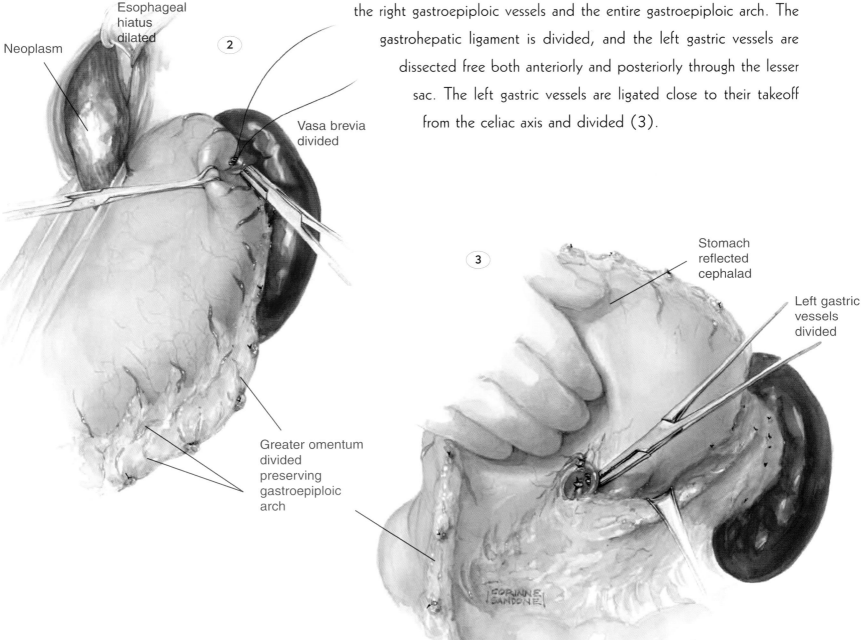

Esophageal hiatus dilated

Neoplasm

2

Vasa brevia divided

Greater omentum divided preserving gastroepiploic arch

3

Stomach reflected cephalad

Left gastric vessels divided

Duodenum
kocherized

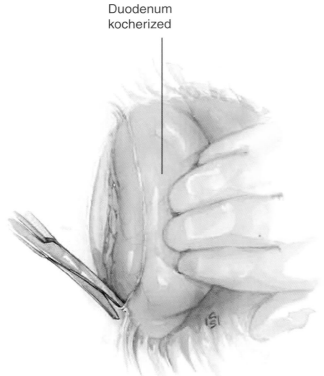

4

The duodenum is extensively kocherized (4), and a pyloromyotomy or pyloroplasty performed, covered with omentum, and marked with small hemoclips (5).

The stomach is now completely mobilized, including the posterior aspect of the cardia and fundus out of the retroperitoneum. The hiatus is widened to allow the surgeon's hand to be inserted into the mediastinum. One may choose to divide the muscle fibers of the hiatus anteriorly. The phrenic vein should be doubly ligated and divided during this process (6). Generally, the triangular ligament is divided, and the left lobe of the liver retracted to the right.

Pylorus opened
horizontaly,
closed transversely

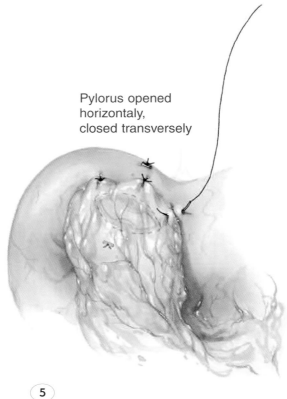

5

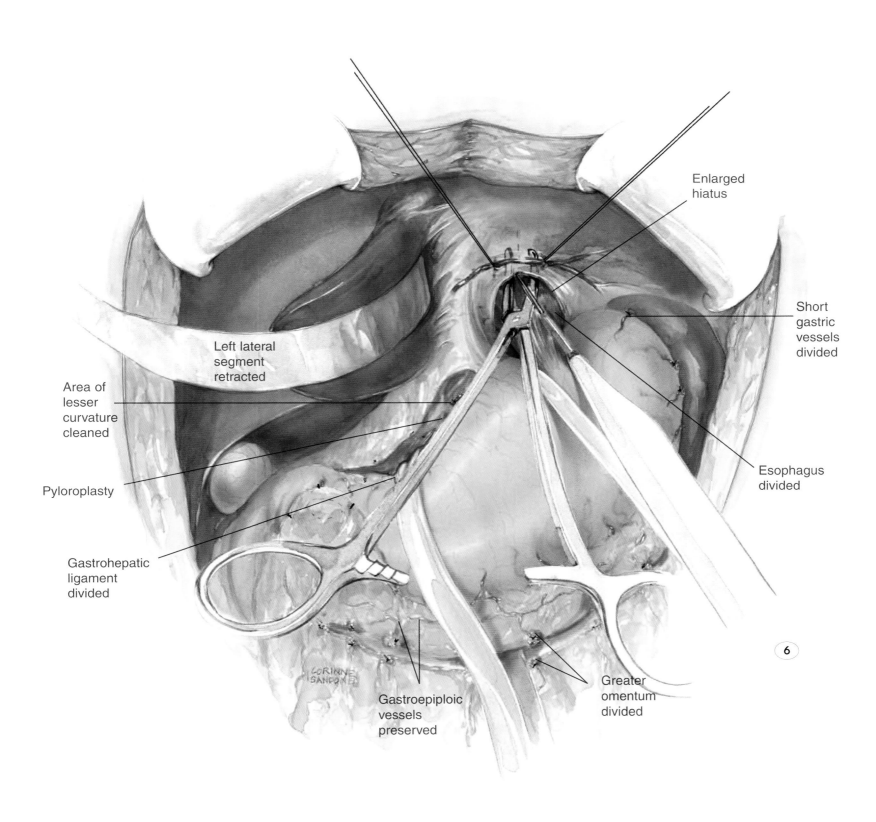

Enlarged
hiatus

Short
gastric
vessels
divided

Left lateral
segment
retracted

Area of
lesser
curvature
cleaned

Esophagus
divided

Pyloroplasty

Gastrohepatic
ligament
divided

Gastroepiploic
vessels
preserved

Greater
omentum
divided

6

The dissection of the distal esophagus continues through the dilated hiatus. By pulling caudally on the Penrose drain passed around the distal esophagus, and by retracting the dilated hiatus with a small Deaver retractor, much of the distal half of the esophagus can be visualized directly. Small vessels can be identified, ligated and divided, or cauterized (7). With both blunt and sharp dissection, under direct vision, much of the distal esophagus can be mobilized without risk of bleeding.

At this point, the cervical esophagus is exposed. A curvilinear incision is made 1 cm above the sternal notch and extended to the left over the midportion of the sternocleidomastoid muscle (8). This is a much more cosmetically appealing incision than one made over the sternocleidomastoid muscle. The platysma is divided and undermined for approximately 1 cm around the edges. The omohyoid muscle usually needs to be divided, as does the middle thyroid vein. The trachea and thyroid are now retracted medially, and the sternocleidomastoid muscle laterally, with a self-retaining retractor, taking care not to put too much stretch on the recurrent laryngeal nerve or the carotid sheath (9). The esophagus with an indwelling nasogastric tube can be easily palpated. The esophagus is mobilized circumferentially and grasped with a Babcock clamp.

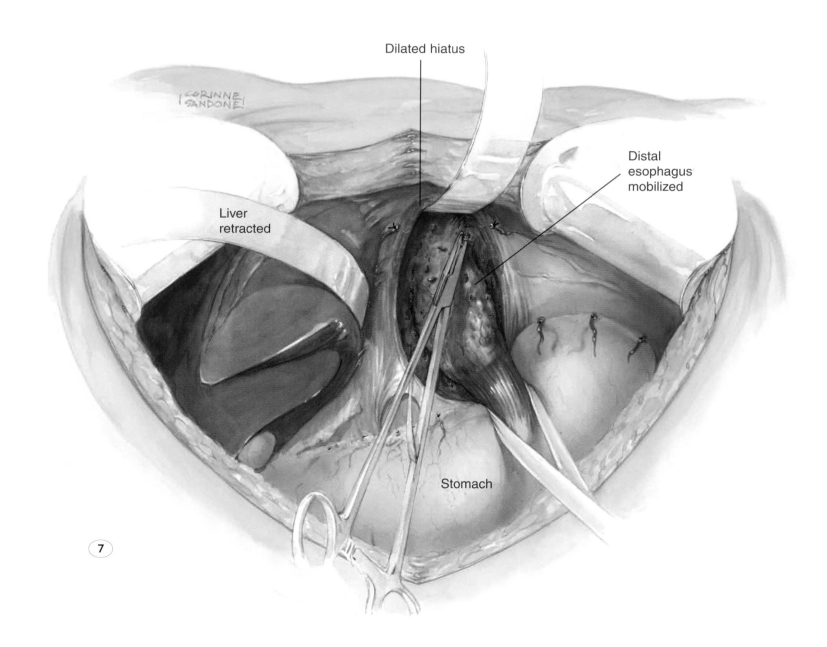

Dilated hiatus

Distal esophagus mobilized

Liver retracted

Stomach

7

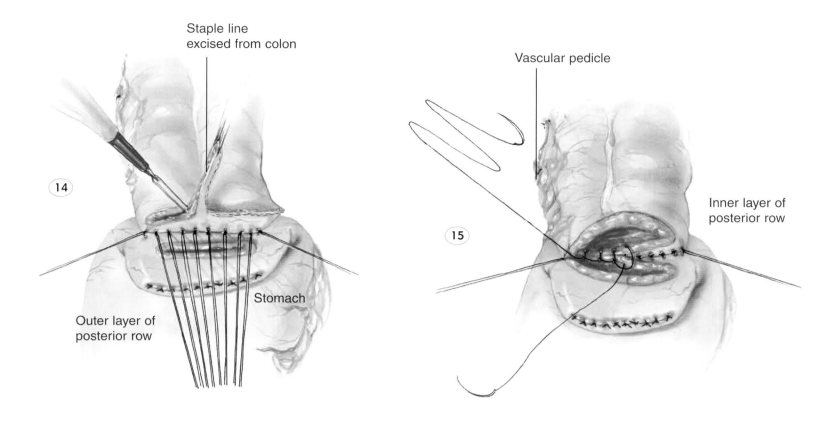

The outer layer of the posterior row is placed first, using interrupted 3-0 silk sutures placed in a Lembert fashion. The staple line is then removed from the colon using the electrocautery (14). A gastrotomy is performed using the electrocautery. The inner layer of the posterior row consists of a continuous locking suture of 3-0 synthetic absorbable material (15). This is brought around anteriorly for the inner layer of the anterior row, in a Connell fashion (16). Prior to closure of the inner anterior row, the nasogastric tube is advanced through the distal part of the colon conduit into the stomach. The cologastrostomy is completed with an outer layer of 3-0 silk Lembert sutures in the anterior row (17).

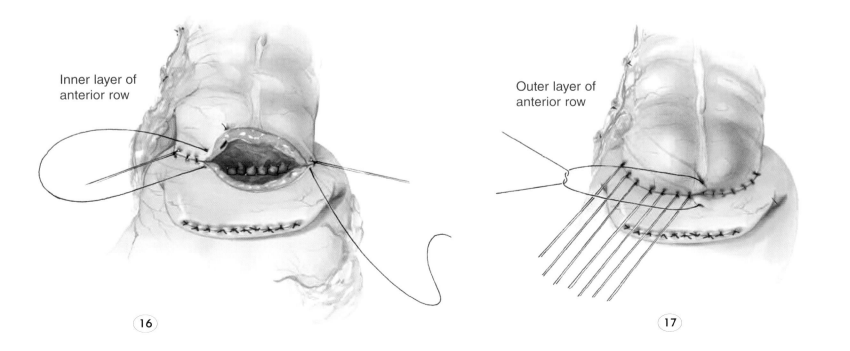

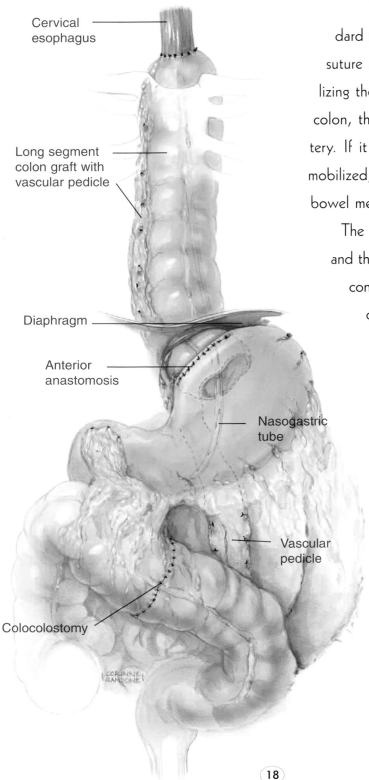

Cervical esophagus

Long segment colon graft with vascular pedicle

Diaphragm

Anterior anastomosis

Nasogastric tube

Vascular pedicle

Colocolostomy

(18)

The right transverse and distal left colon are reanastomosed in a standard two-layer fashion with an inner continuous layer of synthetic absorbable suture and an outer layer of interrupted 3-0 silk (18). Generally, by mobilizing the right colon out of the retroperitoneum and by mobilizing the sigmoid colon, this anastomosis can be made above the root of the small bowel mesentery. If it will not reach without tension, the right colon should be extensively mobilized, turned down, and then anastomosed below the root of the small bowel mesentery.

The long segment colon graft should extend between the cervical esophagus and the posterior body wall of the stomach easily without tension. The pedicle, consisting of the ascending branches of the left colic vessels, passes posterior to the stomach and resides alongside the colon in the mediastinum. A pyloromyotomy (or pyloroplasty) is performed because of the inevitable vagotomy that results from the esophagectomy (19). Alternatively, the cologastrostomy can be performed along the anterior part of the stomach (20). Some surgeons prefer this approach to allow for better emptying of the colon.

A small Penrose drain is left near the anastomosis in the neck, and the neck incision closed in layers. A feeding jejunostomy is placed as described in "Esophagogastrectomy: Separate Abdominal and Thoracic Incisions" above. The abdominal incision is closed without drains.

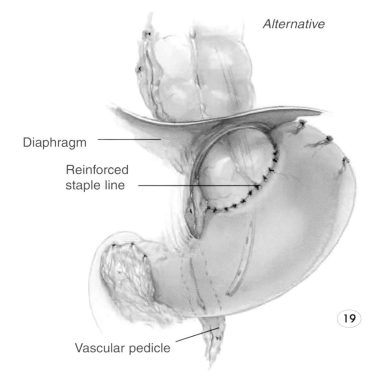

Alternative

Diaphragm

Reinforced staple line

(19)

Vascular pedicle

Esophageal Reconstruction Following Total Laryngopharyngectomy: Pharyngogastrostomy or Reconstruction Utilizing Free Jejunal Graft

Operative Indications

Occasionally malignancies occurring in the neck require laryngectomy, pharyngectomy, and cervical esophagectomy. Such tumors may arise in the cervical esophagus, in the larynx, or in the pharynx, and involve adjacent structures. If such a malignancy is treated by surgical resection, generally the pharynx and cervical esophagus have to be sacrificed. The quickest, easiest, and safest means of restoring enteric continuity following such a major resection is to sacrifice the thoracic esophagus, pull the stomach up into the neck, and anastomose it directly to the pharynx.

A variety of techniques have been used to restore continuity between the thoracic esophagus and pharynx. These have included tubular grafts constructed from skin and other ingenious techniques that were tedious and had a high failure rate. Alternatively, a free jejunal graft can be harvested from the abdomen, and used to interpose between the thoracic esophagus and pharynx. This is a slightly less morbid operation than total esophagectomy and pull-up of a gastric conduit.

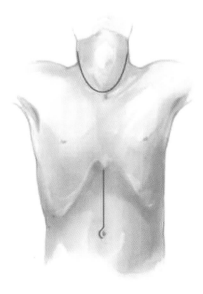

Operative Technique

Gastric Conduit Pull-Up

The patient is placed in the supine position; the abdomen, anterior chest, and neck are prepped and draped appropriately. Generally the cervical resection is performed through a transverse incision. In this presentation, a laryngectomy, pharyngectomy, and right radical neck dissection have been performed, and the specimen has been wrapped

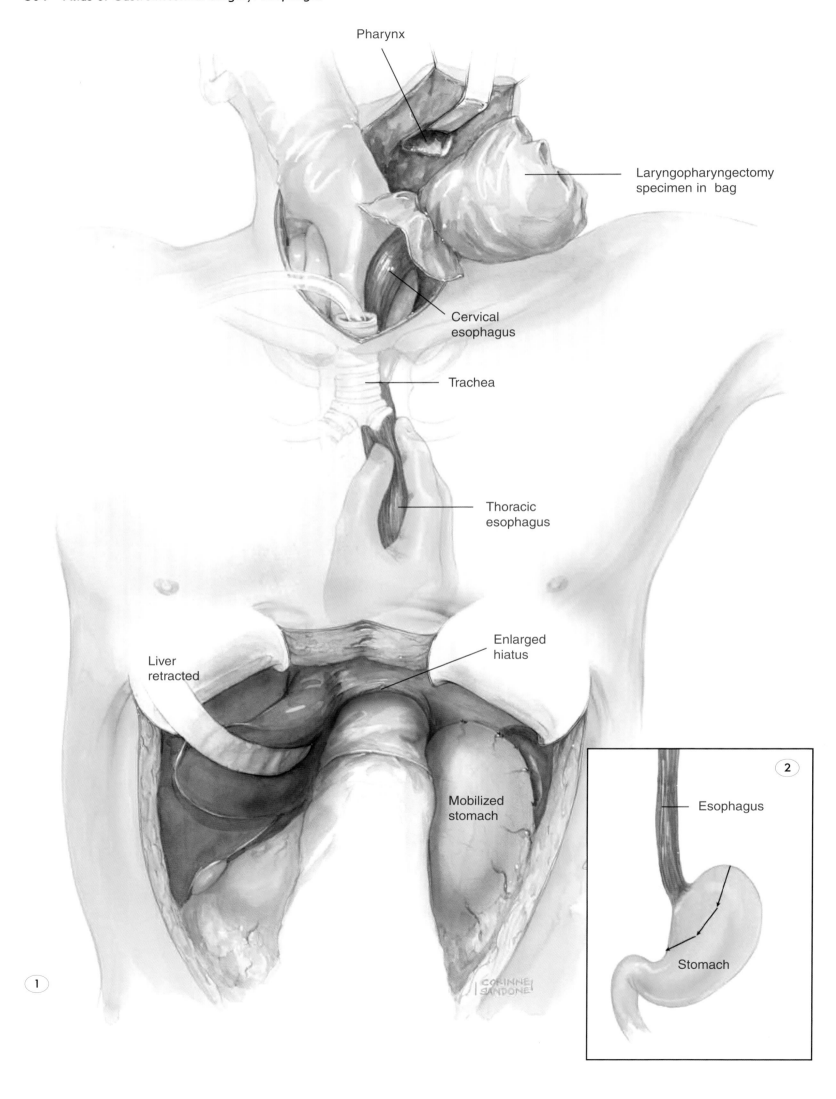

Pharynx

Laryngopharyngectomy
specimen in bag

Cervical
esophagus

Trachea

Thoracic
esophagus

Liver
retracted

Enlarged
hiatus

Mobilized
stomach

Esophagus

Stomach

CORINNE
SANDONE

1

2

in a bag (1). The endotracheal tube has been removed. Ventilation is carried out with a tube placed directly into the transected trachea in the neck wound and passed off the table to the anesthesiologist.

At this point, the abdomen is opened with an upper midline incision. The stomach and esophagus are mobilized similar to that described for a transhiatal esophagectomy in "Transhiatal Blunt Esophagectomy with Esophagogastrostomy" above. Dissection of the esophagus from the neck is much easier with all the cervical components removed (1). Similar to a resection of pathology in the lower esophagus, the gastric conduit is created with serial applications of the linear stapler to create a tube-like structure (2). A pyloromyotomy or pyloroplasty is performed and covered with a patch of omentum (3).

Since the gastric pedicle has to be brought up higher in the neck than with a usual transhiatal blunt esophagectomy, three additional maneuvers are required. First, the tissue along the lesser curvature of the stomach, consisting of remnants of the gastrohepatic ligament and the branches of the left gastric vessels, are divided in two or three areas. This eliminates much of the blood supply from the right gastric artery, but the right gastroepiploic vessels keep the stomach vascularized without difficulty. Dividing this tissue along the lesser curvature allows one to straighten out the lesser curvature and gain additional length (3).

Gastrohepatic
ligament radially
incised along
lesser curvature

3

Secondly, the inner aspect of the duodenal C loop is dissected, removing omentum and transverse mesocolon (4). Finally, the duodenum is extensively Kocherized; in addition, structures along the portal triad are dissected, again to allow maximum mobility in gaining all possible length (5).

The rounded end of a 32 French chest tube is sutured to the fundus on the esophageal side, and the beveled end is sutured to the most cephalad portion of the fundus of the gastric tube. The esophagus and proximal stomach are then pulled up through the mediastinum into the neck, pulling the chest tube behind it. The specimen is then removed from the operative field. With the chest tube as a guide, the stomach conduit is pulled, then pushed, and advanced up through the posterior mediastinum in the bed of the resected esophagus into the cervical wound (6). This should be done with great care so as not to injure the gastroepiploic arcade. The stomach is pushed and guided more with the hand through the hiatal ring in the abdomen than it is pulled with the chest tube.

The anastomosis is carried out between the open pharynx and the most cephalad portion of the fundus of the stomach. This is performed with two layers of interrupted 3-0 silk. The posterior layer is carried out first using an interrupted layer of 3-0 silk Lembert sutures. A gastrotomy is then performed. From the inside, the

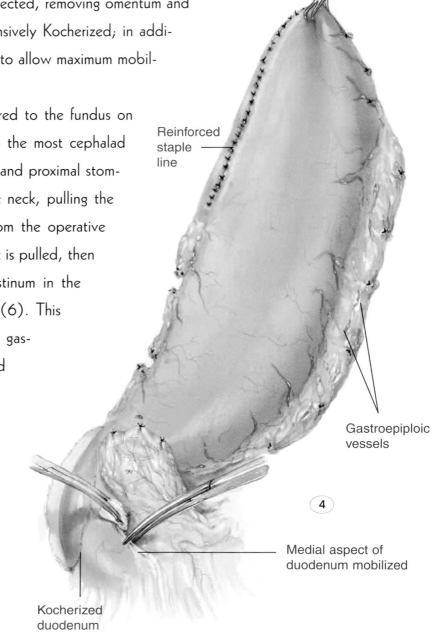

Reinforced staple line

Gastroepiploic vessels

4

Medial aspect of duodenum mobilized

Kocherized duodenum

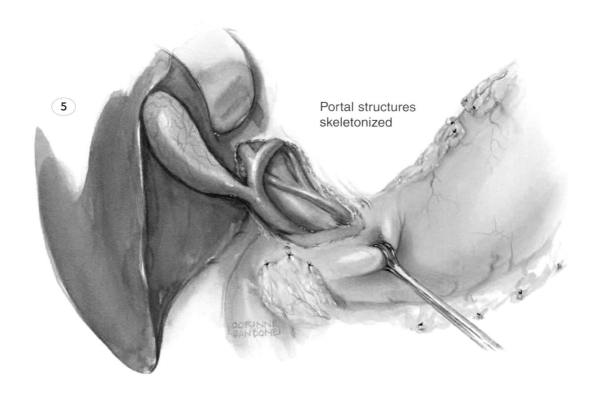

5

Portal structures skeletonized

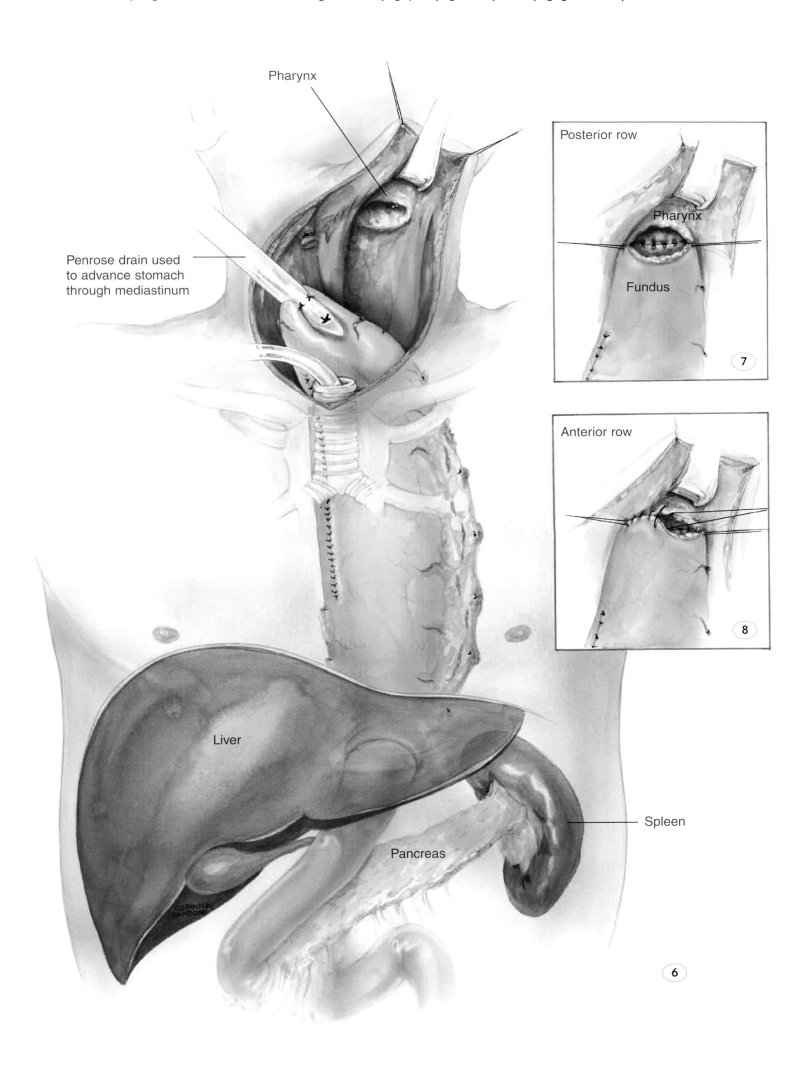

Pharynx

Penrose drain used
to advance stomach
through mediastinum

Posterior row

Pharynx

Fundus

7

Anterior row

8

Liver

Pancreas

Spleen

6

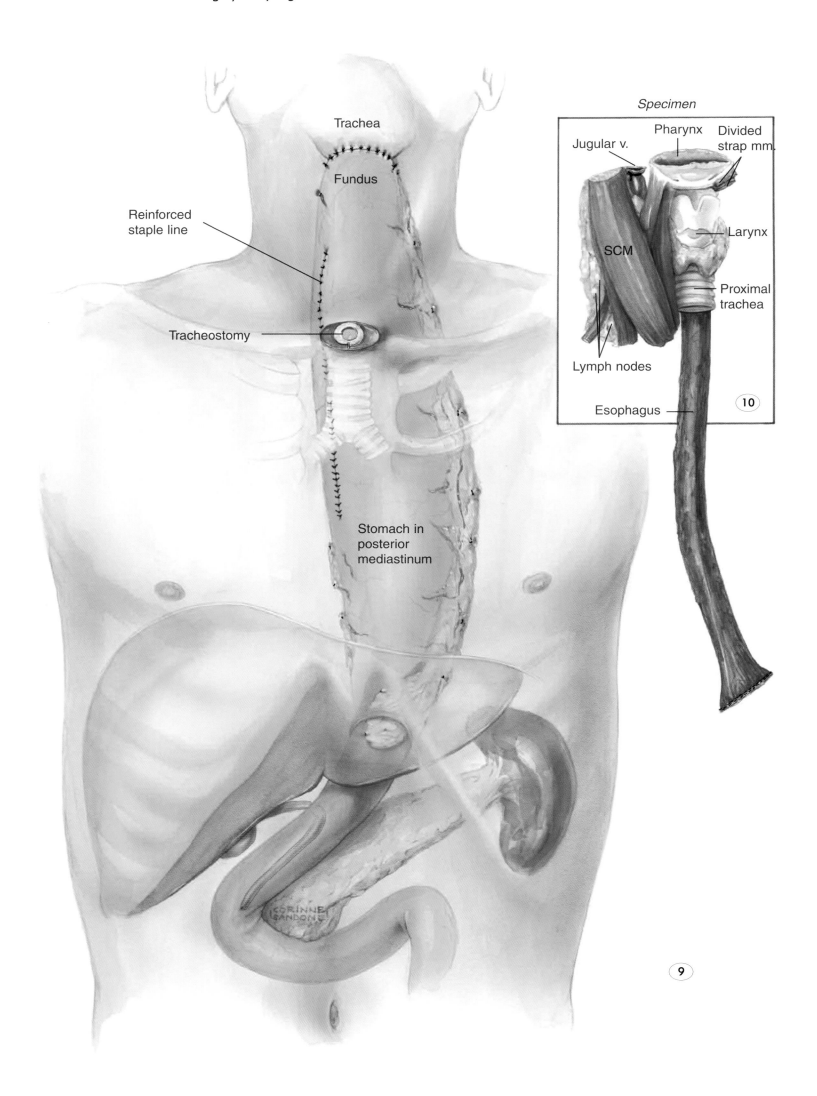

Trachea

Fundus

Reinforced
staple line

Tracheostomy

Stomach in
posterior
mediastinum

Specimen

Jugular v.

Pharynx

Divided
strap mm.

SCM

Larynx

Proximal
trachea

Lymph nodes

Esophagus

10

9

inner layer of the posterior row is placed passing sutures through and through the full thickness of pharynx and stomach (7). The inner layer of the anterior row is performed using 3-0 silk, passing from inside out on the pharynx and outside in on the stomach (8). The anastomosis is completed with the outer layer of the anterior row, using interrupted 3-0 Lembert silk sutures.

After the anastomosis has been completed, virtually all of the stomach is up in the mediastinum and cervical regions (9). The pylorus rests at the esophageal hiatus. Often it is desirable to tack the stomach to the hiatus with interrupted 3-0 silks. A permanent tracheostomy is fashioned, and the neck and abdominal wounds are closed in layers. The pharyngogastrostomy is drained with closed suction drains near the anastomosis. A feeding jejunostomy is placed as described in "Esophagogastrectomy: Separate Abdominal and Thoracic Incisions" above. The abdomen is closed without drains. The specimen consists of the abdominal, thoracic, and cervical esophagus; pharynx; larynx; proximal trachea; and the remnants of a right radical neck dissection (10).

Free Jejunal Transfer Conduit

The patient is placed in the supine position, and the neck, anterior chest and abdomen prepared and draped. The cervical pathology is dissected out and the appropriate structures removed (1). The defect in esophageal continuity is measured with an umbilical tape. A laparotomy incision is performed. A segment of jejunum is chosen approximately 30 cm distal to the ligament of Treitz. The segment of jejunum selected must have a well vascularized arcade and be fed by a single vessel (11).

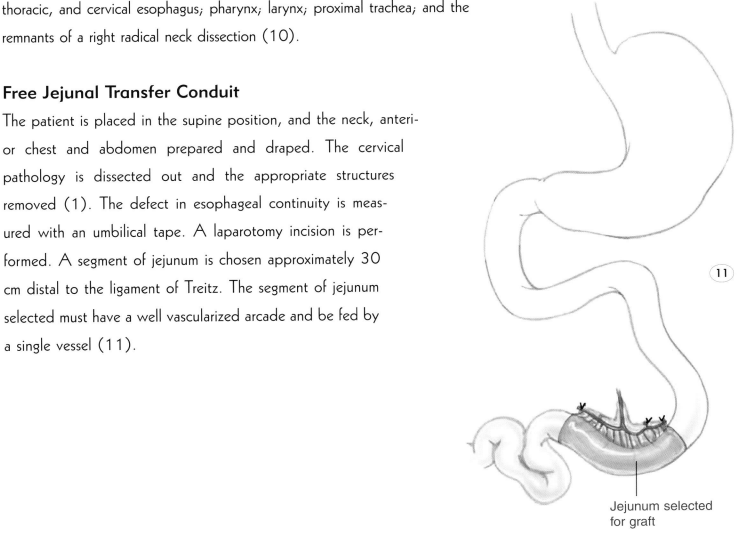

11

Jejunum selected
for graft

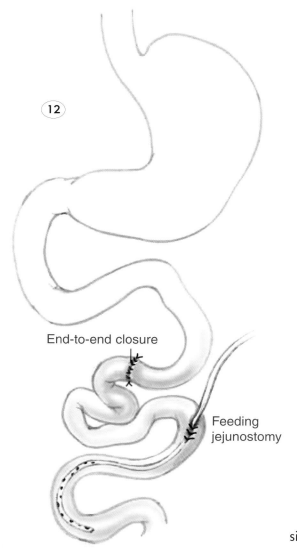

End-to-end closure

Feeding
jejunostomy

The bowel is divided proximally and distally with a linear stapler, taking a segment of jejunum a little longer than that measured with the umbilical tape. The mesentery is divided carefully preserving the vascular arcade. Bulldog clamps are then placed on the mesenteric vascular arcade on both sides of the transected bowel to ensure there is sufficient arterial supply and venous return for that segment. Enteric continuity is restored in a standard end-to-end fashion using two layers: an inner continuous layer of synthetic absorbable suture and an outer layer of interrupted 3-0 silk. A feeding jejunostomy placed at least 30 cm distal to the anastomosis as described in "Esophagogastrectomy: Separate Abdominal and Thoracic Incisions" above (12).

Meanwhile, vessels in the neck are dissected, looking for potential target vessels for arterial inflow and venous return. On the arterial side, potential vessels include the superior thyroid, transverse cervical, and external carotid arteries. Potential venous structures include the external jugular and superior thyroid veins. Once the neck is completely prepared and vessels controlled, the vascular pedicle for the jejunal graft is divided and doubly ligated with 2-0 silk sutures on the proximal side, leaving the distal vessels open. The artery and the vein in the pedicle are separated slightly.

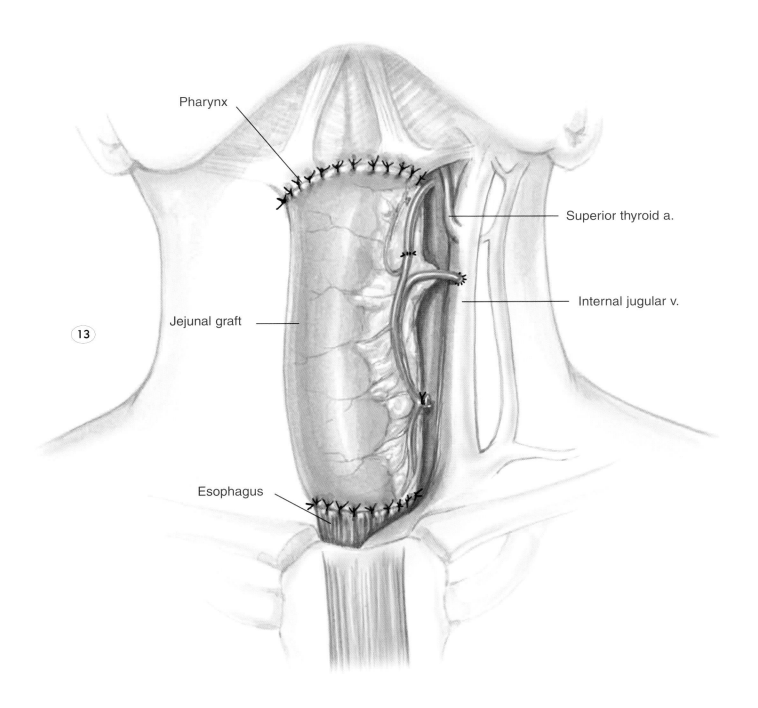

The jejunal graft is then brought to neck, and the arterial anastomosis is performed immediately. Depending upon the vessel, this is done either in an end-to-end or end-to-side fashion using a running 8-0 polypropylene suture. This can be done with magnification, either directly or with a microscope. The venous anastomosis is performed next in the same fashion. In the illustration (13), the superior thyroid artery and the internal jugular vein are the target vessels used, respectively. An audible Doppler probe is used to verify vascular flow in the graft. The bowel viability is monitored during the entire procedure.

Once the vascular anastomoses have been completed the jejunal graft anastomoses are performed. The proximal, then distal, enteric ends are anastomosed in a standard two-layer fashion. The inner layer consists of continuous 3-0 synthetic absorbable suture, and the outer layer consists of interrupted 3-0 silk. The neck is closed, leaving Penrose drains in place next to the proximal and distal anastomoses.

Esophageal Reconstruction Using Substernal Colon

Operative Indications

Placing the colon in the retrosternal position for reconstructing or bypassing the esophagus is used very rarely as a surgical option. The colon may be positioned substernally if the patient has already had the esophagus removed and perhaps had a failed reconstruction, thus obviating the possibility of having the conduit pass through the original esophageal bed.

In rare instances, patients with esophageal neoplasms are best palliated without performing an esophagectomy. Patients with tracheoesophageal fistulas are clearly incurable, and resection of the esophagus presents the surgeon with the almost insurmountable task of repairing the tracheal or bronchial defect. In addition, other patients who do not have a tracheoesophageal fistula, but who on bronchoscopy clearly have tracheal involvement, are also in many instances best palliated without removing the esophagus. Such patients may have complete obstruction; and if a tracheoesophageal fistula is present, they may repeatedly aspirate and develop pneumonia. These patients can be palliated by bypassing the esophagus with a substernal colon, thus palliating the dysphagia and allowing them to eat and drink during the remainder of their disease.

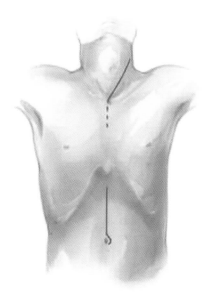

Operative Technique

Patients undergoing a substernal bypass are positioned supine, and the neck, anterior chest, and abdomen are prepped and draped appropriately. The head is rotated to the right. The abdomen is opened through a long midline incision. A long segment colon interposition graft is prepared. This consists of most of the transverse colon, the splenic flexure, and a major portion of the descending colon, all based on the ascending branch of the left colic artery. The omentum is taken off the transverse colon, and the left colon is mobilized out of the retroperitoneum (1). One can tentatively pick points of division of the right transverse colon and descending colon and then measure the length of colon graft with an umbilical tape. Adequate length of the colon is measured, being certain that it will reach the neck with some excess. The viability of the graft, based on the ascending branch of the left colic artery, can be tested by placing Bulldog clamps across the base of the middle colic artery and across the marginal artery proximally and distally at the proposed sites of division. After viability is insured, the marginal artery at each end of the graft is doubly clamped and divided (2). In addition, the middle colic artery proximal to its bifurcation is also ligated and divided. The transverse mesocolon is divided over to the ascending branch of the left colic vessels.

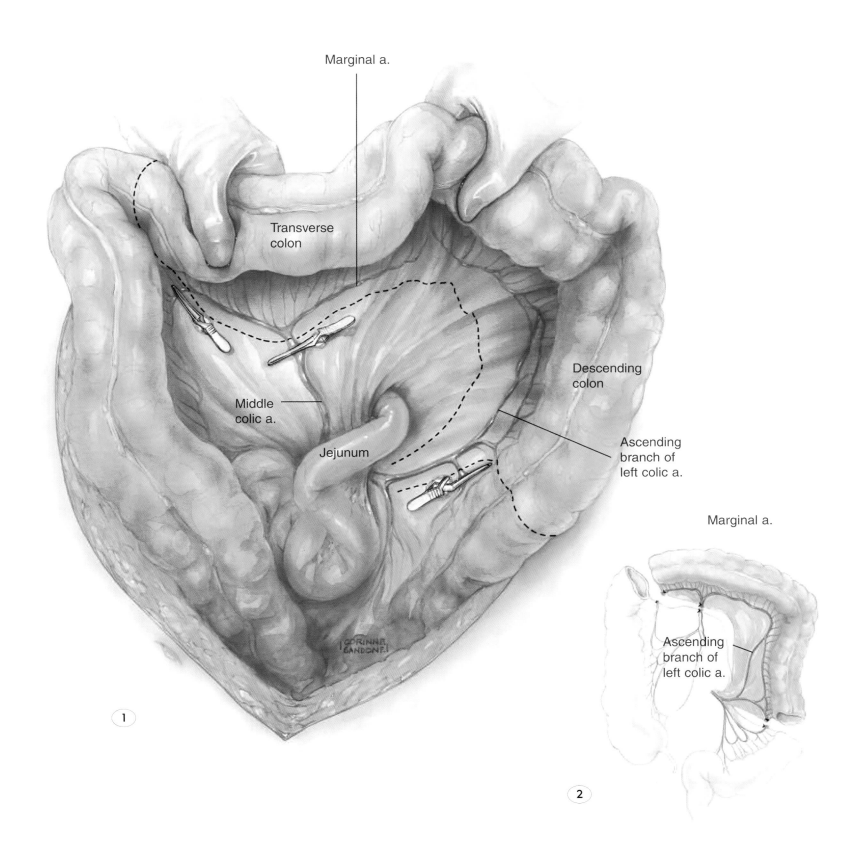

Mobilization of the long segment colon graft is completed by taking down the splenic flexure. The colon is then divided proximally and distally with a linear stapler (3).

If the patient has had no previous cervical incision, a curvilinear incision is made 1 cm above the sternal notch and extended to the left, over the midportion of the sternocleidomastoid muscle. This is a much more cosmetically appealing incision than one along the anterior border of the sternocleidomastoid muscle. The platysma is divided and undermined approximately 1 cm around the edges. The omohyoid muscle and middle thyroid vein

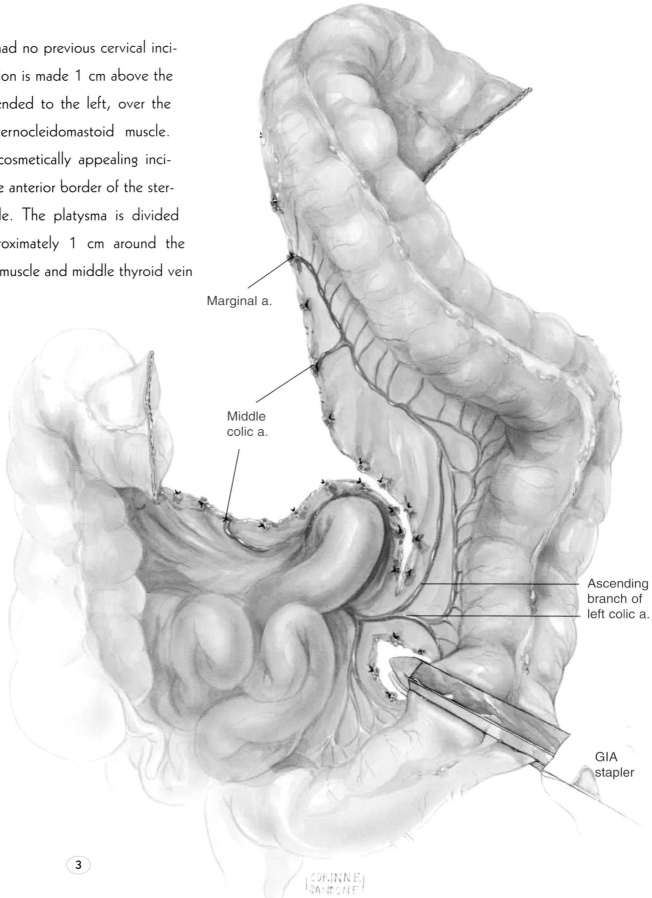

Marginal a.

Middle colic a.

Ascending branch of left colic a.

GIA stapler

(3)

are divided. The trachea and thyroid are retracted medially, and the sternocleidomastoid muscle laterally, with a self-retaining retractor, taking care not to put too much stretch on the recurrent laryngeal nerve or the carotid sheath. The esophagus with an indwelling nasogastric tube can be easily palpated. The esophagus is mobilized circumferentially and grasped with a Babcock clamp. One must be careful, during the dissection of the esophagus, to avoid injury to the recurrent laryngeal nerves. A small Penrose drain is used to encircle the cervical esophagus.

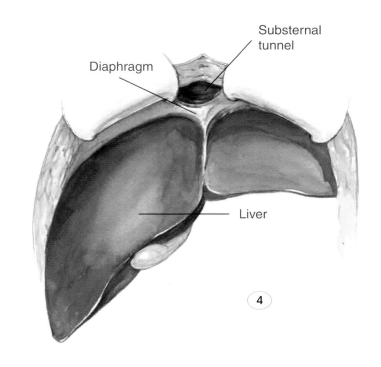

If an esophagostomy is already present, it is dissected away from the surrounding tissues, and the previous cervical incision is opened. Dissection is performed down to the prevertebral fascia.

The substernal tunnel is then developed (4). Inferiorly, if one uses the electrocautery and incises the xiphoid, the space directly adjacent to the periosteum along the posterior sternum is easily entered (5). This potential space is filled only with areolar tissue and is very easily developed from below. The same space is entered from above by developing the space directly posterior to the periosteum of the sternum. By working from above and below, this substernal space can easily be developed, generally without entering either pleural space (6). If the left sternoclavicular head is prominent, it may be necessary to remove it with a bone rongeur or Lebske knife to avoid undue compression on the colon graft (5).

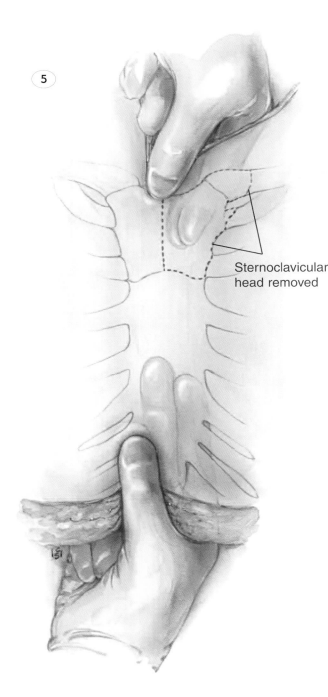

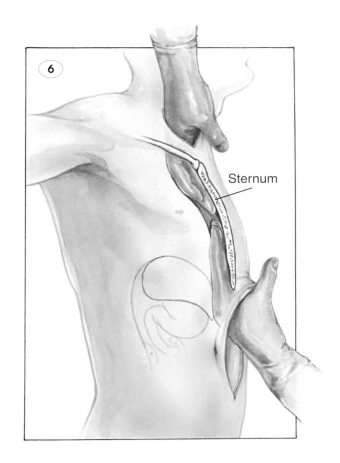

Sternum

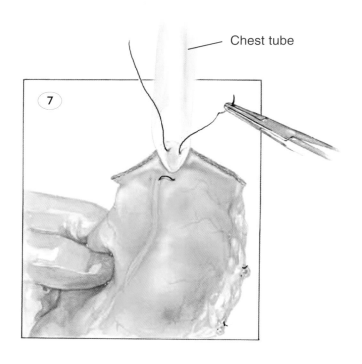

Chest tube

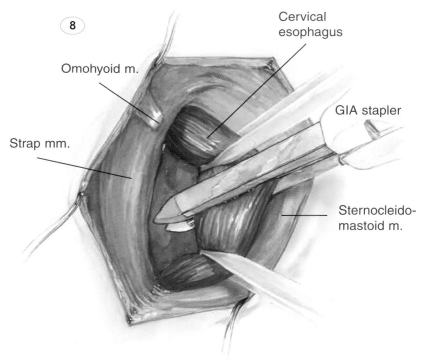

Omohyoid m.

Strap mm.

Cervical esophagus

GIA stapler

Sternocleido-mastoid m.

Once this space is developed, a 32 French chest tube is sutured to the proximal end of the colon graft with interrupted 2-0 silk sutures (7). This will aid in passing the long segment of colon through the substernal space. The chest tube is passed from below through the substernal space and grasped from above. The chest tube and the attached colon graft are gently advanced into the cervical region. When the colon graft is pulled up, it should pass posterior to the stomach so that, subsequently, the vascular pedicle resides posterior to the stomach.

There should be no difficulty in obtaining adequate length for the long segment colonic graft. The esophagus is divided with a linear stapler (8) just above the thoracic inlet. The colon should rest comfortably in the neck incision and a tension-free end-to-end esophagocolostomy performed; this is accomplished with two layers of interrupted 3-0 silk. The outer posterior layer of interrupted 3-0 silks is placed before dividing the esophagus. The staple lines from both the esophagus and colon are removed (9). The inner layer of the posterior row is placed, passing the 3-0 silk sutures through and through the full thickness of esophagus and colon. Prior to completing the anterior layer, a nasogastric tube is passed from the esophagus through the colon, to be positioned later into the stomach (10). The inner layer of the anterior row is placed using interrupted 3-0 silk sutures passing inside out on the colon and outside in on the esophagus. The outer layer of the anterior row is completed with a series of 3-0 silk Lembert sutures (11).

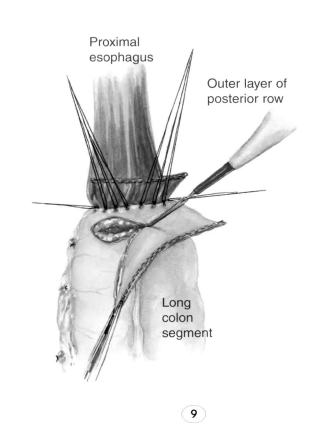

Proximal esophagus

Outer layer of posterior row

Long colon segment

9

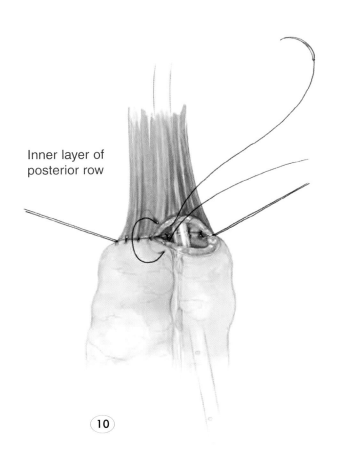

Inner layer of posterior row

10

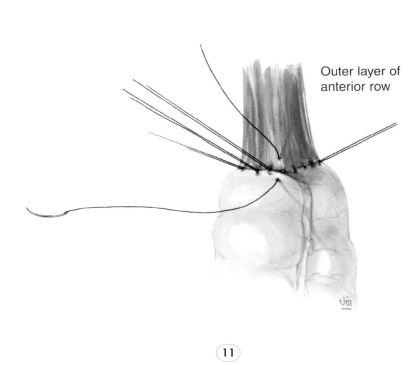

Outer layer of anterior row

11

The cologastrostomy is performed next, on the posterior body of the stomach. Any excess length of colonic graft should be excised before performing the distal anastomosis. A standard two-layer anastomosis is performed between the colon and stomach with an outer interrupted layer and an inner continuous layer. The outer layer of the posterior row is placed first, using interrupted 3-0 silk sutures in a Lembert fashion. The staple line is then removed from the colon and a gastrotomy is performed using the electrocautery (12).

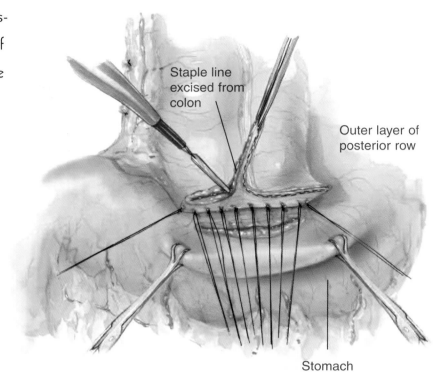

Staple line excised from colon

Outer layer of posterior row

Stomach

(12)

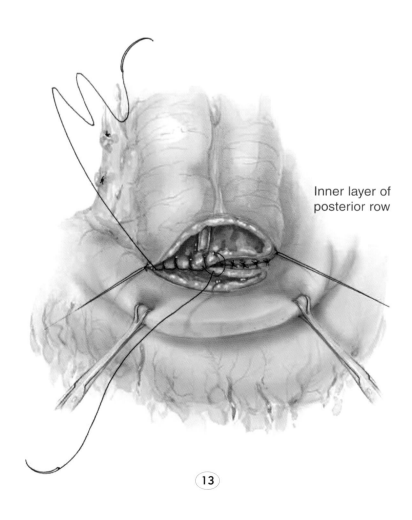

Inner layer of posterior row

(13)

The inner layer of the posterior row consists of a continuous locking suture of 3-0 synthetic absorbable material (13).

This is brought around anteriorly for the inner layer of the anterior row in a Connell fashion (14). Prior to closure of the inner anterior row, the nasogastric tube is advanced through the distal part of the colon conduit into the stomach. The cologastrostomy is completed with an outer layer of 3-0 silk Lembert sutures in the anterior row (15). The completed conduit passes retrosternally in the thorax and posterior to the stomach in the abdomen (17).

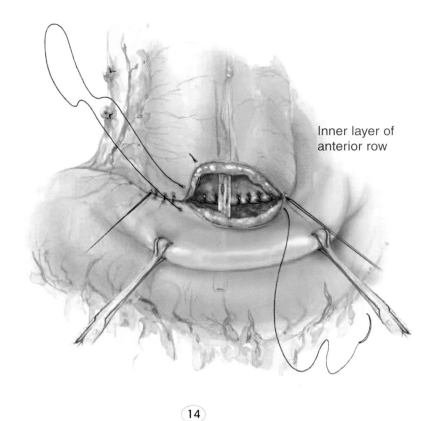

Inner layer of anterior row

14

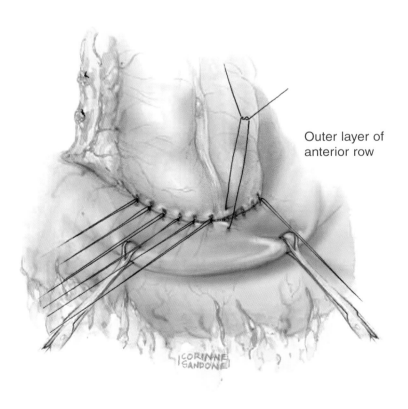

Outer layer of anterior row

CORINNE SANDONE

15

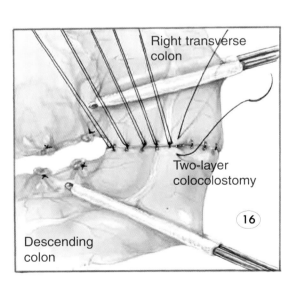

Right transverse colon

Two-layer colocolostomy

16

Descending colon

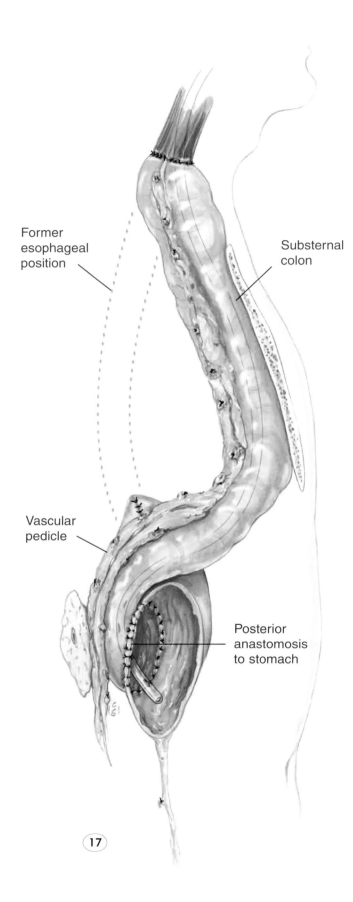

Former
esophageal
position

Substernal
colon

Vascular
pedicle

Posterior
anastomosis
to stomach

(17)

Colonic continuity is reestablished with a colocolostomy (16). The right transverse and distal left colon are reanastomosed in a standard two-layer fashion. Generally, by mobilizing the right colon out of the retroperitoneum and by mobilizing the sigmoid colon, this anastomosis can be performed above the root of the small bowel mesentery. If it will not reach without tension, the right colon should be extensively mobilized, turned down, and then anastomosed below the root of the small bowel mesentery.

One has several options in performing a substernal colon bypass and excluding the thoracic esophagus. If the esophagus is still in place and has been excluded (18), it is an unusual occurrence, but occasionally, the isolated segment of esophagus between the neck and obstructing tumor can rupture at its proximal staple line. A mediastinal infection may result. If this is a concern, a small French catheter can be left in the proximal esophageal segment, and the esophagus secured around it with a purse-string suture of 3-0 silk. The catheter is brought out through the neck and left as a decompression port (19).

One may also want to ligate the gastroesophageal junction with a piece of umbilical tape, particularly if a patient has a tracheoesophageal fistula. This maneuver prevents gastroesophageal reflux up into the proximal esophagus and potentially through the tracheoesophageal fistula into the lungs (20). If one does this, the vagal nerves should be dissected off the distal esophagus, and the umbilical tape placed within the vagal nerves for their preservation. If there is concern that the vagal nerves have been interrupted during the proximal or distal esophageal dissections or are involved with tumor, a pyloromyotomy or pyloroplasty can be performed through the abdominal incision. A feeding jejunostomy is placed as described in "Esophagogastrectomy: Separate Abdominal and Thoracic Incisions" above. The neck incision is closed in layers, leaving a small Penrose drain near the esophagocolostomy anastomosis. The abdomen is closed without drains.

Boerhaave's Syndrome: Esophageal Exclusion, Diversion and Closure

Operative Indications

Most patients with Boerhaave's syndrome who are seen early can be managed with thoracotomy, surgical débridement and closure of the esophagus, with reinforcement using a pleural flap. In some patients who are seen several days after the perforation and who undergo thoracotomy, the esophagus is obviously not reparable with any hopes of primary healing. In such patients, primary closure and reinforcement have a high likelihood of failure. These patients usually are critically ill and are candidates for diversion and exclusion of the esophagus. In addition, other patients who have initially been treated with esophageal closure and reinforcement will break down and develop a fistula. These patients are also candidates for this operative procedure. This operation is performed in the critically ill patient as a lifesaving procedure. If the patient recovers, esophageal replacement of at least the distal esophagus will probably be required.

Operative Technique

The patient is placed in the supine position and the abdomen and left neck are prepped and draped appropriately. The cervical incision is made anterior to the border of the left sternocleidomastoid muscle. The incision is deepened through the platysma. The omohyoid and middle thyroid vein are divided. The carotid sheath is retracted laterally, and the trachea and thyroid medially. The esophagus is identified. The cervical esophagus is dissected free, taking care not to injure either recurrent laryngeal nerve. Once the esophagus has been mobilized, it is divided with a TA stapler just above the thoracic inlet. The proximal end is brought out as an end cervical esophagostomy (1). Subsequently, when the neck incision is closed, two 3-0 silk sutures are placed on the distal end of the divided esophagus and brought out through the cervical incision. Later, these sutures will help the surgeon quickly identify the distal end of the esophagus when the ends are reanastomosed. In the past, surgeons have been reluctant to divide the cervical esophagus, thinking that an end-to-end reanastomosis could

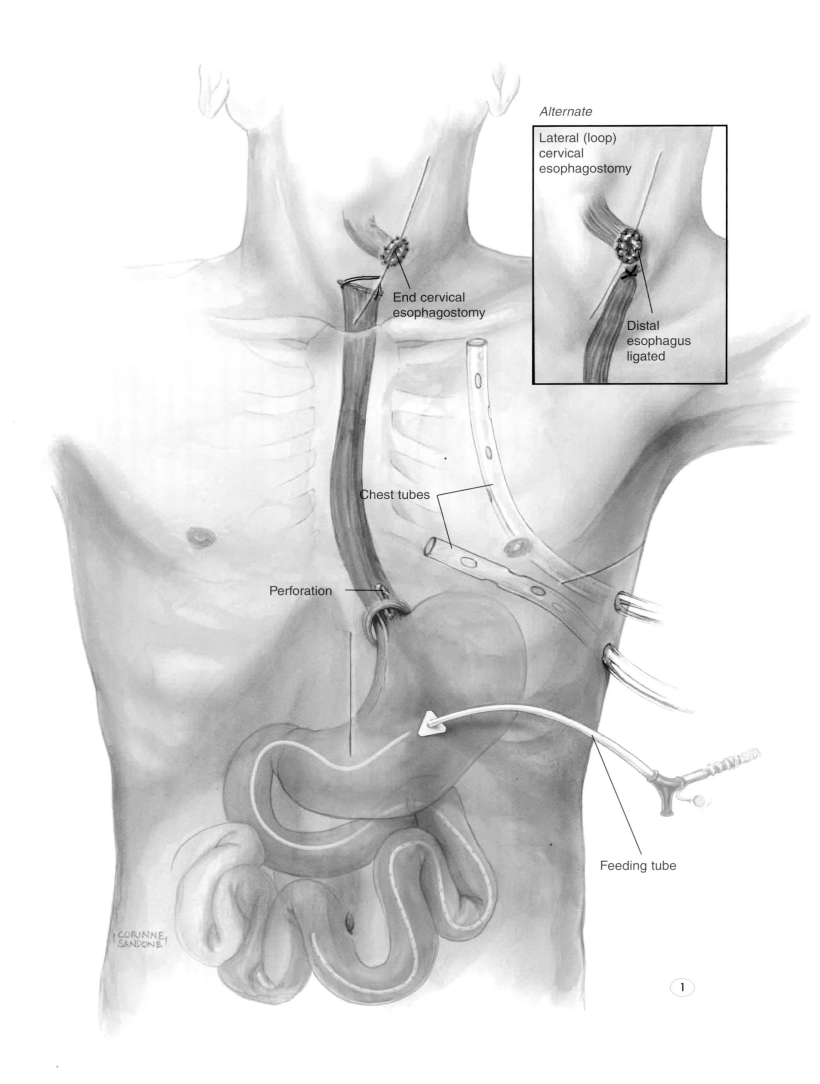

Alternate

Lateral (loop) cervical esophagostomy

Distal esophagus ligated

End cervical esophagostomy

Chest tubes

Perforation

Feeding tube

1

not subsequently be performed. With adequate mobilization, however, it is now recognized that an end-to-end cervical esophagostomy can be carried out subsequently.

An alternative, however, is to mobilize the cervical esophagus, bring it to the skin, and perform a lateral side cervical (loop) esophagostomy, ligating the distal esophagus with heavy (No. 0 or No. 1) synthetic absorbable suture (fig 1 inset). This alternative is often favored because it is easier to close later (when the patient has recovered) by opening the distal suture with dilators (Maloney or cervical) followed by closure of the ostomy in two layers.

After the cervical esophagostomy has been performed, the neck wound is irrigated with antibiotic-containing solution, and the incision is closed in layers. At the same setting, a small upper abdominal midline incision is made, a gastrostomy tube is inserted, and a feeding jejunostomy tube is placed. In addition, some surgeons advocate mobilizing the intra-abdominal esophagus, elevating both vagus nerves, and placing a ligature around the distal esophagus to prevent gastroesophageal reflux. This ligature should be of heavy synthetic absorbable suture material. Some surgeons believe that merely placing the gastrostomy is sufficient to prevent gastroesophageal reflux; in most instances, however, ligating the intra-abdominal esophagus is preferable. The abdomen is irrigated with antibiotic-containing solution, and the wound closed.

The patient is then repositioned in the lateral thoracotomy position with the left chest up. The left chest is entered through the sixth or seventh interspace. The left chest generally will be contaminated and should be irrigated copiously with antibiotic-containing solution. The mediastinal pleura is opened widely, and the mediastinum is débrided. Occasionally, due to extensive contamination and inflammatory changes, the site of perforation is not found. However, if the injury is identified, necrotic tissue is débrided and the perforation is closed in two layers as described in "Boerhaave's Syndrome: Esophageal Repair" above. Two chest tubes are left. One should be in the lower chest close to the esophageal perforation. A second chest tube is left in the apex of the chest. The pleural cavity is once again copiously irrigated with antibiotic-containing solution and closed in layers.

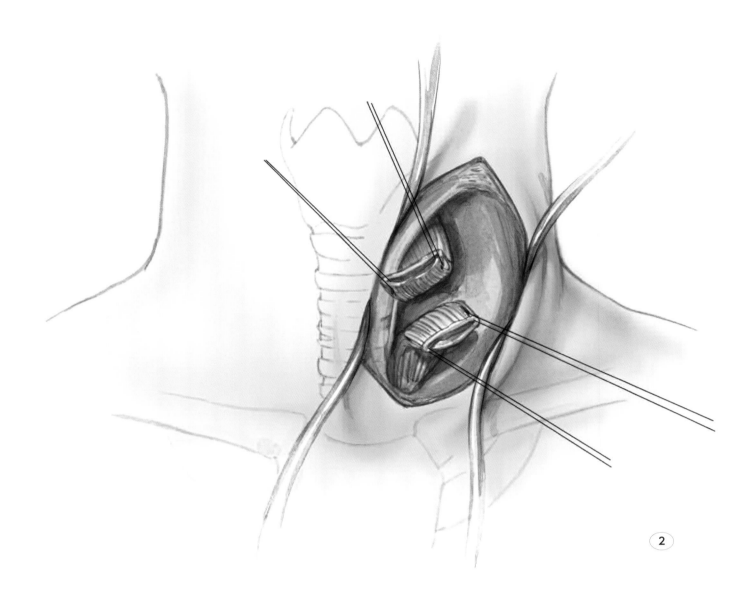

(2)

Esophagostomy Closure Technique

Several months after the patient has recovered and the injury has healed, the diverting esophagostomy is closed. Depicted is closure of a formal end esophagostomy with formal division of the esophagus distally. The previous neck incision is opened along the sternocleidomastoid muscle (2). The proximal esophagostomy is mobilized circumferentially from the skin and dissected down to the prevertebral fascia. The redundant skin epithelium is cut away from the proximal end of the ostomy. Traction sutures of 2-0 synthetic absorbable material are placed on either side for retraction. The distal end of the esophagus, which has been easily identified because of the 3-0 silk sutures previously left as tags, is dissected from the mediastinum. Once found, similar traction sutures are placed to elevate the esophagus out of the mediastinum. Care is taken not to dissect too much of the surrounding tissues to prevent devascularization of the esophageal segment. Occasionally, the upper manubrium has to be split in the midline in order to gain access to the esophagus and to perform the anastomosis if the esophagus was previously divided too low in the neck in the mediastinum.

Repair of Thoracic Esophageal Perforation

Operative Indications

Perforation of the thoracic esophagus during esophagoscopy or during dilatation of an esophageal stricture is generally a surgical emergency. Patients may be treated nonoperatively if they are relatively asymptomatic, afebrile, and not septic, and, on water-soluble contrast media swallow, the perforation is well contained by the mediastinal pleura and drains back into the esophagus. In the majority of instances, however, these patients present as surgical emergencies.

A variety of surgical options is available for the surgeon. The esophageal pathology and perforation can be resected, the stomach pulled up into the chest, or into the neck, and an esophagogastrostomy performed as described in previous sections. Another option is to resect the distal esophagus and to reconstruct with a short segment colon interposition. Each of these procedures is an option, but both are fairly extensive operations. Both would have to be carried out on a patient with unprepped bowel, and the patient may be too ill to undergo such a procedure. A third option is to repair the esophageal perforation from a thoracic exposure, which, compared to the other options, may be the easiest and quickest procedure to perform on a very ill patient.

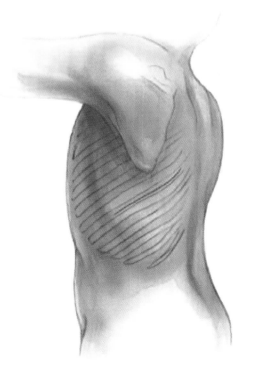

Operative Technique

The patient is placed in the lateral thoracotomy position with the left chest up. The left pleural cavity is entered through the sixth or seventh interspace. Pleural contamination may be considerable, and thorough irrigation with an antibiotic containing solution should be carried out. The mediastinal pleura should be opened widely. The esophagus is identified and mobilized.

The area of pathology (in this instance, a long stricture with perforation) is identified (1). The area of the perforation is débrided, and then the opening in the esophagus is extended through the entire length of the stricture (2).

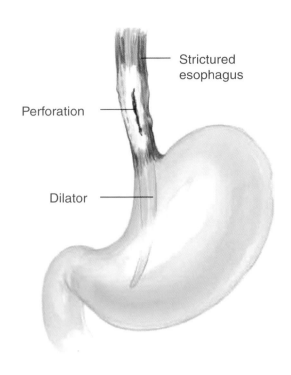

Strictured esophagus

Perforation

Dilator

(1)

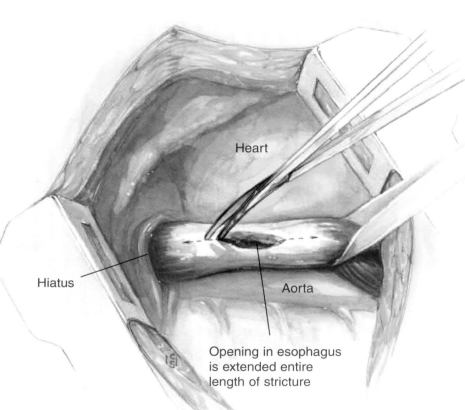

Heart

Hiatus

Aorta

Opening in esophagus is extended entire length of stricture

(2)

The hiatus is dilated, and the fundus is delivered into the chest; this requires division of several of the vasa brevia along the greater curvature, as well as branches of the left gastric vessels along the lesser curvature (3).

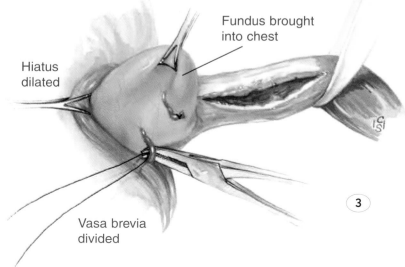

Fundus brought into chest

Hiatus dilated

Vasa brevia divided

(3)

Once the fundus of the stomach has been sufficiently mobilized, it is used to close the esophageal defect. This closure is carried out by suturing the fundus of the stomach to both walls of the opened esophagus. A single layer of interrupted synthetic nonabsorbable suture material is passed full thickness through the esophageal wall and through the seromuscular layer to include the submucosa on the gastric wall. The two rows of sutures on the fundus are placed approximately 1 to 2 cm apart, to restore normal diameter to the esophagus (4).

Once the gastric patch has been sutured to the esophageal opening, the mobilized fundus is wrapped circumferentially around the esophagus to complete a fundoplication (5, 6).

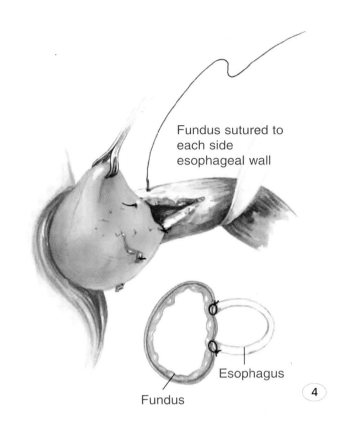

Fundus sutured to each side esophageal wall

Esophagus

Fundus

4

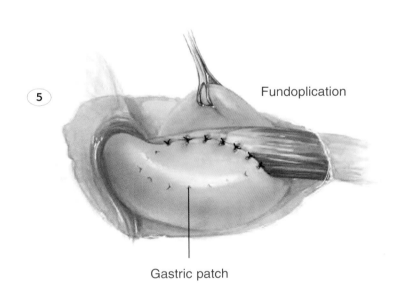

5

Fundoplication

Gastric patch

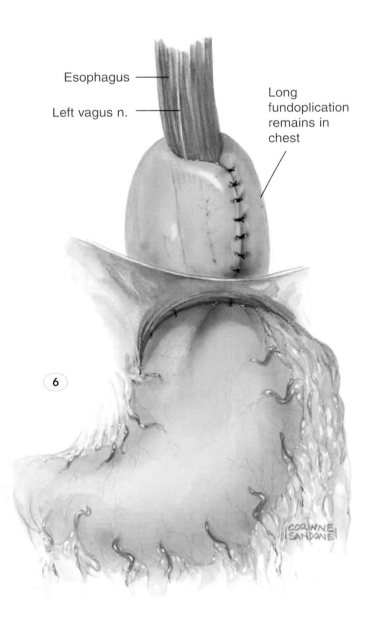

Esophagus

Left vagus n.

Long fundoplication remains in chest

6

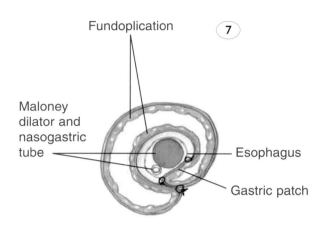

Fundoplication ⑦

Maloney dilator and nasogastric tube

Esophagus

Gastric patch

The fundic wrap is generally much longer than the usual Nissen fundoplication performed through the abdomen for gastroesophageal reflux. This long wrap necessitates leaving the fundoplication in the chest. It is recognized that this carries subsequent risks; some patients subsequently develop gastric ulceration or gastritis in the thoracic portion of the stomach. If the hiatus is dilated sufficiently so that no stasis exists in the gastric fundus, this risk is thought to be acceptable because of the patient's life-threatening situation. The stomach is sutured to the dilated hiatus with interrupted 3-0 silks (6). The fundoplication should be performed with a nasogastric tube and a 46 French Maloney dilator in place, so that one is certain not to narrow the esophageal lumen (7, 8). The thoracic cavity is irrigated copiously with antibiotic-containing solution; two chest tubes are placed: one in the apex of the chest, and a second near the esophageal perforation. The chest is closed in layers.

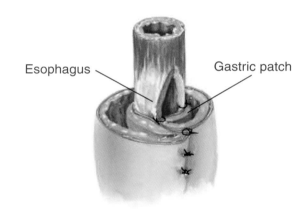

Esophagus

Gastric patch

⑧

Repair of Acquired Tracheoesophageal Fistula

Operative Indications

Most acquired tracheoesophageal fistulas are due to pressure necrosis at the site of a cuffed tracheostomy tube. Other less common causes include blunt or penetrating trauma, granulomatous infections, foreign bodies, or complications from prior surgery of the spine, neck, or esophagus. Spontaneous closure is rare, and in the appropriate patient, surgical repair is highly effective. To help ensure successful repair, the patient should be weaned off mechanical ventilation, be hemodynamically stable, have adequate nutrition, and minimized gastroesophageal reflux. A cervical approach is reserved for those lesions at least 3 cm above the carina.

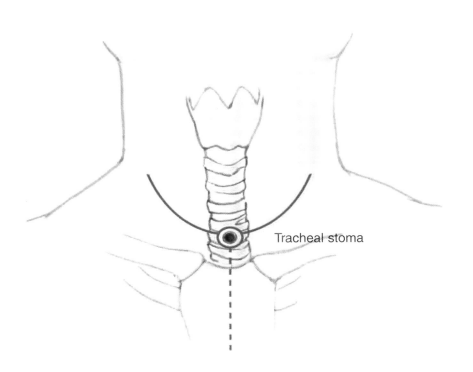

Tracheal stoma

Operative Technique

The patient is placed in the supine position with a small roll behind the shoulders, and the neck hyperextended. Flexible esophagoscopy and bronchoscopy are performed to locate the level of the fistula. The initial incision is a transverse curvilinear incision including the tracheal stoma and staying 2 cm above the sternal notch. The tracheal stoma is excised in an elliptical fashion. Occasionally, it is necessary to T-off of the transverse incision, extending it from the midline inferiorly over the manubrium. This will allow one to perform an upper sternal split, if necessary. The incision is deepened through the platysma, and flaps are created superiorly to the thyroid cartilage notch and inferiorly to the sternum and clavicle. The sternocleidomastoid muscles are retracted laterally, the omohyoid and prethyroid muscles divided. The middle thyroid vein and inferior thyroid artery are ligated and divided. This creates excellent exposure of all the structures in the field and allows identification of the fistula when the structures are moved (1).

The recurrent laryngeal nerve is identified but not dissected. Often, local inflammation makes the nerve and fistula difficult to locate but helps in locating the level of the fistula. Circumferential mobilization of

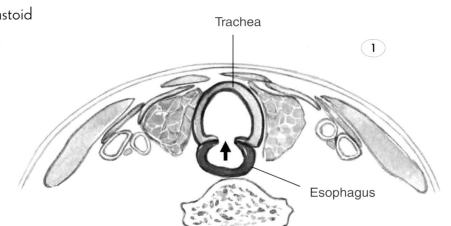

Trachea

Esophagus

1

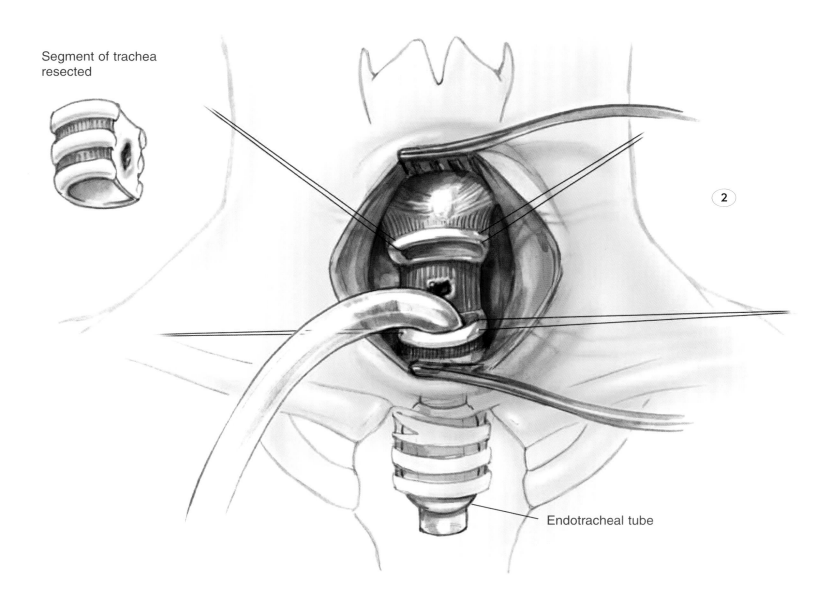

Segment of trachea resected

Endotracheal tube

2

the trachea is required. Once the fistula is located, resection of a short segment of trachea is carried out above and below the fistula tract to expose the esophageal defect. No more than three rings of trachea should be excised. Rarely, the tracheoesophageal fistula can be divided and both defects repaired without resecting the trachea. The distal trachea is intubated with a flexible endotracheal tube placed across the sterile field (2).

The esophageal edges are débrided (3). The mucosal layer is closed with interrupted 3-0 synthetic absorbable sutures, and the muscular layer is closed with interrupted 3-0 silk Lembert sutures (4). The trachea is reanastomosed end-to-end using multiple interrupted 2-0 synthetic nonabsorbable monofilament sutures placed above and below the adjacent tracheal rings. A pedicle of vascularized neck muscle is interposed between the tracheal and esophageal closures and sutured in place with 3-0 silk sutures to prevent fistula reformation (5). A small Penrose drain is left in place, and the neck irrigated and closed in several layers.

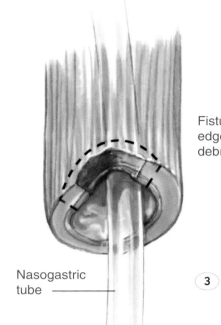
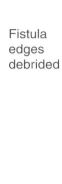

Fistula edges debrided

Nasogastric tube

3

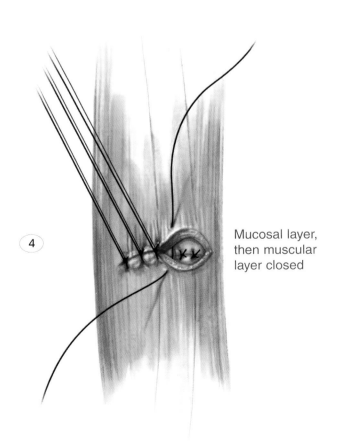

4

Mucosal layer, then muscular layer closed

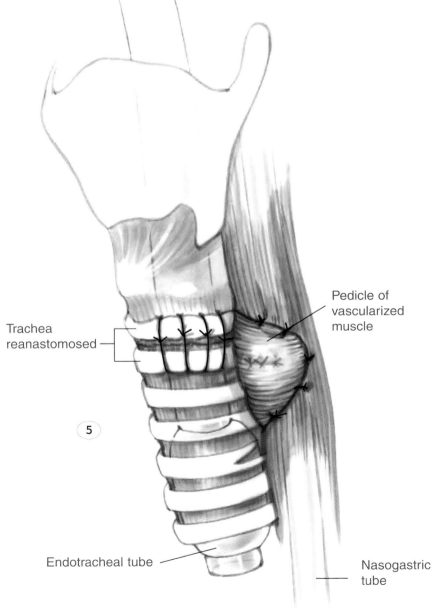

Trachea reanastomosed

Pedicle of vascularized muscle

5

Endotracheal tube

Nasogastric tube

INDEX